Inherited Disorders of
Vitamins and Cofactors

Inherited Disorders of Vitamins and Cofactors

Proceedings of the 22nd Annual Symposium of the SSIEM, Newcastle upon Tyne, September 1984

The combined supplements 1 and 2 of *Journal of Inherited Metabolic Disease* Volume 8 (1985)

edited by
G. M. Addison, K. Bartlett,
R. A. Harkness and R. J. Pollitt

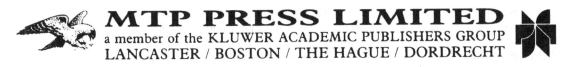

MTP PRESS LIMITED
a member of the KLUWER ACADEMIC PUBLISHERS GROUP
LANCASTER / BOSTON / THE HAGUE / DORDRECHT

Published in the UK and Europe by
MTP Press Limited
Falcon House
Lancaster, England

British Library Cataloguing in Publication Data

Society for the Study of Inborn Errors in Metabolism,
  Symposium (22nd: 1984: Newcastle upon Tyne)
  Inherited disorders of vitamins and cofactors:
  proceedings of the 22nd annual symposium of the
  SSIEM, Newcastle upon Tyne, September 1984.
  1. Metabolism, Inborn errors of—Nutritional
  aspects 2. Avitaminosis
  I. Title II. Addison, G. M. III. Journal of
  inherited metabolic disease
  616.3'9042   RC627.8

Published in the USA by
MTP Press
A division of Kluwer Boston Inc
190 Old Derby Street
Hingham, MA 02043, USA

Library of Congress Cataloging in Publication Data

Society for the Study of Inborn Errors of Metabolism.
  Symposium (22nd: 1984; Newcastle upon Tyne, Tyne
  and Wear)
  Inherited disorders of vitamins and cofactors.

  "The combined supplements 1 and 2 of Journal of
inherited metabolic disease, volume 8 (1985)."
  Includes bibliographies and index.
  1. Metabolism, Inborn errors of—Congresses.
2. Vitamins in human nutrition—Congresses.
I. Addison, G. M. (Gerald Michael) II. Journal of
inherited metabolic disease. III. Title. [DNLM:
1. Avitaminosis—familial & genetic—congresses.
2. Metabolism, Inborn Errors—congresses. 3. Vitamins—
congresses. W3 S05915K 22nd 1984i/WD 205 S678 1984i]
RC627.8.S62 1984 616.3'9 85-13271

ISBN 978-94-011-8021-4   ISBN 978-94-011-8019-1 (eBook)
DOI 10.1007/978-94-011-8019-1

Typeset by Speedlith Photo Litho Limited, Longford Trading Estate, Manchester M32 0JT.

Contents

Section V: Short Communications

Index of Authors

Subject Index

J. Inher. Metab. Dis. 8 Suppl. 1 (1985) 1

Preface

In 1972 the 10th Annual Symposium of the Society for the Study of Inborn Errors of Metabolism was held in Cardiff and the proceedings published in 1973. The meeting was devoted to the treatment of inborn errors of metabolism; in particular the dietary treatment of phenylketonuria and vitamin responsive disorders were reviewed. These two areas have seen notable advances in the intervening years. It has become apparent that a number of variants of PKU are due to defective cofactor metabolism, and, indeed, some patients refractory to simple dietary restriction of phenylalanine respond to the administration of the phenylalanine hydroxylase cofactor biopterin or related compounds. Biopterin, normally synthesized *de novo*, in some individuals has become a 'vitamin'. Secondly, a number of enzyme defects have been described which can be partly or wholly corrected by the administration of supranormal amounts of the vitamins which are the precursors of their respective cofactors. Thus inborn errors responsive to pyridoxine, biotin, thiamine, riboflavin, cobalamin, and indeed most of the vitamins have been reported. The underlying mechanisms of these effects have been the object of intensive study and we now know that a number of different biochemical aetiologies can give rise to a clinical response by a vitamin. In view of the striking advances in our understanding it was appropriate that the 22nd Annual Symposium of the Society, held in Newcastle upon Tyne, should be concerned with defects of cofactors and vitamins.

A highlight of the 1972 Cardiff Symposium was the Milner lecture, delivered by Professor C. R. Scriver on the subject of vitamin-responsive inborn errors of metabolism. It was therefore fitting that the opening lecture of a meeting devoted to this topic should be presented by Professor Scriver, who reviewed the place of vitamins in evolution and provided a backdrop for the rest of the proceedings. Then followed papers on vitamin physiology by Drs Bates and Rose.

The Raine Memorial Lecture was delivered by Professor Kaufman who provided an invaluable introduction to a session devoted to inborn errors of biopterin metabolism. This was succeeded by presentations from Drs Curtius, Niederweisser and Smith, together with short communications from members to provide a valuable overview of the current status of this field. The difficulty in establishing an unequivocal clinical response to vitamin treatment was discussed by Dr Leonard. The papers on biotin-responsive combined carboxylase deficiency presented by Drs Bartlett, Wolf and Baumgartner emphasized the widely differing mechanisms which may underline apparently similar clinical responses. In particular biotinidase deficiency appears to be a unique defect of cofactor recycling. Riboflavin, thiamine, and pyridoxine responsive disorders were succinctly reviewed by Drs Gregersen, Duran and Fowler, again interspersed with relevant short communications from members. Two papers by Drs Muller and Jackson were concerned with the role of vitamin E in the prevention of oxidative damage in a number of conditions and illustrated an unusual application of vitamin therapy.

In such a complex and diverse field some selection of subject matter is inevitable but the 22nd Symposium of the Society gave a fascinating account of some current developments. The success of the meeting was ensured by the efforts of a number of people; in particular our President for 1984 Professor Brandt, the Meetings Secretary Mrs Anne Green and the Chairman Dr Holton. In addition Anthony Causey, Paul Griffiths, Hiliary Wastell and Janet Stirk are thanked for their hard work before and during the Symposium. The expert secretarial help of Julie Crilly and Josephine Jepson and the editorial assistance of Philip Johnstone and Valerie Baker are gratefully acknowledged. We thank the University and City of Newcastle for their unstinting hospitality. The Wellcome Foundation, Newcastle District and the Northern Regional Health Authorities are thanked for their financial support. In particular the Society acknowledges Mr Brian Gill and Scientific and Hospital Supplies Ltd. of Liverpool for their continuing general financial support and for sponsorship of the Raine Memorial Lecture.

G. M. Addison
R. A. Harkness

K. Bartlett
R. J. Pollitt

J. Inher. Metab. Dis. 8 Suppl. 1 (1985) 2–7

Vitamins: An Evolutionary Perspective

C. R. SCRIVER

*Center for Human Genetics, and Departments of Biology and Pediatrics, McGill University and
Division of Medical Genetics, McGill University-Montreal Children's Hospital Research Institute,
2300 Tupper Street, Montreal, Quebec H3H 1P3, Canada*

Access to vitamins and the genetic endowment to utilize them maintain vitamin-dependent metabolic homeostasis in heterotrophs. Whereas the extent of adverse nutritional experiences has declined in modern human societies, phenocopies of deficiency diseases persist; accordingly, they have high heritability. The "vitamin-responsive hereditary metabolic diseases" identify DNA that specifies conserved apoenzyme domains interacting with coenzyme and the cellular processes providing access to coenzymes. Could heterozygosity at those loci also be a determinant of disease (or health) under certain circumstances?

Vitamins fascinate people and Lipmann opined: "Doctors like to prescribe vitamins and millions of people take them but it requires a good deal of biochemical sophistication to understand why they are needed and how the organism uses them" (quoted in Stryker, 1981). Geneticists have a helpful point of view here: they know that certain mutations are useful markers of the ways that organisms use vitamins and what functions they serve. Geneticists are also sensitive to the evidence that "vitamins serve nearly the same role in all forms of life, but higher animals have lost the capacity to synthesize them" (Stryker, 1981). Implicit therein is the idea that domains of apoenzymes which interact with coenzymes were conserved while new loci evolved to accommodate the essential interactions between nature (organism) and nurture (environment). When such interesting biological perspectives happen also to have implications for the everyday health of people, one might say that "discovery of the vitamins and their life-saving value in the prevention and cure of nutritional deficiency diseases is one of the most important contributions of biochemistry to medicine and human welfare" (Lehninger, 1982).

HETEROTROPHS REQUIRE VITAMINS

Discovery of the cause of beriberi comprises a well-known chapter in the history of science; we give credit to Funk for the word "vitamin(e)" and to Hopkins for the concept that vitamins are "accessory food substances" (MRC (UK), 1932). From Peters, his pigeons and his colleagues at Oxford we learned that thiamin serves the oxidation of pyruvate (Thompson, 1983). Together, those discoveries inform about essential linkages between nutrition and metabolism in heterotrophs.

Organisms prosper when requirements for their particular chemical homeostasis are met. Autotrophic organisms, such as plants and some bacteria and

protozoa, are self-supporting; they maintain homeostasis either by photosynthesis or chemosynthesis and their nutritional requirements are met by the simplest inorganic substances. Heterotrophs do not acquire energy directly, either from sunlight or by splitting simple inorganic chemicals; they require organic substances, the catabolism of which provides energy for synthetic processes, growth and differentiation. Simpler heterotrophs are less exacting in their requirements for free living; higher forms are invariably more exacting (Baldwin, 1964). The more exacting the phenotype the higher the constraints on adaptation. On the other hand, the more flexible the adaptation, the more intrinsic the machinery must be for homeostasis. By enhancing catalysis, coenzymes confer an adaptive advantage. Conservation of this function for any particular coenzyme implies that evolution has committed domains of the relevant enzyme to interact with the coenzyme and the substrate; conservation of mechanisms assuring access to coenzymes is also implied.

Homo sapiens, a free-living omnivorous heterotroph, has access to vitamins because of feeding behaviour and the genetic endowment that permits coenzymes to play their roles. It follows that detrimental experiences or mutations that impair coenzyme activity will compromise metabolic homeostasis. The result may be disadaptive, recognizable as a disease.

Access to vitamins: adaptive and disadaptive practices

Man's upright posture and modified dentition were compatible with an omnivorous dietary behaviour. Domestication of animals and sedentary agricultural practices lead to controlled food supply and encouraged population growth. Eventually the tension between population growth and availability of food would have its biological consequences and one can conceive how adaptive practices emerged in response to the phenomenon of unabated natural selection. These, when persistent in modern societies, are sometimes advantageous, but at other times they are not. Some examples illustrate this point of view (Table 1).

This is publication No. 85009 from the McGill University-Montreal
Children's Hospital Research Institute

Journal of Inherited Metabolic Disease. ISSN 0141-8955. Copyright © SSIEM and MTP Press Limited, Queen Square, Lancaster, UK.

Table 1 Adaptive and disadaptive practices affecting vitamin activities

Vitamin activity	Disease associated with deficient activity[1]	Practice Adaptive	Practice Disadaptive
Thiamin	Beriberi Wernicke–Korsakoff psychosis		Milling of grain Alcoholism
Niacin	Pellegra	Soaking cornmeal in lime water	
Ascorbate	Scurvy	Citrous fruits	Exploration
Cholecalciferol	Rickets and osteomalacia	Fair skin[2]	Urbanization

[1]Environmental events may be the most prevalent cause of the disease; however, mutation is likely to be the cause when disadaptive practices are eliminated or appropriate food regulations offset them
[2]An evolutionary rather than behavioural adaptation

The optimal environment achieved through informed dietary practice and food regulations will ensure relative freedom of the collective from many diseases of altered vitamin activity and perhaps that is why the environmentalists are so strident in their aspirations. While one must applaud their effort, it cannot achieve perfection; phenocopies of the deficiency diseases will persist in some individuals; but why? The answer is, of course, mutation.

Study of the causes of rickets in modern communities well protected by adequate food regulations shows that the residual cases are Mendelian disorders of vitamin D, calcium or phosphorus homeostasis. Whereas inadequacies of experience (nurture) and genotype (nature) were both causes of rickets in former times; the former were so prevalent as to make the latter inapparent. As the former were brought under control the latter became more obvious although still infrequent. It follows that heritability of the persisting phenotype has risen relative to earlier times (Scriver and Tenenhouse, 1981). This is an important finding; as a prototype, it serves two viewpoints. First, the relevant mutations will be useful markers for a taxonomy of genes dedicated to homeostasis of coenzymes. Second, heterozygosity at these loci may be a contributing cause of diseases easily recognized early in life in their homozygous forms but less obvious in later life in their "multifactorial" forms. That is to say, what we learn from the rare "vitamin-responsive inborn errors of metabolism" may become relevant to an understanding of some common diseases of later life.

VITAMIN-RESPONSIVE INBORN ERRORS OF METABOLISM: EVOLUTIONARY VIEWPOINT

Since the nutrient vitamin is not necessarily the coenzyme itself, intermediate events must link nutrient with coenzyme; those processes involve either transport or conversion, or both, of precursors and coenzyme. Cellular catalysts (polypeptides) mediate these events; as gene products they are susceptible to mutation. Accordingly, the Mendelian phenotypes, classified as "vitamin-responsive inborn errors of metabolism" (Scriver, 1973a) are markers for the genes that control homeostasis of coenzymes. Previous reviews describe many of the variant phenotypes (diseases) (Scriver, 1973a, b; Rosenberg, 1976, 1981); the underlying

concept seems to have emerged somewhat earlier (Scriver, 1967).

Coenzymes reflect two evolutionary relationships. The first is their catalytic role in relation to apoenzymes. The optimal steric arrangement between polypeptide, substrate and coenzyme is selected by evolution. Since coenzyme and substrate structures are constant but the primary sequence of the polypeptide is unlikely to be so in organisms of different species, there is opportunity here to discern convergent or divergent evolutionary strategies. The second relationship concerns the types of genes and their phenotypes that are dedicated to maintain coenzyme homeostasis in the heterotroph.

Coenzyme, polypeptide interaction

The coenzyme is a small molecule; the polypeptide apoenzyme is a macromolecule with tertiary or quartenary structure under evolutionary constraint. A specific spatial relationship of one to the other enhances the catalytic action of the polypeptide toward its substrate. Alcohol dehydrogenase and its NAD coenzyme illustrate the guiding principles (see Plapp (1982) for details).

Alcohol dehydrogenase is a ubiquitous enzyme found, for example, in fungal, insect and mammalian heterotrophs. Although the primary sequence of the apoenzyme differs greatly in the three classes of organism, hydrophobic residues in the internal regions of the tertiary structure are either conserved, similar or compensated; as a result the critical space-filling dimensions of the apoenzyme serving its catalytic role are comparable, folding patterns are similar and nucleotide (coenzyme) binding domains are equivalent in different species. The findings are compatible with evolutionary conservation, by whatever strategy, of the nucleotide-binding domain and its steric relation to the substrate.

Why does alcohol dehydrogenase have subunits? The mammalian liver enzyme is a dimeric homopolymer; other NAD-requiring dehydrogenases are either dimers (e.g. malate dehydrogenase) or tetramers (e.g. lactate dehydrogenase). It is presumed that the oligomeric structure was selected for an optimal functional relationship. For example, liver alcohol dehydrogenase forms the substrate-binding cleft from amino acid residues in the catalytic domain of one subunit and the NAD-binding domain of the other. This complex arrangement is associated with conformational changes when the holoenzyme (coenzyme bound to apoenzyme) binds substrate to form the ternary complex; catalytic domains rotate relative to NAD-binding domains, the result being a significant spatial change in the active site situated between the domains. Although conformational change upon binding of substrate is a general phenomenon of enzymes, it is not known why they change conformation when they bind substrate, how the transition is accomplished or whether it is essential for catalysis.

Specific amino acid residues are involved in binding NAD to alcohol dehydrogenase (Figure 1). For example, the lysine at residue 228, when substituted, alters coenzyme binding and consequently alters the reaction rate; cationic amino acids other than lysine at position 228, can enhance binding of NAD and thus slow the reaction which is an ordered BiBi mechanism. Arginine residues 47 and 369 have an ionic interaction with the NAD pyrophosphate group; mutation substituting histidine at residue 47 impairs binding affinity for NAD. An aspartate residue at position 223 in the liver enzyme is invariant at the equivalent position in all mammalian, yeast and Drosophila alcohol dehydrogenases studied so far; its apparent role is to block the binding of NADP and to accept only NAD. The selective advantage attached to this residue is readily apparent.

NAD is the coenzyme form used primarily in energy pathways whereas NADP is the form used almost exclusively in reductive biosynthesis. Alcohol dehydrogenase serves energy metabolism.

The substrate is bound tightly in a hydrophobic pocket with the alcohol oxygen ligated directly to the zinc atom at the active site. The metal is positioned by two sulfurs from cysteine residues and by one histidine residue. Substitution of one or other of these residues largely inactivates the enzyme.

The catalytic process involves transfer of the pro-*R* hydrogen on carbon 1 of the alcohol to carbon 4 on the *re*-face of the NAD ring, with removal of the proton on the hydroxyl group of ethanol to form acetaldehyde. While the exact mechanism is unknown, it seems likely that a proton relay is formed by the hydroxyl group of serine 48, the 2'-hydroxyl group of nicotinamide ribose and the imidazole group of histidine 51 of the protein in the pocket adjacent to the coenzyme.

From this overview of an interaction between a coenzyme, an apoenzyme and its substrate, it is apparent how specificity of the polypeptide phenotype, and therefore the genotype, determines optimal coenzyme-binding and catalytic function. It is equally clear that point mutations could alter coenzyme-binding through substitution of residues in the specific domain, or by modifying the position of the domain relative to the catalytic site.

Mendelian probes of coenzyme dishomeostasis in man

Mutations offer a working taxonomy of the mechanisms serving coenzyme homeostasis. They can be divided into mutants that affect binding of coenzymes, their processing and the transport of precursors or coenzymes themselves (Figure 2). A catalogue is not intended here; only examples are given to illustrate the concepts.

Binding mutants

Mutations that affect binding must occur in coding sequences that determine domains or residues of apoenzyme (see above). Accordingly, such mutations will map at apoenzyme loci (and not at putative regulatory loci). Their phenotype is expected to alter the affinity of coenzyme-binding. Whether the quantitative phenotype that might be delineated *in vitro* with purified apoenzyme is a true measure of the phenotype *in vivo* is a more remote matter of speculation. Autosomal alleles affect, for example, pyridoxal-5-phosphate-binding by cystathionine β-synthase and cystathioninase in homocystinuria and cystathioninuria, respectively (see Mudd and Levy (1983) for details); and binding of thiamine pyrophosphate to branched chain α-ketoacid dehydrogenase in a thiamine-responsive form of MSUD (Chuang *et al.*, 1982).

The phenotypic effects of "binding" mutations are of genetic and clinical interest. First the enzyme phenotypes, by definition, are cross-reacting-material positive. Second, the metabolic dishomeostasis associated with the variant catalyst may be reparable when sufficient coenzyme is supplied to offset the unfavourable binding kinetics. Third, the impaired catalytic activity may also reflect reduced concentration of apoenzyme because its

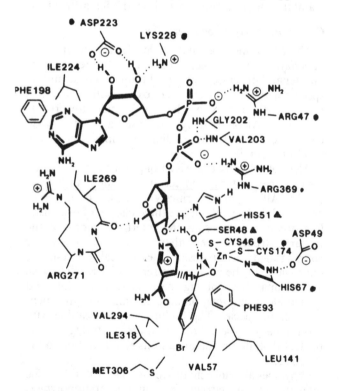

Figure 1 Diagram of the active site of mammalian liver alcohol dehydrogenase. Interactions between critical amino acids in the apoenzyme (indicated by ●, ▲ symbols) and NAD coenzyme, and positioning of the substrate (*p*-bromobenzyl alcohol) are indicated. The pro-*R* hydrogen of the alcohol, is shown in large case; the *re*-face of the nicotinamide ring has the positive charge facing and the carboxamido group away from the viewer (from Plapp, 1982, by permission of Sinauer Associates Inc. Publishers)

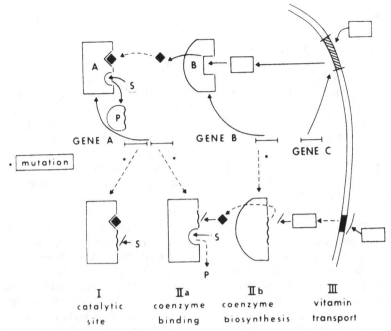

Figure 2 Proposed mechanisms for specific vitamin responsiveness in certain inborn errors of metabolism. Gene A codes for apoenzyme A, which converts a substrate to a product; gene B codes for apoenzyme B, which converts a vitamin to its active coenzyme form. Gene C codes for a membrane transport protein responsible for vitamin (or coenzyme) uptake by the cell. Coenzyme must interact with apoenzyme A for normal catalysis. Mutation at gene locus A (model IIa) perturbs the normal interaction of coenzyme with apoenzyme. If mutation affects only substrate-binding (model 1) the depressed residual enzyme function might be augmented by saturating the mutant apoenzyme with coenzyme to reduce its turnover and raise holoenzyme concentration. Mutation at gene locus B blocks synthesis of coenzyme. A partial block (K_m) might be offset by increasing the vitamin concentration. Mutation at gene locus C impairs entry of vitamin (or coenzyme) into the cell, a circumstance that may be offset by higher extracellular concentrations of vitamin (from Scriver, 1973b, by permission of Grune & Stratton, Inc.)

turnover is likely to be increased when undersaturated with coenzyme (Mudd and Levy, 1983). Fourth, the likelihood of many "binding" alleles is high, judging from empirical evidence; thus many different homozygous and compound phenotypes are likely, implying that a spectrum of clinical responsiveness to a pharmacologic dose of vitamin is probable. That is to say, each proband (and pedigree) in outbred societies, where the segregating alleles are many, could have its own phenotype.

Processing mutants
The apoenzyme must have access to coenzyme. Therefore it is dependent on events that attach the coenzyme covalently when it is not ionically bound (e.g. biotin), synthesise it from precursors, and transport it or the precursor form.

(i) *Attachment.* Biotin is a novel coenzyme; it is attached covalently to the epsilon amino group of a specific lysine residue in four mammalian carboxylating enzymes to form their prosthetic groups. The biotinyllysine residue, called biocytin, is the active form of biotin. Formation of biocytin requires a "ligase" (holocarboxylase synthetase); release of biotin during turnover and degradation of carboxylases requires "biotinidase". Any mutation impairing "ligase" activity is disadaptive since it affects multiple carboxylase activities and homeostasis of the relevant metabolic pathways for propionyl-CoA, β-methylcrotonyl-CoA, and pyruvate in mitochondria; and for conversion of acetyl-CoA to malonyl-CoA in cytosol (see Rosenberg (1983) for details). Any mutation

impairing biotinidase activity affects homeostasis of biotin itself by increasing its turnover and loss; the carboxylase enzymes are affected secondarily. "Ligase"- and "biotinidase"-deficient phenotypes are described elsewhere in this symposium but some caution will still be required to interpret the corresponding clinical phenotypes since access to biotin is also dependent on transcellular (and perhaps intracellular), transport processes prior to synthesis of biocytin and abnormalities of these steps could and may occur. It is still not known whether cytosol and mitochondrial "ligase" enzymes are identical nor where biotinidase plays its principal role.

One wonders whether lipoic acid is attached to and removed from the E_2 component of pyruvate, α-ketoglutarate, and branched chain ketoacid dehydrogenases by analogous ligating and cleavage enzymes. Work on this topic is in progress (B. Wolf, personal communication, 1984).

(ii) *Synthesis.* Many coenzymes are the product of conversion pathways for which the precursor substrate is a vitamin. The pathway for synthesis and maintenance of tetrahydrobiopterin is of special relevance in this symposium. Even though the precursor substance is not a vitamin, the product of the pathway functions as a cofactor. Tetrahydrobiopterin represents an adaptation of a pterine for a particular role in catalysis different, for example, from the use of pterines in pigment metabolism among insects. A complicated sequence to which several genes are committed yields the precursor of tetrahydrobiopterin; a single locus product (dihydropteridine reductase) conserves tetrahydrobiopterin homeostasis during the stoichiometric expenditure of cofactor in the hydroxylations of phenylalanine, tyrosine and tryptophan. There is adaptive economy here; activity of the reductase ensures that the product of the biosynthetic pathway is used efficiently. Any mutation that impairs synthesis or conservation of tetrahydrobiopterin is likely to have a profoundly disadaptive effect, in view of the role played by the relevant hydroxylases in development and function of the central nervous system; the corresponding Mendelian phenotypes in man bear out this view.

The pathways for converting vitamin B_{12} activity to its coenzyme forms (methylcobalamin serving homocysteine methylation; adenosylcobalamin serving methylmalonyl-CoA isomerization) are now well understood (Rosenberg, 1983); mutation proved to be a powerful probe to identify the essential steps in the human pathways (Rosenberg, 1981). Probands with deficient methylmalonyl-CoA mutase activity reveal a general principle of clinical relevance for all patients with vitamin-responsive inborn errors of metabolism. When mutation occurs at the mutase locus and causes complete loss of catalytic activity (mut° phenotype), the clinical prognosis is poor (Figure 3); all patients, regardless of efficiency in diagnosis and treatment, either die or have impaired development. On the other hand, probands with cobalamin-responsive mutase deficiency, associated with disorders of adenosylcobalamin synthesis (cbl A and cbl B phenotypes) or with only partial loss of enzyme activity (mut⁻ phenotype) have a better prognosis (Figure 3); up to 70% of such patients in a given category are alive and "well" following diagnosis and treatment (Matsui *et al.*, 1983).

(iii) *Transport*. Coenzymes serve many roles that are specifically intracellular. For the vitamin precursor (or coenzyme in the case of ascorbate and biotin) to gain access to the internal milieu it must first traverse the lipid bilayer of plasma membranes. If the water-soluble vitamins entered only by diffusion they would do so

slowly and heterotrophs would be at the mercy of the vitamin content of the external environment. Mediated transport is an adaptive strategy that permits organisms to acquire unique sets of molecules from the larger mixed population, and to attain intracellular homeostasis. When the transport system is coupled to energy metabolism, the organisms can pump its substrate against a transmembrane electrochemical gradient. Such specificity of transport function can be achieved in biological systems only by polypeptides in the membrane; accordingly, if there is a transport mechanism there is a gene (or genes if it is a heteropolymeric structure) to specify the process.

Higher heterotrophs acquire vitamins by absorbing them from the bowel lumen. Water-soluble vitamins require membrane intestinal transport systems; (fat soluble vitamins are absorbed by the different strategies serving lipids). Rose discusses the specific vitamin transport systems elsewhere in this symposium.

Whereas the intestinal transport systems serve nutrient-dependent homeostasis, renal transport serves global homeostasis of the organism by reabsorbing substances that would otherwise be lost in filtrate. The majority of vertebrates have the capacity to synthesize ascorbic acid (Chaterjee *et al.*, 1975) and they also conserve it by renal reabsorption. A specific, sodium ion-coupled, saturable process in brush-border membrane of proximal tubule serves renal transport of ascorbate (Toggenburger *et al.*, 1981). Heterotrophs which have lost the capacity to synthesize ascorbate must obtain it from the environment. They evolved an adaptive strategy; they possess an ascorbate-specific carrier in the brush-border membrane of intestinal epithelium with characteristics that differ slightly from the renal system.

Two questions are raised by these findings. First, is the gene for L-gulonolactone oxidase deleted in *Homo sapiens* or is it a dormant non-transcribed pseudogene? Second, is the gene for the ascorbate transport protein present but suppressed in intestinal cells of oxidase-proficient species; and is it derepressed or a new gene in oxidase-deficient species? The molecular geneticists may find these problems worthwhile to pursue.

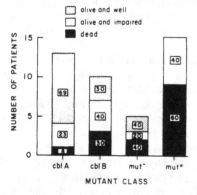

Figure 3 Long-term outcome of patients with methylmalonicaciduria: cb1A, cb1B, are vitamin B_{12} responsive forms of disordered coenzyme (adenosylcobalamin) synthesis. Mut⁻ and mut° are apoenzyme phenotypes, the latter never B_{12}-responsive. "Impaired" indicates retarded development of proband with recurrent metabolic dishomeostasis. Numbers in bars indicate percentage of patients in category (from Matsui *et al.*, 1983, reprinted by permission of the *New England Journal of Medicine*)

THE INBORN ERRORS OF VITAMIN RESPONSIVENESS: A BROADER INTERPRETATION

Discovery of vitamin-responsive inborn errors of metabolism is likely to continue. Tetrahydrobiopterin-responsive forms of hyperphenylalaninaemia are being enumerated; and the putative biotinidase-deficient phenotype has only recently revealed itself. The hereditary phenocopies of vitamin deficiency diseases are recent discoveries for two quite different reasons. First, there is new knowledge that helps us to know more about the molecular basis of coenzyme action; hence we are better prepared to analyze and interpret the associated diseases. Second, the benefits of public health and nutrition practices lead to a remarkable abatement in the flood of deficiency diseases; the "post-deluvian" period leaves only the monadnock-like phenocopies whose shape is molded not by the environment but by the genotype of the individual. Of course, the disadaptive effects of these diseases are not solely determined by the genes and are not just an expression of increased heritability. Whereas genes indeed propose, it is the environment that disposes; in the case of individuals with "inborn errors of vitamin responsiveness" their requirements for vitamin or coenzyme are deviant from normal. In recognizing this, we gain access to treatment; an augmented supply of the relevant vitamin/coenzyme restores metabolic homeostasis, prevents disease and largely neutralizes expression of the mutant gene.

A novel illustration of this view is the Wernicke–Korsakoff syndrome. Chronic alcoholism increases the risk for thiamin deficiency and many alcoholics are deficient, yet only a few develop the syndrome. Most are Caucasian; few are Black. Those with the syndrome appear to have a specific abnormality of thiamin-binding to transketolase (Blass and Gibson, 1977). The latter event, if genetically determined, is a constitutional explanation for the syndrome and its segregation. Accordingly, the risk that a particular alcoholic will develop the syndrome could be measured and thiamin prescribed at pharmacologic dose levels to that particular person. This is specific preventive treatment and more logical than thiamin fortification of all alcoholic beverages to be consumed by the collective (Centerwall and Criqui, 1978).

A fuller awareness of the role of genotype and of the particular interaction with environment that results may be required to explain some forms of human disease. The present catalogue of "inborn errors of vitamin responsiveness" lists only the discontinuous variation associated with homozygous or compound autosomal alleles. They are all rare phenotypes (incidence $< 10^{-5}$ usually). Their rarity may reflect the low frequency of the alleles, or reduced viability of affected fetuses. In either case, the heterozygous phenotype is much more prevalent than the corresponding homozygous/compound form. Do we know whether these individuals are without risk to their health? Is the interaction between the heterozygous phenotype and the environment utterly benign or would certain experiences be disadvantageous to these individuals? For example, acetylation polymorphisms affect vitamin B_6 requirements in patients treated with isoniazid. We might begin with a question of topical interest: Are all humans devoid of a synthetic capacity for ascorbate (Cummings, 1981). This question, and others like it, adorn the major recurring question in medicine: "Why does this patient have (or not have) this disease, at this time?" (King, 1982).

References

Baldwin, E. *An Introduction to Comparative Biochemistry*, 4th Edn., Cambridge University Press, Cambridge, 1964

Blass, J. P. and Gibson, G. E. Abnormality of a thiamine-requiring enzyme in patients with Wernicke–Korsakoff syndrome. *N. Engl. J. Med.* 297 (1977) 1367–1370

Centerwall, B. S. and Criqui, M. H. Prevention of the Wernicke–Korsakoff syndrome. A cost benefit analysis. *N. Engl. J. Med.* 299 (1978) 285–289

Chaterjee, I. B., Majumber, A. K., Nandi, B. K. and Subramanian, N. Synthesis and some major functions of vitamin C in animals. *Ann. N.Y. Acad. Sci.* 258 (1975) 24–46

Chuang, D. T., Ku, L. S. and Cox, R. P. Thiamin-responsive maple-syrup-urine disease: Decreased affinity of the mutant branched-chain alpha-keto acid dehydrogenase for alpha-ketoisovalerate and thiamin pyrophosphate. *Proc. Natl. Acad. Sci. USA* 79 (1982) 3300–3304

Cummings, M. Can some people synthesize ascorbic acid? (Letter). *Am. J. Clin. Nutr.* 34 (1981) 297–298

King, L. S. *Medical Thinking. A Historical Preface*, Princeton University Press, Princeton, 1982, pp. 187–203

Lehninger, A. *Principles of Biochemistry*, Worth Publishing, New York, 1982, p. 249

Matsui, S. M., Mahoney, M. J. and Rosenberg, L. E. The natural history of the inherited methylmalonic acidemias. *N. Engl. J. Med.* 308 (1983) 857–861

Medical Research Council (UK). Vitamins: A survey of present knowledge. Special Report Series, No. 167 (1932)

Mudd, S. H. and Levy, H. L. Disorders of transsulfuration. In Stanbury, J. B., Wyngaarden, J. B., Fredrickson, D. S., Goldstein, J. L. and Brown, M. S. (eds.) *The Metabolic Basis of Inherited Disease*, 6th Edn, McGraw-Hill, New York, 1983, pp. 552–559

Plapp, B. V. Origins of protein structure and function. In *Perspectives on Evolution*, Sinauer Assocs., Sunderland, MA, 1982

Rosenberg, L. E. Vitamin-responsive inherited metabolic disorders. In Harris, H. and Hirschhorn, K. (eds.) *Advances in Human Genetics*, Plenum Press, New York, Vol. 6, 1976, pp. 1–74

Rosenberg, L. E. The inherited methylmalonicacidemias: A model system for the study of vitamin metabolism and apoenzyme-coenzyme interactions. In Belton, N. R. and Toothill, E. (eds.) *Transport and Inherited Disease (Proc. 17th Symp. Soc. Study Inborn Errors Metab.)*, MTP Press, Lancaster, 1981, pp. 3–32

Rosenberg, L. E. Disorders of propionate and methylmalonate metabolism. In Stanbury, J. B., Wyngaarden, J. B., Fredrickson, D. S., Goldstein, J. L. and Brown, M. S. (eds.) *The Metabolic Basis of Inherited Disease*, 5th Edn., McGraw-Hill, New York, 1983, pp. 474–497

Scriver, C. R. Treatment in medical genetics. In Crow, J. F. and Neel, J. V. (eds.) *Proc. Third Int. Congr. Hum. Genet. (Chicago, September 1966)*, The Johns Hopkins Press, Baltimore, 1967, pp. 45–56

Scriver, C. R. Vitamin-responsive inborn errors of metabolism (the hereditary vitamin dependencies). In Seakins, J. T., Saunders, R. A. and Toothill, C. (eds.) *Treatment of Inborn Errors of Metabolism (Proc. 10th Symp. Soc. Study Inborn Errors Metab.)*, Churchill Livingstone, Edinburgh, 1973a, pp. 127–148

Scriver, C. R. Vitamin responsive inborn errors of metabolism (progress in endocrinology and metabolism). *Metabolism* 22 (1973b) 1319–1344

Scriver, C. R. and Tenenhouse, H. S. On the heritability of rickets, a common disease (Mendel, mammals and phosphate). *Johns Hopkins Med. J.* 149 (1981) 179–187

Stryker, L. *Biochemistry*, 2nd Edn., W. H. Freeman, San Francisco, 1981

Thompson, R. H. S. Thiamine and the metabolism of pyruvate. *Trends Biochem. Sci.* 8 (1983) 460–461

Toggenburger, G., Hausermann, M., Mutsch, B., Genoni, G., Kessler, M., Weber, F., Hornig, D., O'Neill, B. and Semenza, G. Na$^+$-dependent, potential-sensitive L-ascorbate transport across brush-border membrane vesicles from kidney cortex. *Biochim. Biophys. Acta* 646 (1981) 433–443

J. Inher. Metab. Dis. 8 Suppl. 1 (1985) 8–12

Normal Vitamin Requirements in Neonates and Infants

C. J. BATES

MRC Dunn Nutrition Laboratory, Milton Road, Cambridge CB4 1XJ, UK

Information about vitamin requirements by neonates and infants has been derived from studies of the composition of breast milk, from feed–response trials, from the occurrence of overt deficiency in infants fed damaged milk formulae, and by extrapolation from experimental deficiency studies on adult humans and on animals. Our knowledge is far from complete, however, and dietary recommendations have been formulated for only about half the known vitamins in the UK. In the near future, studies with stable isotope-labelled vitamins should help to define pool sizes and turnover rates that are associated with particular intakes and thus give firmer evidence about requirements.

The term 'vitamin requirements' applied to human populations or groups can have at least two different meanings in different contexts. One of these is the *minimum* amount needed to support normal physiological function and prevent signs and symptoms of overt deficiency in otherwise healthy, normal and adequately nourished subjects. This defines the borderline below which the average individual would eventually exhibit overt deficiency. An alternative definition refers to the amount needed to satisfy the requirements, for physiological and biochemical 'normality', of the *majority* of individuals within a population or group. The latter definition forms the basis of tables of recommended dietary amounts of vitamins, and other nutrients, compiled by expert committees in most countries (Truswell *et al.*, 1983).

Whereas vitamin requirements of experimental animals have been defined very accurately by controlled feeding trials using deficient diets, this investigative approach has rarely been possible with human subjects and the available evidence about minimum requirements, especially for young babies, is therefore very limited. Of the thirteen substances generally recognised as vitamins for humans, only six have been ascribed daily intake recommendations in the UK (Table 1) because information about requirements for the remainder is currently considered inadequate. The USA recommendations (Table 1) include a figure for all thirteen, but three of these are listed separately as 'safe and adequate' intakes, since the criteria for estimation of minimum requirements could not be met. The purpose of the recommendations is the planning of food supplies and of special diets for groups of individuals and it is important to recognise that individual requirements for some vitamins may vary widely even between genetically normal individuals and that the failure of a particular

Table 1 Recommended dietary amounts in mg day^{-1} of vitamins for term infants in the first year of life

	UK (DHSS, 1979)	USA (National Research Council, 1980)
Thiamine (B$_1$)	0.3	0.3–0.5
Riboflavin (B$_2$)	0.4	0.4–0.6
Pyridoxine (B$_6$)		0.3–0.6
Niacin equivalents[†]	5.0	6.0–8.0
Total folacin	(50 × 10^{-3})[‡]	30–45 × 10^{-3}
Vitamin B$_{12}$		0.5–1.5
Biotin		35–50 × 10^{-3} [§]
Pantothenate		2–3 [§]
Vitamin C	20	35
Vitamin A (retinol equivalents)	0.45	0.42–0.40
Vitamin D	7.5 × 10^{-3}	10 × 10^{-3}
Vitamin E		3.4
Vitamin K		10–20 × 10^{-3} [§]

* Where two figures are given, they are for 0–6 months and 6–12 months, respectively
† Niacin equivalents = mg niacin + (mg tryptophan/60)
‡ UK folacin value subsequently withdrawn
§ "Safe and adequate intakes"

Journal of Inherited Metabolic Disease. ISSN 0141–8955. Copyright © SSIEM and MTP Press Limited, Queen Square, Lancaster, UK.

individual to reach the recommended intake does not necessarily imply imminent functional deficiency. However, the greater the proportion of a population who receive less than the recommended amount, and the further below that they fall, the greater is the probability of overt deficiency.

Since, by definition, a vitamin-responsive inborn error in metabolism shows a beneficial response at intakes many-fold greater than the normal requirement or amount obtained from a balanced but unsupplemented diet, it will always be necessary to identify and treat these cases separately. The theory that mega-vitamin supplementation is likely to confer benefits outweighing its dangers and disadvantages for genetically normal subjects has not been proved and may be dangerous in some instances. The fat-soluble vitamins A and D are particularly noted for their toxicity at moderately high doses and some undesirable pharmacological effects have also been reported after prolonged high intakes of certain water-soluble vitamins. The long-term significance of high doses of vitamins given to infants has not been investigated adequately, and this consideration is especially relevant to the feeding of preterm and low birth weight infants, who frequently receive large doses of vitamins as a prophylactic measure during the first few weeks of life. Since neither the composition of such supplements nor the timing of their introduction are securely based on adequate information about risk:benefit ratios, more information is urgently needed.

The evidence on which available estimates of infant vitamin requirements is based comes from several sources:

(a) The range of concentrations in human milk (Table 2) and the occurrence, if any, of deficiencies or inadequate status in fully breast-fed infants. For most practical purposes, and in particular for the design of infant formula milk, human milk is the ultimate yardstick of nutrient provision and it also contains specific proteins which may facilitate the utilisation of certain vitamins: e.g. folate-binding protein (Colman *et al.*, 1981) and bile salt-stimulated lipase for vitamin A (Fredrikzon *et al.*, 1978). Despite the fact that milk from different individuals may vary widely in its vitamin content, the fact that milk at different stages of lactation shows important changes in composition, and the fact that milk from malnourished mothers contains smaller amounts of some vitamins than the milk from well-nourished mothers (Table 2), nevertheless there are very few well-documented instances of overt vitamin deficiency arising in normal, fully breast-fed babies even in the most poorly-nourished communities (with the possible exception of vitamin D and vitamin K which are special cases).

(b) Information about requirements has also been obtained from records of cases where infants have been accidentally fed damaged or maltreated milk products. Certain vitamins, notably vitamin A, riboflavin, vitamin C, folate and vitamin B_6, are very susceptible either to heat, to light, or to oxidation, and the procedures involved in producing condensed or evaporated milk are particularly harmful to these vitamins. Although the events which resulted in infantile scurvy, vitamin B_6 deficiency convulsions or folate deficiency megaloblastic anaemia were unintentional and therefore uncontrolled, they have demonstrated the susceptibility of human infants to vitamin deficiency syndromes and have given an order-of-magnitude indication of the minimum requirement.

(c) Epidemiological studies in poorly nourished populations have given some information about minimum requirements, although considerable effort and ingenuity is usually needed to collect adequate dietary data, and to interpret clinical deficiency signs which may be complicated by multiple nutrient deficiencies and exacerbated by local infections. The magnitude of the response to controlled supplements of

Table 2 Vitamin content of mature human milk (mgl^{-1})

Vitamin	Kon and Mawson (1950)	DHSS (1977)	Ford et al. (1983)	Belavady and Gopalan (1959)	Macy et al. (1950)
Thiamine (B_1)	0.27	0.16	0.18	0.15	0.14
Riboflavin (B_2)	0.24	0.31	0.31	0.17	0.37
Pyridoxine (B_6)		0.06	0.11		0.18
Niacin	1.83	2.3	1.82	0.57	1.8
Niacin equivalents		6.2			
Total folacin		0.05	0.04		0.04
Vitamin B_{12}		0.1×10^{-3}	0.23×10^{-3}		
Biotin		7.6×10^{-3}	5.3×10^{-3}		8×10^{-3}
Pantothenate		2.6	2.6	2.3	2.5
Vitamin C	35	38		26	52
Vitamin A	0.47	0.60			0.65
Vitamin D		0.25×10^{-3}			
Vitamin E		3.4			
Vitamin K*		2.1×10^{-3}			

Values are means obtained from groups of normal mothers during full lactation, expressed in mg l^{-1}. The first three studies were in the UK; the fourth was in India, and the fifth in the USA
* The vitamin K value was obtained in the UK by Haroon *et al.* (1982)

single nutrients can give further valuable information in this context.

(d) Controlled depletion–repletion studies have proved to be by far the most useful and accurate sources of information on vitamin requirements of adults but this approach is not, of course, directly applicable to infants. Some information about infant requirements has been derived by extrapolation from observations on adults and the relationship between adult and infant requirements has been studied extensively in experimental animals. Preterm infants represent, in some respects, a "naturally" depleted group, whose low body stores coupled with rapid growth predispose them to deficiency, despite an apparently 'adequate' intake, even when they are well. Studies of their nutritional requirements and special problems are just beginning to emerge and are currently of considerable interest.

Comparison between different groups of infants receiving different diets in feed–response trials is an ethically acceptable alternative to controlled depletion. This has been especially applicable in studies on premature infants who have low body stores of some vitamins at birth and a rapid growth rate, necessitating rapid accretion of nutrients. The combination of this approach with the use of stable isotope-labelled vitamins should, be capable in the near future, of measuring body pool sizes, turnover rates and other kinetic parameters. This will permit the estimation of 'acceptable' nutrient intakes on the basis of dynamic indices of status which promise to be more comprehensive and relevant than the indices currently available.

(e) Extrapolation from studies on experimental animals may be feasible, provided the animals' course of development and maturation is similar to that of the human infant. However, interspecies differences in absorption, refection, storage efficiency, turnover rate and requirements at the molecular level make it unwise to rely too heavily on this approach.

Not surprisingly, the magnitude of daily vitamin requirements of young infants changes markedly as they grow and mature. Provided these changes are proportional to the changes in energy and protein requirement the quality of the diet has no need to change. The problem becomes more complex, however, when the requirement for micronutrients changes in relation to the requirement for energy. Examples are the need for additional vitamin C to prevent abnormal tyrosine metabolism (Irwin and Hutchins, 1976) and the possible need for dietary carnitine by preterm infants (Borum, 1981).

There follows below a brief discussion of the requirements for certain individual vitamins.

THIAMINE

Early studies (Knott *et al.*, 1943) indicated that thiamine requirements of infants were similar to those of adults on an energy basis: 0.27 mg/1000 kcal. Thiamine deficiency in infants is still being reported from some developing countries (Pongpanich *et al.*, 1974; Neumann *et al.*, 1979). There is little information about the requirements of preterm infants.

RIBOFLAVIN

Lack of meat and dairy products in the diet make riboflavin deficiency one of the commonest nutrient deficiencies in developing countries. Infants whom we have studied in a rural community in The Gambia, for instance, were born biochemically deficient and improved only slightly during suckling (Bates *et al.*, 1982). Weaning on the local gruels which provided only *ca.* 0.2 mg riboflavin day^{-1} produced further deterioration of status, whereas a supplementary weaning food which ensured an intake of 0.4 mg day^{-1} (equal to the UK recommended amount) eliminated the biochemical abnormality.

Even in Western society, biochemical riboflavin deficiency occurs transiently during the first 2 weeks of life in term or preterm infants who are fed solely on human milk (Hovi *et al.*, 1979; Lucas and Bates, 1984). Accidental exposure of milk to sunlight, ward lighting or phototherapy lights exacerbates the problem by destroying riboflavin. The possible physiological implications of this subclinical deficiency are currently being investigated.

VITAMIN B$_6$

Damaged cow's milk preparations caused neonatal convulsions, attributable to vitamin B$_6$ deficiency in the USA (Bessey *et al.*, 1957; American Academy of Pediatrics, 1966). Protection was provided by 0.26 mg vitamin B$_6$ day^{-1}, and the vitamin B$_6$-dependent tryptophan catabolism pathway was also normalised by an intake of 0.3 mg vitamin B$_6$ day^{-1}. The central role of vitamin B$_6$ in amino acid catabolism is reflected by a close correlation between vitamin B$_6$ requirements and protein intake; an intake ratio of 0.015 mg vitamin B$_6$ g protein^{-1} is currently recommended for infant formulae (American Academy of Pediatrics, 1966).

NIACIN

There are no data on niacin requirements of infants, nor has their ability to convert tryptophan to niacin been studied. Human milk contains *ca.* 1.8–2.3 mg niacin l^{-1}, and can in theory yield about a further 4 mg l^{-1} from tryptophan.

FOLACIN

Since several studies have shown that low birth weight or premature infants fed evaporated cow's milk preparations may develop folate-responsive megaloblastic anaemia (Rodriguez, 1978; Strelling *et al.*, 1979), the adequacy of folate nutrition, which is critical for normal cell division, has become a cause for concern for certain at-risk groups. In fresh milk, folate is protected by ascorbate (Ford and Scott, 1968), and fully breast-fed term infants are reported to have adequate folate status (Ek and Magnus, 1979).

Asfour *et al.* (1977) reported that 3.6 µg folate kg body wt^{-1} day^{-1} was adequate in term infants to ensure maximum haemoglobin levels and weight gain. Strelling *et al.* (1979) have recommended 50 µg day^{-1} as a safe and desirable prophylactic intake for preterm infants below a 2 kg body weight; the current recommended dietary amount in the USA is 30–45 µg day^{-1}. Intakes of 100 µg are most commonly recommended for premature infants, and it is not uncommon for hospitals to give as much as 1–2 mg daily. Gandy and Jacobson (1977) demonstrated beneficial effects of 5 mg daily supplements of folate for erythroblastotic infants, and Jacobson (personal communication) has indicated that the intellectual performance of infants who are moderately deficient in folate during the time of most rapid brain development, may be retarded or impaired.

BIOTIN

Infants below 6 months old sometimes show a seborrhoeic dermatitis which responds to biotin supplements; the mild form may represent a simple nutrient deficiency, whereas a more severe form known as Leiner's Disease, appears to have a genetic component (Bonjour, 1977; Roth, 1981). No estimates of minimum requirements are currently available, however.

VITAMIN B$_{12}$ AND PANTOTHENIC ACID

Both of these vitamins are supplied in adequate amounts by all 'natural' diets, or by normal intestinal flora, making the development of a purely nutritional deficiency apparently extremely rare. In contrast, the development of pernicious anaemia, through failure of intrinsic factor or other facets of the B$_{12}$ transport and delivery system, is relatively common, and an important cause of morbidity.

CARNITINE

Although not usually classified as a vitamin for humans, there are preliminary indications that carnitine synthesis from lysine may be inadequate in some preterm infants (Warshaw and Curry, 1980; Borum, 1981; Schmidt-Sommerfeld et al., 1982).

VITAMIN C

This is one of the most labile nutrients in milk and infant formulae, whose destruction caused the characteristic and potentially fatal syndrome of infantile scurvy in nineteenth century Britain. Estimates of the daily requirement vary widely, especially for preterm infants (Irwin and Hutchins, 1976), perhaps reflecting the variety of proposed biological functions and criteria of adequacy that this vitamin has attracted.

Prevention of abnormal tyrosine metabolism has tended to dominate the subject of infant requirements, whereas the function of vitamin C in collagen biosynthesis is perhaps more relevant to the clinical signs of scurvy and the development of rapidly growing tissues.

FAT-SOLUBLE VITAMINS

Liver stores of vitamin A are likely to be low in preterm infants because the transfer of vitamin A from mother to fetus normally takes place most rapidly during the last few weeks of intrauterine life. While this is unlikely to result in overt deficiency in Western society, where food sources of vitamin A are generally plentiful, it is possible that the premature infant might be at increased risk of developing a florid deficiency during preschool years in those countries where dietary vitamin A deficiency is endemic.

Vitamin D deficiency is still relatively common in Britain, especially among Asian immigrants (Brooke, 1983), and the current dietary recommendation for vitamin D for infants (Table 1) is far higher than the amount found in breast milk (Table 2) reflecting the fact that 'pharmacological' amounts in the diet are needed to counteract the inadequacy of *de novo* synthesis in the skin. However, the long-term implications of dietary vitamin D in the immediate postnatal period need further study, in view of its potential toxicity and the fact that the calcium/phosphate ratio may after all be the main critical factor in rickets of prematurity. The optimum amounts of calcium and phosphate in infant feeds, especially those for premature infants, are currently being reinvestigated.

Vitamin E-responsive cases of edema and anaemia have been observed in low birth weight infants fed milk formulae which were rich in polyunsaturated fatty acid, but low in vitamin E. The American Academy of Pediatrics (1977) has recommended that each gram of linoleic acid in milk formulae should be accompanied by at least 0.6 mg α-tocopherol or its equivalent. New interest in the vitamin has recently been stimulated by the discovery of a potential for preventing damage from retrolental fibroplasia (Hittner and Kretzer, 1983), although there is some concern about the possibility of deleterious effects involving necrotising enterocolitis.

Injection of vitamin K at birth is standard practice where there is a significant risk of neonatal haemorrhage. The very low vitamin K content of human milk (Shearer et al., 1982) is responsible for vitamin K deficiency in some breast-fed infants, which has led, in a few instances, to serious sequelae such as intracranial haemorrhage (Payne and Hasegawa, 1984).

In conclusion, there is still a great deal to be learned about normal infant vitamin requirements, especially for preterm and low birth weight infants. Paradoxically, those vitamins for which vitamin-responsive inborn errors are most common are among those for which there is least information about normal requirements. The study of inborn errors may help to provide a window on the definition of normal requirements, e.g. by providing information about physiological responses to marginal deficiency states. Likewise, a better understanding of the range and limits of normal requirements and responses will facilitate the identification of abnormalities in genetic variants.

References

American Academy of Pediatrics. Committee on nutrition: vitamin B$_6$ requirements in man. *Pediatrics* 38 (1966) 1068–1076

American Academy of Pediatrics. Committee on nutrition:

Nutritional needs of low birth-weight infants. *Pediatrics* 60 (1977) 519–530

Asfour, R., Wahbeh, C. I., Waslien, C. I., Guindi, S. and Darby, W. J. Folacin requirements of children II. Normal infants. *Am. J. Clin. Nutr.* 30 (1977) 1098–1105

Bates, C. J., Prentice, A. M., Paul, A. A., Prentice, A., Sutcliffe, B. A. and Whitehead, R. G. Riboflavin status in infants born in rural Gambia, and the effect of a weaning food supplement. *Trans. R. Soc. Trop. Med. Hyg.* 76 (1982) 253–258

Belavady, B. and Gopalan, C. Chemical composition of human milk in poor Indian women. *Ind. J. Med. Res.* 47 (1959) 234–245

Bessey, O. A., Adam, D. J. and Hansen, A. E. Intake of vitamin B_6 and infantile convulsions: a first approximation of requirements of pyridoxine in infants. *Pediatrics* 20 (1957) 33–44

Bonjour, J. P. Biotin in man's nutrition and therapy: a review. *Int. J. Vit. Nutr. Res.* 47 (1977) 107–118

Borum, P. R. Possible carnitine requirement of the newborn and the effect of genetic disease on the carnitine requirement. *Nutr. Rev.* 11 (1981) 385–390

Brooke, O. G. Supplementary vitamin D in infancy and childhood. *Arch. Dis. Child.* 58 (1983) 573–574

Colman, N., Hettiarachchy, N. and Herbert, V. Detection of a milk factor that facilitates folate uptake by intestinal cells. *Science* 211 (1981) 1427–1428

Department of Health and Social Security. The composition of mature human milk. Report on Health and Social Subjects, No. 12, HMSO, London (1977)

Department of Health and Social Security. Recommended daily amounts of food energy and nutrients for groups of people in the U.K. Report on Health and Social Subjects, No. 15, Report by the Committee on Medical Aspects of Food Policy, HMSO, London (1979)

Ek, J. and Magnus, E. M. Plasma and red blood cell folate in breast-fed infants. *Acta Paediatr. Scand.* 68 (1979) 239–243

Ford, J. E. and Scott, K. J. The folic acid activity of some milk foods for babies. *J. Dairy Res.* 35 (1968) 85–89

Ford, J. E., Zechalko, A., Murphy, J. and Brooke, O. G. Comparison of the B vitamin composition of milk from mothers of preterm and term babies. *Arch. Dis. Child.* 58 (1983) 367–372

Fredrikzon, B., Hernell, O., Blackberg, L. and Olivecrona, T. Bile salt-stimulated lipase in human milk; evidence of activity *in vivo* and a role in the digestion of milk retinol esters. *Pediatr. Res* 12 (1978) 1048–1052

Gandy, G. and Jacobson, W. Influence of folic acid on birthweight and growth of the erythroblastotic infant. 1. Birthweight. 2. Growth during the first year. 3. Effect of folic acid supplementation. *Arch. Dis. Child.* 52 (1977) 1–21

Haroon, Y., Shearer, M. J., Rahim, S., Gunn, W. G., McEnery, G. and Barkhan, P. The content of phylloquinone (vitamin K_1) in human milk, cows' milk and infant formula foods, determined by high pressure liquid chromatography. *J. Nutr.* 112 (1982) 1105–1107

Hittner, H. M. and Kretzer, F. L. Vitamin E and retrolental fibroplasia: ultrastructural mechanism of clinical efficacy.

Ciba Foundation Symp. 101 (1983) 165–185

Hovi, L., Hekali, R. and Siimes, M. A. Evidence of riboflavin depletion in breast-fed newborn: and its further acceleration during treatment of hyperbilirubinemia by phototherapy. *Acta Paediatr. Scand.* 68 (1979) 567–570

Irwin, M. I. and Hutchins, B. K. A conspectus of research on vitamin C requirements of man. *J. Nutr.* 106 (1976) 834–879

Knott, E. M., Kleiger, S. C. and Schulz, F. W. Is breast milk adequate in meeting thiamine requirements of infants? *J. Pediatr.* 22 (1943) 43–49

Kon, S. K. and Mawson, E. H. *Human Milk*, Special Report Series of the Medical Research Council, No. 269, HMSO, London 1950

Lucas, A. and Bates, C. J. Transient riboflavin deficiency in premature infants: occurrence, prevention and reversal. *Arch. Dis. Child.* 59 (1984) 837–841

Macy, I. G., Kelly, H. J. and Sloan, R. E. The composition of milks. National Research Council Publication, No. 254, National Academy of Sciences, Washington D.C. (1950)

National Research Council, Food and Nutrition Board, Committee on Dietary Allowances. *Recommended Dietary Allowances*, 9th Edn., National Academy of Sciences, Washington D.C. (1980)

Neumann, C. G., Swendseid, M. E., Jacob, M., Stiehm, E. R. and Dirige, O. V. Biochemical evidence of thiamin deficiency in young Ghanaian children. *Am. J. Clin. Nutr.* 32 (1979) 99–104

Payne, N. R. and Hasegawa, D. K. Vitamin K deficiency in newborns: A case report of α-1-antitrypsin deficiency and a review of factors predisposing to hemorrhage. *Pediatrics* 73 (1984) 712–716

Pongpanich, B., Srikrikkrich, N., Dhanmitta, S. and Valyaseri, A. Biochemical detection of a thiamin deficiency in infants and children in Thailand. *Am. J. Clin. Nutr.* 27 (1974) 1399–1402

Rodriguez, M. S. A conspectus of research on folacin requirements of man. *J. Nutr.* 108 (1978) 1983–2103

Roth, K. S. Biotin in clinical medicine—a review. *Am. J. Clin. Nutr.* 34 (1981) 1967–1974

Schmidt-Sommerfeld, E., Penn, D. and Wolf, H. Carnitine blood concentrations and fat utilisation in parenterally alimented premature newborn infants. *J. Pediatr.* 100 (1982) 260–264

Shearer, M. J., Rahim, S., Barkhan, P. and Stimmler, L. Plasma vitamin K_1 in mothers and their newborn babies. *Lancet* 2 (1982) 460–463

Strelling, M. K., Blackledge, D. G. and Goodall, H. B. Diagnosis and management of folate deficiency in low birthweight infants. *Arch. Dis. Child.* 54 (1979) 271–277

Truswell, A. S., Irwin, T., Beaton, G. H., Suzue, R., Haenel, H., Hejda, S., Hou, X-C., Leveille, G., Morava, E., Pedersen, J. and Stephen, J. M. L. Recommended dietary intakes around the world. Report by Committee 1/5 of the International Union of Nutritional Sciences (1982). *Nutr. Abstr. Rev.* 53 (1983) 939–1015

Warshaw, J. B. and Curry, E. Comparison of serum carnitine and ketone body concentrations in breast and formula-fed newborn infants. *J. Pediatr.* 97 (1980) 122–125

J. Inher. Metab. Dis. 8 Suppl. 1 (1985) 13–16

Intestinal Transport of Vitamins

R. C. ROSE

Departments of Physiology and Surgery, The Milton S. Hershey Medical Center, The Pennsylvania State University, P.O. Box 850, Hershey, PA 17033, USA

Animals rely on acquiring through their diet, certain micronutrients required to support metabolism that we refer to as vitamins. The water-soluble vitamins are absorbed in the intestine only slowly by simple diffusion; specific mechanisms of transport have evolved that normally insure complete availability of each substrate to the organism. Secondary genetic errors that result in the impairment of an intestinal transport mechanism may become debilitating.

Plants and animals alike use a variety of organic factors that assist in enzyme-catalyzed reactions. Early in evolution, animals lost the ability to synthesize several of these coenzymes. These inborn errors of metabolism dictated that the animal acquire some form of the coenzyme in the diet. We refer to these factors as vitamins.

Animal species differ in their dietary requirements for the vitamins. Ascorbic acid is used by all animal species as an antioxidant and in a variety of other biochemical conversions. Most animal species have the enzymatic mechanism to synthesize ascorbic acid from glucose in the liver. However, the guinea-pig, man, and lower primates have genetically lost the enzyme L-gulonolactone oxidase necessary for ascorbic acid production. Scurvy is averted only by including ascorbic acid in diet. The process by which ascorbic acid is absorbed in these species will serve as one example of vitamin transport in the intestine. It might be of interest that similar transport mechanisms exist for the same substrate in cell membranes of the kidney, central nervous system, hepatocytes and other body components.

The lumen of the gastrointestinal tract is separated from the circulation and the rest of the body by a nearly contiguous array of epithelial and other cells. These cells severely restrict passage by simple diffusion of the large water-soluble vitamins, which are the focus of this presentation. Certain sections of the small intestine have acquired components, usually of protein composition, within the cell membrane that specifically bind to each of the vitamins and aid in their absorption.

ABSORPTION OF ASCORBIC ACID

Several experimental techniques have been useful in elucidating the details of vitamin absorption. Patterson *et al.* (1982) removed the distal ileum from guinea-pigs anaesthetized with sodium pentobarbital. The segment was opened by a longitudinal incision along the antimesenteric border. The tissue was rinsed and a separation of mucosa from smooth muscle was achieved using glass microscope slides. The mucosa was then cut into 2.5 cm lengths (50–100 mg) and placed in a physiologic buffer solution at 37°C. Transport properties were evaluated by including ^{14}C-ascorbic acid

($8 \mu mol\, l^{-1}$) in the bathing medium. The presence of ^{3}H-inulin permitted the quantity of extracellular water to be estimated under the assumption that inulin is excluded from the intracellular space and is distributed in the extracellular water at the same concentration as in the bathing solution. Tissue water was confirmed to be approximately 80% of tissue weight. Extracellular ^{14}C-ascorbic acid was calculated from the inulin space and subtracted from total ^{14}C-ascorbic acid. The remaining ^{14}C-ascorbic acid is considered to be uniformly dissolved in the cellular water. The identity of the ^{14}C-label was determined by homogenizing tissue samples in 5% metaphosphoric acid, centrifuging and injecting a sample of the extract onto an HPLC column. The column effluent was collected and assayed on a scintillation spectrometer.

The importance of the normal intracellular electrolyte content in accumulation of ascorbic acid was evaluated by incubating mucosal strips of distal ileum in physiologic buffer that contained ouabain at a concentration that effectively inhibits activity of the Na–K ATPase activity (Figure 1) and results in the intracellular fluid acquiring the ionic composition of the bathing medium. Tissue exposed to ^{14}C-ascorbic acid and ouabain ($0.1 \, mmol\, l^{-1}$) from the time zero had a much lower rate of ascorbic acid uptake over 50 min of incubation. In addition, tissue samples that were allowed to accumulate ascorbic acid under control conditions for 20 min showed net loss of the vitamin when exposed to ouabain during the following 30 min. The final ascorbic acid concentration in this tissue was approximately the same as the concentration in the bathing solution throughout the study. Similar results were obtained when the tissue was exposed to cyanide ($1 \, mmol\, l^{-1}$) instead of ouabain. Under control conditions ascorbic acid accumulated within the intracellular water to a concentration approximately 10 times that in the bathing solution.

The mechanism of ascorbic acid transport was further investigated by evaluating accumulation of the vitamin with various concentrations of Na in the bathing solution. Buffers were prepared by replacing NaCl with Tris-Cl. Incubations were performed for 25 min on ileal mucosa from five guinea-pigs. The cellular concentration of ascorbic acid (Figure 2) was linearly related to bathing media Na concentration. In Na-free

Journal of Inherited Metabolic Disease. ISSN 0141–8955. Copyright © SSIEM and MTP Press Limited, Queen Square, Lancaster, UK.

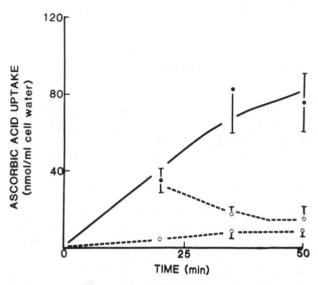

Figure 1 Uptake of ascorbic acid in guinea-pig ileal mucosa. Tissue was exposed to ^{14}C-ascorbic acid ($8\,\mu mol\,l^{-1}$). Solid circles represent control conditions. Open circles represent tissue exposed to ouabain ($10^{-4}\,mol\,l^{-1}$) either from time zero or after 20 min under control conditions. Values are means $\pm$ SEM of five–six determinations. (From Patterson *et al.*, 1982, with permission)

media, the final cellular concentration was significantly less than bathing media concentration.

The dependence of ascorbic acid uptake on intact cellular metabolic energy was evaluated. Strips of mucosa were incubated under control conditions or in physiologic buffer that contained cyanide ($1\,mmol\,l^{-1}$) or rotenone ($2.5\,mmol\,l^{-1}$) or under anoxic conditions. The results indicate that the ability of tissue to take up ascorbic acid against a concentration gradient is impaired in cells depleted of metabolic energy (Table 1; see also Stevenson and Brush, 1969).

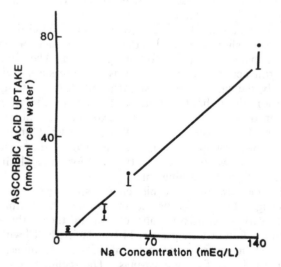

Figure 2 Effect of bathing media sodium concentration on ascorbic acid uptake into guinea-pig ileal mucosa. Tissue was incubated 25 min in Ringer or in buffer with reduced sodium concentrations (Tris replacement). ^{14}C-Ascorbic acid was present at $8\,\mu mol\,l^{-1}$. Values are means $\pm$ SEM from four animals. (From Patterson *et al.*, 1982, with permission)

Table 1 Effect of metabolic inhibition on uptake of ^{14}C-ascorbic acid by guinea-pig ileal mucosa

Control	Rotenone ($2.5\,mmol\,l^{-1}$)	Cyanide ($1\,mmol\,l^{-1}$)	N_2
51.5 ± 10.9	10.8 ± 1.05	16.9 ± 3.5	17.4 ± 3.7

Strips of mucosa were incubated 20 min with ^{14}C-ascorbic acid present at $8\,\mu mol\,l^{-1}$. Values are means $\pm$ SEM in $\mu mol\,l^{-1}$. All values are significantly different from control ($p < 0.05$)
(From Patterson *et al.*, 1982, with permission)

Additional characteristics of ascorbic acid uptake were evaluated by measuring substrate movement from the mucosal bathing solution across the brush-border membrane into absorptive cells of the ileum (Mellors *et al.*, 1977). A segment of the intestine was mounted as a flat sheet mucosal surface up in a lucite chamber that exposed six individual sections of 0.29 cm of the mucosal surface only to a Ringer-type solution stirred by a fine stream of O_2/CO_2. A test solution containing ^{14}C-ascorbic acid and ^3H-inulin bathed the mucosal surface for specified times at 37°C.

The test solution was removed, and the exposed tissue was cut out with a steel punch, washed briefly in cold buffer, blotted and extracted in 0.1 N HNO_3 at 4°C for 18 h. Aliquots of the tissue extract and test solution were assayed for ^{14}C and ^3H. The cumulative uptake of ^{14}C-ascorbic acid is linear with time, which indicates that the resultant data are a reliable measure of unidirectional influx.

The possibility of carrier-mediated entry of ascorbic acid across the brush-border membrane was evaluated by measuring influx from test solutions that contain $0.2-8.6\,mmol\,l^{-1}$ ascorbic acid. Influx was determined with test solutions that had sodium concentrations of 0, 50, and 140 $mmol\,l^{-1}$ (Figure 3). At Na concentrations of 50 and 140 $mmol\,l^{-1}$, influx is not a linear function of the initial ascorbic acid concentration but shows a tendency towards saturation. These results indicate that

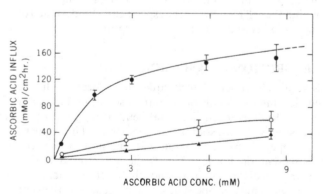

Figure 3 Ascorbic acid influx into guinea-pig ileal mucosa from mucosal ascorbic acid concentrations of $0.28-8.6\,mmol\,l^{-1}$. Exposure times were 5 min. Test solution contained Na = 140 ($\bullet$), 50($\circ$), or 0 ($\blacktriangle$) $mmol\,l^{-1}$. Dashed line extends toward data points at ascorbic acid concentrations of 14.2 and 28.2 $mmol\,l^{-1}$ and has a slope of 7.2 ($\times 10^{-3}\,cm\,h^{-1}$). (From Mellors *et al.*, 1977, with permission)

a carrier mechanism exists for ascorbic acid at the brush-border membrane. In Na-free media the data points do not vary from linearity and no evidence exists for a carrier-mediated process.

Isolated vesicles made from the brush-border membrane of enterocytes have been useful in elucidating the transport mechanism of several substrates. Siliprandi *et al.* (1979) were successful in demonstrating counter-flow of L-ascorbate in vesicles of guinea-pig ileum and in performing kinetic studies which demonstrated a K_m very close to the value determined on the basis of influx studies in intact tissues. In addition, sodium-dependent ascorbate transport was confirmed and shown to be electrically neutral; it was concluded that transport of the monovalent ascorbate anion and a single sodium ion takes place.

CONTROL OF SUBSTRATE TRANSPORT RATES

The rate of intestinal transport of certain nutrients (e.g. Ca) (Krawitt, 1976), thiamine (Hoyumpa *et al.*, 1976), is regulated by specific events at the brush-border membrane brought about by some signal from the body, such as circulating levels of the substrate. Thus, it was of interest to determine if guinea-pigs that are fed diets with ascorbic acid contents higher than normal respond with alterations in the uptake rate of ascorbic acid from the mucosal bathing solution into the tissue.

It was considered necessary to measure the influx of a second water-soluble substance into intestinal mucosa to determine whether any effect of dietary manipulations on ascorbic acid transport is specific for that substance rather than being a generalized membrane permeability response. Thus, the influx of ^{14}C-choline was measured in two samples of each intestine used and the influx of ^{14}C-ascorbic acid was measured in four samples of mucosa from the same intestine (Rose and Nahrwold, 1978). Choline has been shown to be absorbed by a carrier-mediated transport mechanism at the brush-border membrane (Kuczler *et al.*, 1977). There was no significant effect on the influx of choline or ascorbic acid due to the presence of the alternate compound in the test solution. Thus, it is concluded that choline and ascorbic acid have separate transport mechanisms at the brush border.

Guinea-pigs fed diets that contained 5 or 25 times the control level of ascorbic acid for 14 or 28 days had rates of ascorbic acid uptake 32–52% lower than control animals (Table 2). Choline influx was not significantly altered by diets of high ascorbic acid content. Because high oral doses of ascorbic acid specifically limit the transport of ascorbic acid into ileal mucosa, it appears that the receptor activity is under negative feed-back control. To the extent that these studies on guinea-pigs apply in general, to intestinal transport properties of vitamins in man, it may be concluded that individuals who consume high quantities of a particular vitamin might have a reduced capacity for intestinal transport of that vitamin. If this individual then assumed a diet low in content of that vitamin, he would be left with both a

Table 2 **Influx of ascorbic following diets of high and low ascorbic acid content**

Diet	14 day	28 day
Control	10.7 ± 0.7 (20)	10.4 ± 0.3 (20)
5X	7.3 ± 0.7 (12)*	5.9 ± 0.9 (11)*
25X	5.7 ± 0.4 (12)*	5.0 ± 0.5 (12)*

Guinea-pigs were fed for 14 or 28 days either the control diet, or diets having 5 or 25 times the control content of ascorbic acid. Results are in nmol cm^{-2} h^{-1} ± SEM. Number of observations is in parentheses
* Indicates statistically significant differences when compared with control ($p < 0.01$). Test solution contained ^{14}C-ascorbic acid (95 μmol l^{-1})
(From Rose and Nahrwold, 1978, with permission)

diminished transport capacity and less vitamin availability.

The results on ascorbic acid absorption are consistent with the Na-gradient hypothesis of Crane (1962) that rather satisfactorily explains the active transport of many nutrients in intestine.

THIAMINE ABSORPTION

The literature on thiamine absorption was recently reviewed by Rose *et al.* (1984) who cited evidence of active transport of thiamine similar to the Na-gradient model discussed above. In addition, however, thiamine might be trapped in the intestinal mucosa by intracellular phosphorylation (Ferrari *et al.*, 1982), and this phosphorylation process might be rate limiting. However, other major differences between transport and phosphorylation characteristics suggest little interrelationship between the two processes (Ferrari *et al.*, 1971; Komai *et al.*, 1974).

NICOTINAMIDE ABSORPTION

Intestinal absorption of nicotinamide represents a second example in which rapid metabolism of a nutrient to an impermeant form serves to trap and promote absorption (Schuette and Rose, 1983). Uptake and metabolism by chick intestine were studied in isolated epithelial cells and in isolated loops of intestine *in situ*. Nicotinamide was studied at a physiologic concentration of 11.7 μmol l^{-1}. Nicotinamide was taken up rapidly from the bathing media and largely metabolized to NAD by the isolated cells (Table 3). Total accumulation of the substrate was dependent on intact cellular metabolic energy and was saturable at concentrations of nicotinamide up to 351 μmol l^{-1}. Nicotinamide rapidly equilibrated within the intracellular space at all levels of extracellular substrate concentration. Nicotinamide was converted directly to NAD via the intermediate, nicotinamide mononucleotide. In isolated loops, *in vivo* nicotinamide was rapidly absorbed. Exogenous nicotinamide mononucleotide reduced nicotinamide entry into the mucosal cells both *in vivo* and *in vitro*. This is the only suggestion to date that nicotinamide entry might proceed by some form of a specialized transport process.

Table 3 ^{14}C-Nicotinamide uptake and metabolism at $11.7\,\mu\,mol\,l^{-1}$

		Intracellular ^{14}C-label appearing as:			
NMN	*NARP*	*NAm*	*NAD*	*NADP*	*NAAD*
9.4 ± 2.7	1.1 ± 0.3	44.6 ± 5.5	60.6 ± 15.8	0.9 ± 0.3	1.7 ± 0.6

Values are means $\pm$ SE ($n = 3$) in pmol mg protein^{-1}. Time of incubation was 2 min
Abbreviations used: NAm, nicotinamide; NAD, nicotinamide adenine dinucleotide; NMN, nicotinamide mononucleotide; NARP, nicotinic acid ribonucleotide or nicotinic acid mononucleotide; NADP, nicotinamide adenine dinucleotide phosphate; NAAD, nicotinic acid adenine dinucleotide
(From Schuette and Rose, 1983, with permission)

CONCLUSION

The earliest view that water-soluble vitamins are absorbed in the intestine by simple diffusion has been modified as a result of more recent studies that indicate specific transport and metabolic processes for each of the nutrients. The complex carriers and enzymes are under genetic control and subject to malfunction through inherited disorders of metabolism. Just as laboratory investigations on the mechanisms of vitamin absorption throughout the body have helped us to understand related inherited disorders, so observations on vitamin-responsive disorders have helped to stimulate our inquiry into the mechanisms by which the body handles vitamins. Additional progress on each front is anticipated.

References

Crane, R. Hypothesis for mechanism of intestinal active transport of sugars. *Fed. Proc.* 21 (1962) 891

Ferrari, G., Patrini, C. and Rindi, G. Intestinal thiamin transport in rats. *Pflugers Arch.* 393 (1982) 37–41

Ferrari, G., Ventura, U. and Rindi, G. The Na-dependence of thiamine intestinal transport *in vitro*. *Life Sci.* 10 (1971) 67–75

Hoyumpa, A. M., Nichols, S., Schenker, S. and Wilson, F. A. Thiamine transport in thiamine-deficient rats. Role of the unstirred water layer. *Biochim. Biophys. Acta* 436 (1976) 438–447

Komai, T., Kawai, K. and Shindo, H. Active transport of thiamine from rat small intestine. *J. Nutr. Sci. Vitaminol.* 20 (1974) 163–177

Krawitt, E. L. Calcium uptake by isolated intestinal brush border membranes following dietary calcium restriction. *Life Sci.* 19 (1976) 543–548

Kuczler, F. J., Nahrwold, D. L. and Rose, R. C. Choline influx across the brush border of guinea pig jejunum. *Biochim. Biophys. Acta* 465 (1977) 131–137

Mellors, A. J., Nahrwold, D. L. and Rose, R. C. Ascorbic acid flux across the mucosal border of guinea pig and human ileum. *Am. J. Physiol.* 2 (1977) E374–E379

Patterson, L. T., Nahrwold, D. L. and Rose, R. C. Ascorbic acid uptake in guinea pig intestinal mucosa. *Life Sci.* 31 (1982) 2783–2791

Rose, R. C., Hoyumpa, A. M., Jr, Allen, R. H., Middleton, H. M., Henderson, L. M. and Rosenberg, I. H. Transport and metabolism of water-soluble vitamins in intestine and kidney. *Fed. Proc.* 43 (1984) 2423–2429

Rose, R. C. and Nahrwold, D. L. Intestinal ascorbic acid transport following diets of high or low ascorbic acid content. *Int. J. Vit. Nutr. Res.* 48 (1978) 383–386

Schuette, S. A. and Rose, R. C. Nicotinamide uptake and metabolism by chick intestine. *Am. J. Physiol.* 245 (1983) G531–G538

Siliprandi, L., Vanni, P., Kessler, M. and Semenza, G. Na-dependent, electro-neutral L-ascorbate transport across brush border membrane vesicles from guinea pig small intestine. *Biochim. Biophys. Acta* 552 (1979) 129–142

Stevenson, N. and Brush, M. Existence and characteristics of Na-dependent active transport of ascorbic acid in guinea pig. *Am. J. Clin. Nutr.* 22 (1969) 318–326

J. Inher. Metab. Dis. 8 Suppl. 1 (1985) 17–19

Evaluation of Cofactor Responsiveness

J. V. LEONARD and P. DAISH
Institute of Child Health, 30 Guilford Street, London WC1N 1EH, UK

The response to cofactor therapy in inborn errors of metabolism may be dramatic with complete resolution of the clinical illness but more commonly the response is absent or partial. When assessing cofactor responsiveness clinical and biochemical findings as well as the natural history of the disorder must be taken into account.

Several inborn errors of metabolism are characterised by defects in cofactor transport or metabolism. Much attention has been focused on those disorders in which the defect may be overcome by administration of the cofactor (or a precursor) in pharmacological doses. In some disorders (for example, biotinidase deficiency, congenital B_{12} malabsorption) the response to cofactor administration is dramatic with rapid and complete resolution of the clinical illness. However, in many conditions the response is less clear-cut; careful evaluation of clinical and biochemical data is then necessary to avoid erroneous classification of a non-responsive patient as responsive and vice versa. In this paper we will discuss some of the problems that may be encountered in the assessment of the response to cofactor therapy.

DEFINITION

A patient has a cofactor-responsive disorder if there is a substantial and sustained clinical and biochemical improvement following administration of the cofactor (or a precursor).

METHODS OF ASSESSMENT OF COFACTOR RESPONSIVENESS

We shall discuss the methods of assessment as follows:

Laboratory studies:
  enzyme activities and complementation groups
  metabolite concentrations
  response to loading tests.

Clinical measurements:
  growth and development
  degree of dietary restriction.

It should be emphasised that undue reliance on isolated biochemical data may be misleading. Similarly the natural history of the non-responsive disorder must be taken into account when assessing clinical data.

LABORATORY STUDIES

Enzyme and complementation studies

It is well recognised that the demonstration of enhanced enzyme activity following cofactor supplementation *in vitro* does not necessarily correlate with *in vivo* responsiveness (Kaye *et al.*, 1974; Wilcken *et al.*, 1977). This is found particularly with the cbl mutants of methylmalonic acidaemia (McKusick 25110, 25111). Classification by complementation studies may have prognostic significance with regard to cofactor responsiveness. In a survey of patients with methylmalonic acidaemia Matsui *et al.* (1983) found that out of 14 cbl A mutants, 13 showed significant falls in plasma and urinary methylmalonate with cofactor therapy whereas only four out of 11 cbl B mutants were cofactor-responsive.

METABOLITE CONCENTRATIONS

The measurement of changes in metabolite concentrations in body fluids provides an important means of assessing cofactor responsiveness. Evaluation of results is simple if the patient is metabolically in a steady state (or nearly so) before and during cofactor administration. Substantial or complete resolution of biochemical abnormalities following cofactor therapy suggests cofactor responsiveness. However, assessment under non-steady state conditions leads to difficulties. This is particularly true when cofactors are given to critically sick newly diagnosed patients; in these circumstances it may be impossible to separate the effects of cofactor therapy from those of other forms of treatment given at the same time. Figure 1 shows the progress of a baby girl with maple syrup urine disease (McKusick 28460) who was admitted at age 10 days. In addition to routine measures such as assisted ventilation, high carbohydrate intake and protein restriction she also received thiamine 60 mg daily. Her plasma branched chain amino acid concentration fell rapidly and over the next few days the leucine intake (in the form of natural protein) necessary to sustain adequate plasma leucine concentrations rose to $200\,\text{mg}\,\text{kg}^{-1}\,\text{day}^{-1}$—the upper range for *normal* neonates (Francis, 1974). These findings could have been interpreted as a manifestation of cofactor responsiveness. However, her leucine requirements subsequently fell to low levels despite continued thiamine supplementation. At the age of 1 year (by which time thiamine had been discontinued) her leucine intake was $27\,\text{mg}\,\text{kg}^{-1}\,\text{day}^{-1}$.

Journal of Inherited Metabolic Disease. ISSN 0141-8955. Copyright © SSIEM and MTP Press Limited, Queen Square, Lancaster, UK.

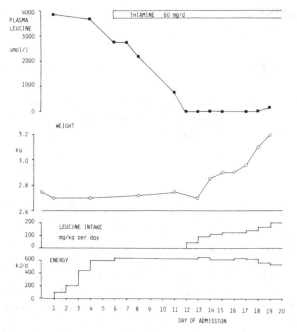

Figure 1   Maple syrup urine disease and thiamine. There was a marked fall in plasma leucine concentrations concurrent with thiamine supplementation; however, tolerance of the high protein intake was not sustained once catch-up growth had been completed

LOADING TESTS

Patients with milder or intermittent disease may have biochemical abnormalities only during illness. Thus, in order to demonstrate that cofactor therapy is of benefit, it may be necessary to induce biochemical abnormalities by stressing the patient. Loading tests before and during cofactor therapy are commonly employed for this purpose. For example, isoleucine may be given as a single oral load (100 mg kg^{-1}) to stress the metabolism of propionate. Meaningful comparisons between the responses to the isoleucine loads before and during cofactor therapy cannot be made unless several conditions have been satisfied. Of these the most important is that the patient be in a steady state prior to the loads and that these be carried out under near identical metabolic conditions. Results obtained otherwise will be misleading. Barnes *et al.* (1970) performed isoleucine loads on a male infant with propionic acidaemia. On the first occasion there was an appreciable and sustained rise in plasma propionate. After 5 days oral biotin therapy the isoleucine load was repeated. This time not only was the preload plasma propionate lower but also the rise in plasma propionate smaller and less prolonged. It was suggested from these data that he might be biotin-responsive. We have had the opportunity to review his subsequent progress. Biotin did not lead to increased tolerance of dietary protein nor was there a reduction in the frequency or severity of ketoacidaemic episodes. He eventually died at the age of 4 years. It should be noted that prior to both loads he was "stabilised" on a diet containing only 0.1 g protein kg^{-1} day^{-1}.

Our experience of single dose isoleucine loading tests

indicates that reliable interpretation of results is extremely difficult. For this reason we suggest they be employed with great caution, if at all.

Longer term loading tests (over several days) are probably more reliable but also potentially dangerous since they may precipitate life-threatening keto-acidaemic episodes in susceptible patients.

CLINICAL AND DIETETIC MEASUREMENTS

Long-term evaluation of cofactor responsiveness in-cludes clinical and dietetic measurements. Cofactor therapy in a responsive patient will be associated with fewer and less severe metabolic crises, normal or improved growth and development, and tolerance of a normal or near-normal diet. However, when seeking evidence of cofactor responsiveness the natural history of the non-responsive disorder must be taken into account, as must the effects of other forms of therapy.

During periods of rapid growth in the neonatal period or early infancy a larger proportion of the protein intake will be used for growth leaving less to be catabolised (see Figure 1). A higher protein requirement also occurs during catch up growth later in infancy or early childhood. Patients with methylmalonic acidaemia commonly present at several months of age with failure to thrive. Once on a high energy–low protein diet they improve and during the period of increased growth may tolerate a relatively high natural protein intake of about 2–2.5 g kg^{-1} day^{-1} (Figure 2). If vitamin B$_{12}$ be given during this growth spurt improvement may be falsely attributed to the effect of the vitamin.

Episodes of ketoacidaemia in patients with organic acidaemias such as methylmalonic acidaemia and propionic acidaemia occur unpredictably. Despite the brittleness of their condition some patients will have prolonged periods of good metabolic control. The patient with methylmalonic acidaemia whose progress is shown in Figure 3 had numerous admissions with ketoacidaemia during his first 2.7 years of life. After being placed in a special day nursery he had no further admissions for 10 months, an improvement that might

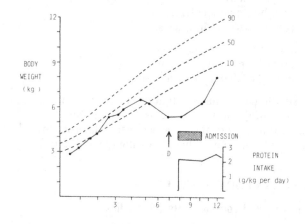

Figure 2   Methylmalonic acidaemia. Increased protein requirements during a period of rapid catch-up growth following admission to hospital. D = diagnosis

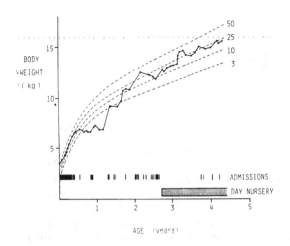

Figure 3 Methylmalonic acidaemia. Regular attendance at a special day nursery and the frequency and duration of admissions to hospital

easily have been attributed to other treatment. It is important to recognise that environmental factors may profoundly alter the course of these disorders.

In other inborn errors with intermittent symptoms such as late-onset propionic acidaemia or disorders of fat oxidations it may be particularly difficult to assess the value of cofactors. For this reason such patients may require prolonged follow-up before a definitive assessment of the value of cofactor therapy can be made.

EMERGENCY ADMINISTRATION OF VITAMINS

Many authors (for example, Buist *et al.*, 1984) recommend the use of megavitamin therapy when a seriously ill child is thought to have a metabolic disorder. The therapy often includes vitamin B_{12}, thiamine, pyridoxine, folate, biotin, nicotinamide and ascorbate. Although there is no obvious contra-indication to such therapy it is essential to reassess its importance at a later date.

CONCLUSIONS

A trial of cofactor therapy is warranted in patients with specific inborn errors of metabolism. Although the response in some patients will be unequivocal it is often less clear-cut and will require careful assessment in the light of the natural history of the disorder and of other forms of treatment given at the same time. Decisions regarding cofactor responsiveness must take into account all the available clinical and biochemical data.

References

Barnes, N. D., Hull, D., Balgobin, L. and Gompertz, D. Biotin-responsive propionicacidaemia. *Lancet* ii (1970) 244–245

Buist, N. R. M. and Kennaway, N. G. Metabolic disorders. In Forfar, J. O. and Arneil, G. C. (eds.) *Textbook of Paediatrics*, 3rd Edn., Churchill Livingstone, Edinburgh, 1984, pp. 1200–1234

Francis, D. E. M. *Diets for Sick Children*, 3rd Edn., Blackwell Scientific, Oxford, 1974, p. 348

Kaye, C. I., Morrow, G. and Nadler, H. L. *In vitro* "responsive" methylmalonic acidaemia: a new variant. *J. Pediatr.* 85 (1974) 55–59

Matsui, S. M., Mahoney, M. J. and Rosenberg, L. E. The natural history of the inherited methylmalonic acidemias. *N. Engl. J. Med.* 308 (1983) 857–861

Wilcken, B., Kilham, H. A. and Faull, K. Methylmalonic aciduria: a variant form of methylmalonyl coenzyme A apomutase deficiency. *J. Pediatr.* 91 (1977) 428–430

J. Inher. Metab. Dis. 8 Suppl. 1 (1985) 20–27

Raine Memorial Lecture

Hyperphenylalaninaemia Caused by Defects in Biopterin Metabolism

S. KAUFMAN

Laboratory of Neurochemistry, National Institute of Mental Health, 9000 Rockville Pike, Bethesda, MD 20205, USA

The hepatic phenylalanine hydroxylating system consists of three essential components, phenylalanine hydroxylase, dihydropteridine reductase and the non-protein coenzyme, tetrahydrobiopterin. The reductase and the pterin coenzyme are also essential components of the tyrosine and tryptophan hydroxylating systems. Recent studies have shown that there are three distinct forms of phenylketonuria or hyperphenylalaninaemia, each caused by the lack of one of these essential components. The variant forms of the disease that are caused by the lack of dihydropteridine reductase or tetrahydrobiopterin are characterized by severe neurological deterioration, impaired functioning of tyrosine and tryptophan hydroxylases and the resultant deficiency of tyrosine- and tryptophan-derived monoamine neurotransmitters in brain.

THE PHENYLALANINE HYDROXYLATING SYSTEM

Ever since phenylketonuria (PKU) was discovered by Fölling in 1934 (Fölling, 1934), our understanding of many aspects of this disease has been intimately related to our knowledge of phenylalanine metabolism. Indeed, on the assumption that this relationship would hold, we decided some years ago to try to learn something about PKU by studying the hepatic phenylalanine hydroxylating system.

One of the first things that we learned about the system was that it was complex, consisting of at least three essential components, two enzymes and a non-protein coenzyme. We isolated the non-protein factor from rat liver extracts on the basis of its ability to stimulate the conversion of phenylalanine to tyrosine in the presence of the two enzymes (Kaufman, 1958a; Kaufman and Levenberg, 1959) and proved that it was the reduced form of the unconjugated pterin, 2-amino-4-hydroxy-6-(1,2-dihydroxypropyl-(L-erythro)-pteridine (Kaufman, 1963), whose trivial name is biopterin ("pterin" is the name for a 2-amino-4-hydroxypteridine). The structure for tetrahydrobiopterin (BH_4), the active form of the coenzyme, is shown in Figure 1. Although biopterin had been isolated previously from human urine (Patterson *et al.*, 1956), its function, if any, in mammals was obscure. In fact, we now know that biopterin itself is probably not a naturally occurring consituent of mammalian tissues; in urine at least it has been shown to be a breakdown product derived from the compound that is naturally occurring, namely BH_4 (Milstien *et al.*, 1980). The demonstration that BH_4 is an essential component of the phenylalanine hydroxylating

system established the first metabolic role for any unconjugated pterin and the first coenzyme role for BH_4.

In addition to the naturally occurring coenzyme, several synthetic tetrahydropterins, such as 6-methyl-tetrahydropterin (6-MPH_4) and 6,7-dimethyltetra-hydropterin ($DMPH_4$), were shown to be active with the phenylalanine hydroxylating system (Kaufman and Levenberg, 1959).

The other essential components of the phenylalanine hydroxylating system are phenylalanine hydroxylase (EC 1.14.16.1) and dihydropteridine reductase (EC 1.6.99.7) (DHPR). The reactions catalyzed by these two enzymes are illustrated in Figure 2 with 6-MPH_4 as the coenzyme. As can be seen, phenylalanine hydroxylase catalyzes a coupled reaction in which L-phenylalanine is oxidized to L-tyrosine and the tetrahydropterin is oxidized to an extremely unstable quinonoid dihydropterin; molecular oxygen is the electron acceptor and is normally reduced to water. The second essential enzyme of the system, DHPR, catalyzes the reduction of the quinonoid dihydropterin back to the tetrahydro level, utilizing a reduced pyridine nucleotide as the electron donor (Kaufman, 1971). This reaction serves to regenerate the active form of the pterin coenzyme and thus allows the coenzyme to function catalytically. Once the roles for BH_4 and DHPR had been established in the

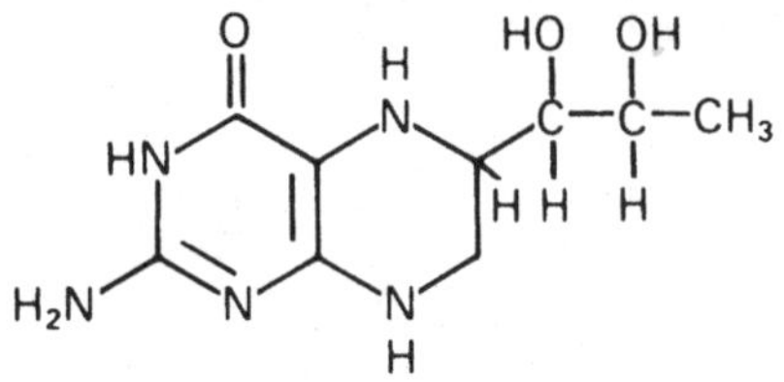

Figure 1 The structure of tetrahydrobiopterin

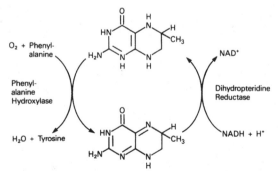

Figure 2 Pterin transformation during the enzymatic conversion of phenylalanine to tyrosine

phenylalanine hydroxylating system, it was shown that they are also essential components of the tyrosine (Brenneman and Kaufman, 1964; Shiman *et al.*, 1971) and tryptophan (Friedman *et al.*, 1972) hydroxylating systems.

CLASSICAL PKU (McKUSICK 26160)

With the demonstration that the hepatic phenylalanine hydroxylating system consists of at least three essential components, phenylalanine hydroxylase, DHPR and BH$_4$, it became evident that the lack of any one of them could lead to an inactive phenylalanine hydroxylating system and could consequently cause PKU (Kaufman, 1967). This biochemical work, therefore, not only led to the expectation that there might be three distinct molecular varieties of PKU but it also reopened an issue that appeared to be settled, namely, the identity of the missing component in classic PKU. This issue appeared to be finally settled when quantitative determinations of the levels of phenylalanine hydroxylase, DHPR and BH$_4$ in biopsy samples from several PKU patients proved that they all suffered from a lack of only a single component, phenylalanine hydroxylase (Kaufman, 1958b). Furthermore, in these early studies no phenylalanine hydroxylase activity could be detected in liver biopsy samples from classic PKU patients, findings that were consistent with the possibility that this form of the disease is caused by a deletion mutation of the structural gene for the hydroxylase. With the use of more sensitive assays for the enzyme, however, residual phenylalanine hydroxylase activity, equal to about 0.30% of the normal activity, was detected in a liver sample from a patient with classic PKU. Furthermore, the properties of the enzyme in this patient's liver were different from those of the normal enzyme, suggesting the presence of a structurally-altered hydroxylase (Friedman *et al.*, 1973). More recently, residual hydroxylase activity was detected in liver samples from two patients with classic PKU; in 13 other classic PKU patients, no phenylalanine hydroxylase activity was detected (Bartholomé *et al.*, 1975).

HYPERPHENYLALANINAEMIA CAUSED BY DHPR DEFICIENCY (McKUSICK 26163)

The prediction that variant forms of PKU might exist that are caused by defects in one of the other essential components of the phenylalanine hydroxylating system appeared to languish until about 10 years ago. During the period 1974–1975, several preliminary reports appeared describing a new form of PKU with progressive neurological illness that was unresponsive to dietary restriction of phenylalanine (Bartholomé, 1974; Smith, 1974; Smith *et al.*, 1975). Since the activity of phenylalanine hydroxylase in liver biopsy samples appeared to be within the normal range in two of those patients, it was suggested that they suffered from a defect in another component of the complex phenylalanine hydroxylating system. The evidence available at that time, however, left open the possibility that these patients lacked an enzyme involved in phenylalanine catabolism, such as phenylalanine transminase, that is not part of the phenylalanine hydroxylating system.

In 1975, the first case of PKU or hyperphenylalaninaemia caused by the demonstrated lack of a component of the phenylalanine hydroxylating system, other than phenylalanine hydroxylase itself, was reported (Kaufman *et al.*, 1975a). Despite excellent control of blood phenylalanine levels from the third week of life, seizures and other signs of neurological deterioration became evident in this infant at seven months of age. An analysis of the components of the phenylalanine hydroxylating system in a liver biopsy sample obtained when the patient was 14 months old showed that the levels of phenylalanine hydroxylase and the hydroxylation cofactor were adequate but that no DHPR activity was detectable under conditions where 1% of the normal activity could have been detected. DHPR activity was also undetectable in a sample of frontal cortex obtained from the patient, whereas it was present in comparable samples from control patients. The conclusion that this patient's hyperphenylalaninaemia was caused by a lack of DHPR was confirmed by results of antibody studies in which it was shown that an antiserum against pure sheep liver DHPR, which gave a single precipitin line with extracts from control human liver, gave no precipitin line with an extract from the patient's liver (Kaufman *et al.*, 1975a; Milstien and Kaufman, 1975).

The first procedure that was used to diagnose hyperphenylalaninaemia caused by a deficiency of DHPR was based on the quantitative determination of DHPR activity in fibroblasts cultured from patient's skin (Kaufman *et al.*, 1975a). More recently, it has been diagnosed by the determination of DHPR activity in various blood cells including lysed erythrocytes, as well as in blood dried on filter paper (Narisawa *et al.*, 1981). This disease can also be diagnosed by a determination of the state of reduction of biopterin in urine. In normals, most of the biopterin is present as BH$_4$, whereas little or none is present as BH$_4$ in DHPR-deficient patients (Milstien *et al.*, 1980).

Since DHPR is essential not only for phenylalanine hydroxylation, but also for tyrosine (Brenneman and Kaufman, 1964; Shiman *et al.*, 1971) and tryptophan (Friedman *et al.*, 1972) hydroxvlation, patients lacking DHPR would be expected to ffer from at least three distinct metabolic lesions, namely impaired rates of hydroxylation of phenylalanine, tyrosine, and tryptophan. Furthermore, since the possibility exists that DHPR may be involved in still other enzyme systems that have not yet been characterized, these patients may suffer from other metabolic abnormalities. In this regard, it is known that pterins and presumably DHPR are involved in the oxidative cleavage of glyceryl ethers (Tietz *et al.*, 1964). This reaction, however, has not yet been examined in DHPR-deficient patients. It has been shown that DHPR may function to keep folate in the active, tetrahydro form (Pollock and Kaufman, 1978), a role that could explain the low serum folate levels that were reported in one of these DHPR-deficient patients (Kaufman *et al.*, 1975a).

It has been proposed that most if not all of the neuropathology that is seen in patients with hyperphenylalaninaemia due to a deficiency of DHPR is caused by the impaired functioning of the tyrosine and tryptophan hydroxylating systems consequent to the lack of DHPR (Kaufman *et al.*, 1975a). Since these hydroxylases are believed to catalyze the rate-limiting steps in biosynthesis of the neurotransmitters norepinephrine (and dopamine) and serotonin, respectively, it seemed likely that the neurological deterioration was due to a relative lack of these neurotransmitters. This proposal was supported by the demonstration, mentioned earlier, that DHPR was detectable in brain samples from control patients, but was not detectable in a brain biopsy sample obtained from a DHPR-deficient patient. Data from subsequent studies carried out on this patient and on others with DHPR deficiency confirmed the idea that their synthesis of the biogenic amine neurotransmitters in both brain and peripheral tissues is impaired. Thus, low urinary and CSF levels of homovanillic acid (HVA), vanillyl mandelic acid (VMA), and 5-hydroxyindoleacetic acid (5-HIAA), metabolites of dopamine, norepinephrine, and serotonin, respectively have been found in most of these patients (Butler *et al.*, 1978, 1981; Brewster *et al.*, 1979).

THERAPY FOR HYPERPHENYLALANINAEMIA CAUSED BY DHPR DEFICIENCY

There are in theory a variety of different approaches to therapy of hyperphenylalaninaemia due to DHPR deficiency. In practice, unfortunately, the possibilities are much more limited. Since the established role for DHPR is to keep biopterin in the tetrahydro form (Kaufman, 1971; see Figure 2), a role that makes it an essential component of the phenylalanine, tyrosine and tryptophan hydroxylating systems, adminstration of BH_4 or one of the synthetic analogues with high cofactor activity such as $6\text{-}MPH_4$ or $DMPH_4$ might appear to offer an attractive route to therapy. Indeed, Smith *et al.* (1975) suggested this possibility and recommended a starting dose of $0.5\text{--}1.0\,\text{mg}\,\text{kg}^{-1}$. The general problems inherent in this type of treatment for DHPR deficiency and the specific problem that is raised by the recommendation that doses in the range of $0.5\text{--}1.0\,\text{mg}\,\text{kg}^{-1}$ might be effective have been discussed (Kaufman *et al.*, 1975a; Kaufman, 1975). A more realistic estimate of the dose of BH_4 that would be required, which takes into account the relationship between BH_4 and phenylalanine metabolism, indicates that a dose of $300\text{--}500\,\mu\text{mol}\,\text{kg}^{-1}\,\text{day}^{-1}$ of tetrahydropterin (equal to $70\text{--}120\,\text{mg}\,BH_4\,\text{kg}^{-1}\,\text{day}^{-1}$) would have to be supplied merely to keep pace with the daily conversion of phenylalanine to tyrosine. It should be noted that these figures represent the minimum dose. If significant amounts of the BH_4 were excreted or degraded via mitochondrial oxidation, an even larger amount would be required. On the other hand, if some residual DHPR was present a smaller dose would probably be needed. At the current price for BH_4 (about $\$165\,\text{g}^{-1}$), BH_4 therapy for DHPR deficiency would be prohibitively expensive.

When the prospects for pterin therapy for this variant form of PKU were first evaluated, there was an additional reason for being pessimistic about its use,

namely the evidence that in rats intravenously administered BH_4 does not readily enter the brain even when given at a dose of $125\,\text{mg}\,\text{kg}^{-1}$ (Kettler *et al.*, 1974). As will be discussed, however, more recent results have shown that the blood–brain barrier against BH_4 entry into the brain is not as impenetrable as was indicated by the results of Kettler *et al.* (1974). Based on the finding that the levels of neurotransmitters dopamine and serotonin and their metabolites were low in children with hyperphenylalaninaemia due to a documented deficiency of DHPR (Butler *et al.*, 1978; Brewster *et al.*, 1979), a therapy for this disease was proposed which, in addition to control of the hyperphenylalaninaemia by dietary restriction of phenylalanine, involves the oral administration of L-DOPA and 5-hydroxytryptophan, the metabolic products that bypass the impaired activities of tyrosine and tryptophan hydroxylases, respectively (Kaufman *et al.*, 1975a; Butler *et al.*, 1978; Bartholomé and Byrd, 1975). With the addition of carbidopa, an inhibitor of peripheral aromatic amino acid decarboxylase, it was found that lower doses of DOPA could be used (Bartholomé *et al.*, 1977). The effectiveness of this treatment with neurotransmitter precursors has been found to vary with the time at which it is initiated, being most effective when started shortly after birth (Bartholomé *et al.*, 1977; Rey *et al.*, 1977; Butler *et al.*, 1978; Gröbe *et al.*, 1978; Brewster *et al.*, 1979). In view of the low serum folates found in some of these patients (Kaufman *et al.*, 1975a) and the finding that DHPR may play a role in keeping folate in the tetrahydro form (Pollock and Kaufman, 1978), it is reasonable that the therapy for these patients include the administration of a source of tetrahydrofolate, such as N^5-formyltetrahydrofolate or N^5-methyltetrahydrofolate.

HYPERPHENYLALANINAEMIA DUE TO DEFECTS IN BH_4 SYNTHESIS (McKUSICK 26164)

The work reviewed above established the existence of a variant form of hyperphenylalaninaemia caused by the lack of the second essential enzyme in the phenylalanine hydroxylating system, DHPR. The first hint that still another form of the disease exists was provided by reports that not all hyperphenylalaninaemic patients with progressive neurological disease suffered from DHPR deficiency. Thus, in two patients of this type, hepatic activities of both phenylalanine hydroxylase and DHPR were reported to be in the normal range (Kaufman *et al.*, 1975b; Rey *et al.*, 1976). The metabolic defect in this variant form of hyperphenylalaninaemia was delineated when it was shown by Kaufman and his co-workers that the total biopterin levels in liver, blood and urine in these patients was low (Milstien *et al.*, 1977; Bartholomé *et al.*, 1977; Kaufman *et al.*, 1978). In the last patient, apparently normal levels of pterin cofactor were found by an enzymatic assay, but very low hepatic levels of pterins related to biopterin were detected by a microbiological assay (Leeming and Smith, 1979; Kaufman *et al.*, 1979). Although liver biopterin levels were not determined, the detection of low amounts of biopterin in plasma and urine of several other patients suggested that they also suffered from hyperphenylalaninaemia due to biopterin deficiency (Leeming *et al.*, 1976; Rey *et al.*, 1977).

The finding of low biopterin levels in these patients indicated that this form of hyperphenylalaninaemia was due to either a block in the biosynthesis of BH_4 or to an increased degradation of the compound. Strong evidence in favor of the former possibility was provided by results of high performance liquid chromatographic (HPLC) quantitative analysis of pterins, which showed that one of these patients had markedly elevated neopterin to biopterin (N/B) ratios in liver, urine and blood (Kaufman, 1979; Nixon *et al.*, 1980). Since, as can be seen in Figure 3, a neopterin derivative is a normal intermediate in BH_4 synthesis, these results indicated that the metabolic block in this patient was at a step between neopterin and biopterin in the biosynthetic pathway for biopterin.

Additional support for the conclusion that this form of hyperphenylalaninaemia is due to a defect in the *de novo* synthesis of BH_4 came from the observation that, in contrast to normal subjects and classic PKU patients, where it had been shown that blood biopterin levels increase in response to a phenylalanine load (Leeming *et al.*, 1976), this child's blood biopterin levels did not increase after a phenylalanine load (Kaufman *et al.*, 1978). To explain this result, Kaufman and co-workers

postulated that blood BH_4 levels increase in response to phenylalanine because phenylalanine is capable of stimulating BH_4 synthesis. Based on this proposal, the failure to observe a phenylalanine-induced increase in BH_4 was consistent with the conclusion that this patient is blocked in the biosynthetic pathway for BH_4. Furthermore, the subsequent finding that phenylalanine was able to elevate the urinary neopterin concentrations in this patient provided additional evidence for the localization of the metabolic block at a step between neopterin and biopterin (Nixon *et al.*, 1980). The detection by a semiquantitative electrophoretic method of elevated urinary neopterin levels and the failure to detect any biopterin in urine from several other patients suggested that they were also blocked in BH_4 synthesis between neopterin and biopterin (Curtius *et al.*, 1979). Liver concentrations of neopterin and biopterin derivatives, however, were not determined in these patients.

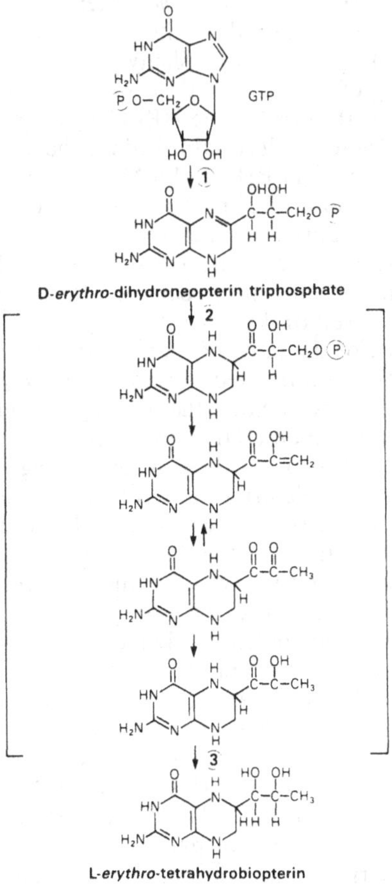

There is still too much uncertainty about the nature of the individual steps in the *de novo* synthesis of BH_4 to permit an exact localization of the metabolic lesion in those patients with abnormally high N/B ratios. Indeed, the previously accepted idea that BH_4 is synthesized through a series of dihydropterin intermediates has been weakened by recent findings. Thus, Nichol *et al.* (1983), Smith and Nichol (1983), and Milstien and Kaufman (1983) have presented strong evidence against the involvement of either sepiapterin or dihydrobiopterin as intermediates in the *de novo* synthesis of BH_4 from GTP catalyzed by enzymes in extracts from bovine adrenal medulla. Subsequent studies with a variety of tissue preparations came to the same conclusion (Heintel *et al.*, 1984; Switchenko *et al.*, 1984). In addition to reporting evidence against the participation of sepiapterin and dihydrobiopterin as intermediates in BH_4 synthesis, Milstien and Kaufman (1983) published data in support of the idea that the pterin intermediates in the pathway beyond dihydroneopterin triphosphate are all tetrahydropterins. Moreover, even though sepiapterin was shown not to be an intermediate, evidence was presented that sepiapterin reductase is involved in the *de novo* biosynthesis of BH_4 (Milstien and Kaufman, 1983). Figure 3 outlines the biosynthetic pathway for BH_4 that incorporates these recent findings. It should be noted that none of the bracketed tetrahydropterins in the scheme have been firmly established as intermediates in the pathway. Indeed, even though, as mentioned above, evidence in favor of the participation of sepiapterin reductase has been published (Milstien and Kaufman, 1983), the precise nature of its substrate in the pathway is not known.

According to the scheme shown in Figure 3, those patients with hyperphenylalaninaemia due to a defect in the *de novo* synthesis of BH_4, who have high neopterin to biopterin ratios, are blocked somewhere between reactions 2 and 3. Given the large number of discreet steps that may be involved, it is possible that not all of these patients lack the same enzyme. Recently, Niederwieser *et al.* (1984) have described a patient who appears to be blocked at the level of GTP cyclohydrolase, the enzyme that catalyzes reaction 1 (Figure 3).

Figure 3 Tentative scheme for the biosynthesis of tetrahydrobiopterin from GTP

Patients lacking this enzyme can be readily distinguished from those who are blocked between neopterin and biopterin because the cyclohydrolase-deficient patients have very low levels of *both* neopterin and biopterin.

THERAPY FOR HYPERPHENYLALANINAEMIA DUE TO DEFECTS IN BH_4 SYNTHESIS

Patients who are blocked in the *de novo* biosynthesis of BH_4, resemble DHPR-reductase-deficient patients in that they also suffer from defects in the synthesis of the neurotransmitters dopamine, norepinephrine, epinephrine, and serotonin, as well as from an impaired ability to hydroxylate phenylalanine (Kaufman *et al.*, 1978; McInnes *et al.*, 1979, 1984). The administration to these patients of BH_4 or a related tetrahydropterin with cofactor activity would, in theory, be a rational therapy for hyperphenylalaninaemia due to defects in *de novo* synthesis of BH_4. The rationale for pterin therapy for this disease is much more compelling than it is for hyperphenylalaninaemia due to lack of DHPR, because patients blocked in the *de novo* synthesis of BH_4, having a normal complement of DHPR would be able to continuously regenerate BH_4, thus allowing the administered BH_4 (or other active tetrahydropterin) to function catalytically in these patients in the same way in which it functions in normal individuals.

Despite the sound theoretical basis for pterin therapy in patients with defects in BH_4 synthesis, the evidence that administered BH_4 does not readily enter the brain from the periphery in either rats (Kettler *et al.*, 1974; Gal *et al.*, 1976) or humans (Danks *et al.*, 1979) appeared to dim the prospects for pterin therapy for this variant form of PKU. Although administration of low doses of BH_4 ($2.5\,mg\,kg^{-1}\,day^{-1}$) has been used in the treatment of this disease (Curtius *et al.*, 1979), its principal effect when given orally at this dosage is to decrease elevated blood phenylalanine levels, thus providing an alternative in this respect to dietary restriction of phenylalanine intake. Oral administration of BH_4 at these low doses is not adequate therapy for the neuropathology that characterizes this disease.

Until recently, the therapy for hyperphenylalaninaemia due to BH_4 synthesis defects was the same as that used with some success in the treatment of hyperphenylalaninaemia due to the lack of DHPR, i.e. restriction of dietary phenylalanine intake and administration of DOPA and 5-hydroxytryptophan in conjunction with inhibition of peripheral aromatic amino acid decarboxylation with carbidopa (Bartholomé *et al.*, 1977; Rey *et al.*, 1977; Kaufman *et al.*, 1978; Curtius *et al.*, 1979; McInnes *et al.*, 1984). In the two patients described in the last two studies, the clinical improvement was only modest. It seems likely, therefore, that just as had been found with DHPR deficiency, neurotransmitter precursor therapy of patients with defective BH_4 synthesis will prove to be most effective when the therapy is initiated as soon as possible after birth.

Recently, the prospects for adequate pterin therapy of hyperphenylalaninaemia due to defective BH_4 synthesis improved notably with the demonstration that high

doses ($20\,mg\,kg^{-1}\,day^{-1}$) of BH_4 when given to rats led to a marked elevation of the concentration of this pterin in the brain. Even higher brain concentrations of $6MPH_4$ were reached when this pterin was given (Kapatos and Kaufman, 1981). This latter compound, a synthetic analogue of BH_4 with high cofactor activity for phenylalanine (Kaufman and Levenberg, 1959), tyrosine (Brenneman and Kaufman, 1964), and tryptophan hydroxylases (Friedman *et al.*, 1972), whose structure is shown in Figure 2, was studied *in vivo* because, being a more hydrophobic compound than BH_4, it was anticipated that it might be able to cross the blood–brain barrier better than the naturally occurring cofactor. As mentioned this expectation was realized (Kapatos and Kaufman, 1981).

Encouraged by these results, the ability of BH_4 and 6-MPH_4 to cross the blood–brain barrier was studied in two patients with defective *de novo* synthesis of BH_4 (Kaufman *et al.*, 1982). With one patient, it was found that the oral administration of $20\,mg\,kg^{-1}\,day^{-1}$ of BH_4 increased his CSF levels of biopterin, determined by HPLC analysis, 20-fold. After the oral administration of 6-MPH_4 at a dose of $20–38\,mg\,kg^{-1}\,day^{-1}$ to another patient, the level of this pterin in CSF was about 100 times higher than the very low levels of BH_4 that were present prior to 6-MPH_4 administration. To confirm the presence of 6-MPH_4 in CSF with an independent assay, and also to determine whether the pterin was present in the cofactor-active tetrahydro form, the amount of tetrahydropterin in CSF was quantitatively. measured by its ability to serve as a cofactor with pure rat liver phenylalanine hydroxylase. The results of the enzymatic assay were in excellent agreement with those of the HPLC assay (Kaufman *et al.*, 1982). These results established for the first time two important facts: (1) BH_4 and 6-MPH_4, when given to humans at a dose of $20\,mg\,kg^{-1}\,day^{-1}$, can enter the brain in amounts that markedly elevate the brain concentration of these tetrahydropterins; and (2) these high brain concentrations can be attained when the pterins are given orally.

Since one of the aims of these pterin studies was to assess the therapeutic effectiveness of 6-MPH_4 and BH_4, it was necessary, before the tetrahydropterins were given, to discontinue DOPA and 5-hydroxytryptophan replacement therapy in these patients long enough to cause a clear deterioration of some aspects of neurological function. It was found that even though high concentrations of these cofactor-active tetrahydropterins were found in the CSF and presumably in the brains of both patients, the therapeutic response was variable. With one patient (T.D.), the administration of BH_4 led to a pronounced improvement in muscle strength and coordination, an increase in physical activity, and a marked decrease in eye-rolling and drooling. Similar improvement in these signs was noted in a separate trial when T.D. was given 6-MPH_4 at the same dose, i.e. $20\,mg\,kg^{-1}\,day^{-1}$ (Kaufman *et al.*, 1982). By contrast, with another patient (R.B.), no persistent effects of pterin administration were apparent, although she had definite periods of increased alertness (Kaufman *et al.*, 1982; McInnes *et al.*, 1984).

A clue to the cause of this variable response was provided by studies of the effects of tetrahydropterins on the cerebral metabolism of monoamine neurotransmitters in these two patients. It was found that the administration to T.D., the responsive patient, of BH_4 and 6-MPH_4 at a dose of $20\,mg\,kg^{-1}\,24\,h^{-1}$ increased the depressed norepinephrine levels in CSF by two-fold to three-fold and increased the plasma norepinephrine levels to a lesser extent. The effect of BH_4 on norepinephrine levels appeared to be greater than that of 6-MPH_4. Neither pterin had any effect on dopamine levels in either CSF or plasma, whereas BH_4 may have increased the normal epinephrine levels to a small extent (Kaufman *et al.*, 1983).

Because of the finding that these two pterins are similar in their ability to increase this patient's low CSF norepinephrine levels, as well as the previously mentioned evidence that peripherally administered 6-MPH_4 enters the brain of rats and humans better than does BH_4, the effects of this synthetic pterin cofactor on various aspects of the patient's neurotransmitter metabolism were studied in greater detail. In some of these studies, doses of 6-MPH_4 as low as $8\,mg\,kg^{-1}$ $24\,h^{-1}$ (one-third of the daily dose given every 8 h) were used because it was shown that this dose was able to increase to normal the patient's exceedingly low physical activity, this response being measured quantitatively with the use of an activity monitor attached to the patient's wrist. The activity level achieved at this dose of 6-MPH_4 coincided with marked clinical improvement in movement, speech, and drooling.

Since changes in CSF concentrations of DOPAC and HVA, and 5-HIAA, the acid metabolites of dopamine, and serotonin, respectively, may reflect altered brain turnover of these monoamine neurotransmitters, their concentrations in CSF were measured before and after a dose of $8\,mg\,kg^{-1}\,day^{-1}$ of 6-MPH_4. As can be seen in Table 1, this dose of the pterin led to a marked increase in the very low levels of all three metabolites. The post-6-MPH_4 levels of these metabolites, however, were still not up to control values. Although this dose of 6-MPH_4 appeared to give a maximum increase in the patient's physical activity, it is possible that a higher dose would be required to raise the CSF level of these biogenic amine metabolites to normal. At the same dose ($8\,mg\,kg^{-1}$ day^{-1}), 6-MPH_4 lowered the patient's elevated levels of phenylalanine in both plasma and CSF to normal levels. These results, together with those in Table 1, indicate

that BH_4 and 6-MPH_4 stimulated the brain activity of both tyrosine and tryptophan hydroxylases and the peripheral activity of phenylalanine hydroxylase.

In sharp contrast to the results obtained with this patient, administration of even higher doses of 6-MPH_4 to R.B. did not increase the very low CSF levels of the biogenic amines or their acid metabolites (McInnes *et al.*, 1984). These results indicate that despite the clear evidence that 6-MPH_4 entered the brain of the patient, it did not stimulate the activities of tyrosine and tryptophan hydroxylases. It did, however, increase the activities of these enzymes in peripheral tissues. Thus, the low urinary excretion rates of the HVA and 5-HIAA, the acid metabolites of dopamine and 5-hydroxytryptophan, respectively, were clearly increased by 6-MPH_4, although they were still well below the normal values. In addition, plasma phenylalanine concentrations were decreased by 70%, from 1.0 to 0.2–0.3 mM, and plasma tyrosine concentrations doubled after administration of $10\,mg\,kg^{-1}$ day^{-1} of 6-MPH_4, providing strong evidence that this dose of 6-MPH_4 had stimulated peripheral activity of phenylalanine hydroxylase (McInnes *et al.*, 1984).

Although it is obvious that conclusions drawn from only two patients must be regarded as tentative, there appears to be a correlation between the severity of the block in BH_4 synthesis and the effectiveness of pterin therapy. In accord with this idea, the block in BH_4 synthesis in the responsive patient is not complete and the response to pterin administration was excellent, whereas in the unresponsive patient the block appears to be more complete and the beneficial effects of pterin administration were minimal (Kaufman *et al.*, 1982). Despite the fact that administered pterins appeared to cross the blood–brain barrier in comparable amounts in both patients, there was a dramatic difference in the ability of these elevated levels of tetrahydropterins to stimulate the activity of brain tyrosine and tryptophan hydroxylases. Thus, in contrast to the ability of 6-MPH_4 to increase the levels and turnover of CSF monoamine neurotransmitters in the responsive patient, there was essentially no effect of the pterin on CSF concentrations of the neurotransmitter metabolites, 5-HIAA and HVA, or on the neurotransmitters, dopamine, norepinephrine, and epinephrine in the unresponsive patient (McInnes *et al.*, 1984).

These results indicate that there may be a correlation between the ability of the administered pterins to stimulate the cerebral synthesis of dopamine, norepinephrine, and serotonin and the ability of the pterins to improve the patient's neuropathology. This last correlation, with its somewhat pessimistic implications for the generality of pterin administration as an adequate therapy in this disease, may reflect a role of BH_4—either via its involvement in monoamine neurotransmitter synthesis, or via some still unknown function—in normal brain development. If BH_4 does prove to be essential for normal brain development, it seems likely that the prospects for successful treatment of hyperphenylalaninaemia due to BH_4 synthesis defects would be improved if pterin therapy, with or without supplementation with DOPA and 5-hydroxy-

Table 1 CSF biogenic amine metabolites before and 2 h after a dose of $8\,mg\,kg^{-1}\,day^{-1}$ of 6-MPH_4 (patient T.D.)*

Metabolite	Before (ng ml^{-1})	After (ng ml^{-1})	Increase (%)
DOPAC	6.41	10.8	69
HVA	8.80	22.2	152
5HIAA	5.73	18.6	225

* Abbreviations used: DOPAC, dihydroxyphenylacetic acid; HVA, homovanillic acid; 5HIAA 5-hydroxyindoleacetic acid Normal values (means ± SEM in ng ml^{-1}). 2–4 years: 5HIAA, 39.6 ± 4.9, HVA, 132.4 ± 10.3 (Seifert *et al.*, 1980)

tryptophan, were initiated as early as possible, perhaps efen prenatally.

In view of the relatively large amounts of either BH_4 or $6\text{-}MPH_4$ that must be administered to a responsive patient in order to see any improvement in neurological signs, we have compared plasma levels of biopterin after BH_4 had been administered to a BH_4-deficient patient by different routes. The data shown in Table 2 demonstrate that the plasma levels of biopterin that are reached after either the intravenous or subcutaneous administration of BH_4 (at a dose of about $12\,mg\,kg^{-1}\,day^{-1}$ in three divided doses) are 50–100 times higher than the levels reached after oral administration. Given the high current cost of BH_4, the subcutaneous route of administration deserves serious consideration for chronic use as a practical and less costly alternative to oral administration.

Table 2 Plasma biopterin levels after the administration of tetrahydrobiopterin by different routes to a patient with defective *de novo* synthesis of tetrahydrobiopterin

Time (min)	Intravenous (ng ml^{-1})	Subcutaneous (ng ml^{-1})	Oral (ng ml^{-1})
0	6.7	5.9	2.8
10	1151	640	
30	611	495	9.4
60	432	410	9.8
120	158	208	10.3
180	130	109	11.0
240	79.2	74.0	16.2
360	27.5	30.0	
480	14.6	17.4	8.8
720	6.3	9.9	

Unpublished results (S. Kaufman, S. Milstien and J. Muenzer)

References

Bartholomé, K. A new molecular defect in phenylketonuria. *Lancet* ii (1974) 1580

Bartholomé, K. and Byrd, D. J. L-DOPA and 5-hydroxytryptophan therapy in phenylketonuria with normal phenylalanine hydroxylase activity. *Lancet* 2 (1975) 1042

Bartholomé, K., Byrd, D. J., Kaufman, S. and Milstien, S. Atypical phenylketonuria with normal phenylalanine hydroxylase and dihydropteridine reductase activity *in vitro*. *Pediatrics* 59 (1977) 757–761

Bartholomé, K., Lutz, P. and Bickel, H. Determination of phenylalanine hydroxylase activity in patients with phenylketonuria and hyperphenylalaninemia. *Pediatr. Res.* 9 (1975) 899–903

Brenneman, A. R. and Kaufman, S. The role of tetrahydropteridines in the enzymatic conversion of tyrosine to 3,4-dihydroxyphenylalanine. *Biochem. Biophys. Res. Commun.* 17 (1964) 177–183

Brewster, T. G., Moskowitz, M. A., Kaufman, S., Breslow, J. L., Milstien, S. and Abroms, I. F. Dihydropteridine reductase deficiency associated with severe neurologic disease and mild hyperphenylalaninemia. *Pediatrics* 63 (1979) 94–99

Butler, I. J., Koslow, S. H., Krumholz, A., Holtzman, N. and Kaufman, S. A disorder of biogenic amines in dihydropteridine reductase deficiency. *Ann. Neurol.* 3 (1978) 224–230

Butler, I. J., O'Flynn, M. E., Siefert, W. E. and Howell, R. R. Neurotransmitter defects and treatment of disorders of hyperphenylalaninemia. *J. Pediatr.* 98 (1981) 729–733

Curtius, H.-Ch., Niederwieser, A., Viscontini, M., Otten, A., Schaub, J., Scheibenreiter, S. and Schmidt, H. Atypical phenylketonuria due to tetrahydrobiopterin deficiency. Diagnosis and treatment with tetrahydrobiopterin, dihydrobiopterin and sepiapterin. *Clin. Chim. Acta* 93 (1979) 251–362

Danks, D. M., Schlesinger, P., Firgaira, F., Cotton, R. G. H., Watson, B. M., Rembold, H. and Hennings, G. Malignant hyperphenylalaninemia. Clinical features, biochemical findings and experience with administration of biopterins. *Pediatr. Res.* 13 (1979) 1150–1155

Fölling, A. Uber Ausscheidung von Phenylbrenztraubensaure in den Harm als Stoffwechselanomalie in Verbindung mit Imbezillitat. *Z. Physiol. Chem.* 227 (1934) 169–176

Friedman, P. A., Fisher, D. B., Kang, E. S. and Kaufman, S. Detection of hepatic phenylalanine 4-hydroxylase in classical phenylketonuria. *Proc. Natl. Acad. Sci. USA* 70 (1973) 552–556

Friedman, P. A., Kappelman, A. H. and Kaufman, S., Partial purification and characterization of tryptophan hydroxylase from rabbit hindbrain. *J. Biol. Chem.* 247 (1972) 4165–4173

Gal, E. M., Hanson, G. and Sherman, A. Biopterin. I. Profile and quantitation in rat brain. *Neurochem. Res.* 1 (1976) 511

Grobë, H., Bartholomé, K., Milstien, S. and Kaufman, S. Hyperphenylalaninemia due to dihydropteridine reductase deficiency. *Eur. J. Pediatr.* 551 (1978) 1–6

Heintel, D., Ghisla, S., Curtius, H.-Ch., Neiderwieser, A. and Levine, R. A. Biosynthesis of tetrahydrobiopterin: Possible involvement of tetrahydropterin intermediates. *Neurochem. Int.* 6 (1984) 141–155

Kapatos, G. and Kaufman, S. Peripherally administered reduced pterins do enter the brain. *Science* 212 (1981) 955–956

Kaufman, S. A new cofactor required for the enzymatic conversion of phenylalanine to tyrosine. *J. Biol. Chem.* 230 (1958a) 931–939

Kaufman, S. Phenylalanine hydroxylation cofactor in phenylketonuria. *Science* 128 (1958b) 1506

Kaufman, S. The structure of phenylalanine hydroxylation cofactor. *Proc. Natl. Acad. Sci. USA* 50 (1963) 1085–1093

Kaufman, S. Unanswered questions in the primary metabolic block in phenylketonuria. In Anderson, J. A. and Swaiman, K. F. (eds.) *Phenylketonuria and Allied Metabolic Diseases*, Proceedings of a Conference held at Washington, D.C., US GPO 6–8 April 1967, pp. 205–213

Kaufman, S. The phenylalanine hydroxylating system from mammalian liver. In Meister, A. (ed.) *Advances in Enzymology*, Vol. 35, John Wiley, New York, 1971, pp. 245–320

Kaufman, S. Pterin administration as a therapy for PKU due to dihydropteridine reductase deficiency. *Lancet* I (1975) 767

Kaufman, S. Biopterin and metabolic disease. In Kisliuk, R. L. and Brown, G. M. (eds.) *Chemistry and Biology of Pteridines*, Elsevier–North Holland, New York, 1979, pp. 117–124

Kaufman, S., Berlow, S., Summer, G. K., Milstien, S., Schulman, J. D., Orloff, S., Spielberg, S. and Pueschel, S. Hyperphenylalaninemia due to a deficiency of biopterin. A variant form of phenylketonuria. *N. Engl. J. Med.* 299 (1978) 673–679

Kaufman, S., Holtzman, N., Milstien, S., Butler, I. J. and Krumholz, A. Phenylketonuria due to a deficiency of dihydropteridine reductase. *N. Engl. J. Med.* 293 (1975a) 785–789

Kaufman, S., Kapatos, G., McInnes, R. R., Schulman, J. D. and Rizzo, W. B. The use of tetrahydropterins in the treatment of hyperphenylalaninemia due to defective synthesis of tetrahydrobiopterin: Evidence that peripherally administered tetrahydropterins enter the brain. *Pediatrics* 70 (1982) 376–380

Kaufman, S., Kapatos, G., Rizzo, W. B., Schulman, J. D., Tamarkin, L. and Van Loon, G. R. Tetrahydropterin therapy for hyperphenylalaninemia caused by defective synthesis of tetrahydrobiopterin. *Ann. Neurol.* 14 (1983) 308–315

Kaufman, S. and Levenberg, B. Further studies on the phenylalanine hydroxylation cofactor. *J. Biol. Chem.* 234 (1959) 2683–2688

Kaufman, S., Milstien, S. and Bartholomé, K. New forms of phenylketonuria. *Lancet* 1 (1975b) 708

Kaufman, S., Milstien, S. and Bartholomé, K. *N. Engl. J. Med.* 300 (1979) 198–199

Kettler, R., Bartholini, G. and Pletscher, A. *In vivo* enhancement of tyrosine hydroxylation in rat striatum by tetrahydrobiopterin. *Nature, Lond.* 249 (1974) 497–477

Leeming, R. J., Blair, J. A., Green, A. and Raine, D. N. Biopterin derivatives normal and phenylketonuric patients after oral loads of L-phenylalanine, L-tyrosine and L-tryptophan. *Arch. Dis. Child.* 51 (1976) 771–777

Leeming R. J. and Smith, I. *N. Engl. J. Med.* 300 (1979) 198–199

McInnes, R., Kaufman, S., Warsh, J. J., Milstien, S., Van Loon, G., Slyper, A. and Sherwood, G. Neurotransmitter metabolites and plasma catechols in biopterin deficiency. *Pediatr. Res.* 13 (1979) 422

McInnes, R., Kaufman, S., Warsh, J. J., Van Loon, G., Milstien, S., Kapatos, G., Soldin, S., Walsh, P., MacGregor, D. and Hanley, W. B. Biopterin synthesis defect. Treatment with L-DOPA and 5-hydroxytryptophan compared with therapy with a tetrahydropterin. *J. Clin. Invest.* 73 (1984) 458–469

Milstien, S. and Kaufman, S. Production of antibodies to sheep liver dihydropteridine reductase: Characterization and use to study the enzyme defect in a variant form of phenylketonuria. *Biochem. Biophys. Res. Commun.* 66 (1975) 475–481

Milstien, S. and Kaufman, S. Tetrahydrosepiapterin is an intermediate in tetrahydrobiopterin biosynthesis. *Biochem. Biophys. Res. Commun.* 115 (1983) 888–893

Milstien, S., Kaufman, S. and Summer, G. K. Hyperphenylalaninemia due to dihydropteridine reductase deficiency. Diagnosis by measurement of oxidized and reduced pterins in urine. *Pediatrics* 65 (1980) 806–810

Milstien, S., Orloff, S., Spielberg, S., Berlow, S., Schulman, J. and Kaufman, S. Hyperphenylalaninemia due to phenyl-alanine hydroxylase cofactor deficiency. *Pediatr. Res.* 11 (1977) 460

Narisawa, K., Arai, N., Hayakawa, H. and Tada, K. Diagnosis of dihydropteridine reductase deficiency by erythrocyte assay. *Pediatrics* 68 (1981) 591–592

Nichol, C. A., Lee, C. L., Edelstein, M. P., Chao, J. Y. and Duch, D. S. Biosynthesis of tetrahydrobiopterin by *de novo* and salvage pathways in adrenal extracts, mammalian cell cultures and rat brain *in vivo*. *Proc. Natl. Acad. Sci. USA* 80 (1983) 1546–1550

Niederwieser, A., Blau, N., Wang, M., Joller, P., Atares, M. and Cardesa-Gareit, J. GTP cyclohydrolase I deficiency, a new enzyme defect causing hyperphenylalaninemia with neopterin, biopterin, dopamine and serotonin deficiencies and muscular hypotonia. *Eur. J. Pediatr.* 141 (1984) 208–214

Nixon, J. C., Lee, C.-L., Milstien, S., Kaufman, S. and Bartholomé, K. Neopterin and biopterin levels in patients with atypical forms of phenylketonuria. *J. Neurochem.* 35 (1980) 898–904

Patterson, E. L., von Saltza, M. H. and Stokstad, E. L. The isolation and characterization of a pteridine required for the growth of *Crithidia fasiculata*. *J. Am. Chem. Soc.* 78 (1956) 5871–5873

Pollock, R. J. and Kaufman, S. Dihydrofolate reductase is present in brain. *J. Neurochem.* 30 (1978) 253–256

Rey, F., Blandin-Savoja, F. and Rey, J. Atypical phenyl-ketonuria with normal dihydropteridine reductase activity. *N. Engl. J. Med.* 295 (1976) 1138–1139

Rey, F., Harpey, J.-P., Leeming, R.-J., Blair, J.-A., Aircardi, J. and Rey, J. Les hyperphenylalaninemies avec activite normale de la phenylalanine-hydroxylase. *Arch. Fr. Pediatr.* 34 (1977) cix–cxx

Seifert, W. E., Foxx, J. L. and Butler, I. J. Age effect on dopamine and serotonin metabolite levels. *Ann. Neurol.* 8 (1980) 38–42

Shiman, R., Akino, M. and Kaufman, S. Solubilization and partial purification of tyrosine hydroxylase from bovine adrenal medulla. *J. Biol. Chem.* 246 (1971) 1330–1340

Smith, G. K. and Nichol, C. A. Tetrahydrobiopterin is synthesized by separate pathways from dihydroneopterin and from sepiapterin in adrenal medulla preparations. *Arch. Biochem. Biophys.* 227 (1983) 272–278

Smith, I. Atypical phenylketonuria accompanied by a severe progressive neurological illness unresponsive to dietary treatment. *Arch. Dis. Child.* 49 (1974) 245

Smith, I., Clayton, B. E. and Wolff, O. H. A variant of phenylketonuria. *Lancet* 1 (1975) 328–329

Switchenko, A. C., Primus, J. P. and Brown, G. M. Intermediates in the enzymatic synthesis of tetrahydro-biopterin in *Drosophila melanogaster*. *Biochem. Biophys. Res. Commun.* 120 (1984) 754–760

Tietz, A., Lindberg, M. and Kennedy, E. P. A new pteridine-requiring enzyme system for the oxidation of glyceryl-ethers. *J. Biol. Chem.* 239 (1964) 4081–4090

J. Inher. Metab. Dis. 8 Suppl. 1 (1985) 28–33

Biosynthesis of Tetrahydrobiopterin in Man

H.-Ch. Curtius, D. Heintel, S. Ghisla[1], Th. Kuster, W. Leimbacher and A. Niederwieser
Division of Clinical Chemistry, Department of Pediatrics, University of Zurich, Switzerland
[1]*Department of Biology, University of Constance, POB 5560, D-7750 Constance, FRG*

The biosynthesis of tetrahydrobiopterin (BH_4) from dihydroneopterin triphosphate (NH_2P_3) was studied in human liver extract. The phosphate-eliminating enzyme (PEE) was purified ~ 750-fold. The conversion of NH_2P_3 to BH_4 was catalyzed by this enzyme in the presence of partially purified sepiapterin reductase, Mg^{2+} and NADPH. The PEE is heat stable when heated at 80 °C for 5 min. It has a molecular weight of 63 000 daltons. One possible intermediate 6-(1'-hydroxy-2'-oxopropyl)5,6,7,8-tetrahydropterin(2'-oxo-tetrahydropterin) was formed upon incubation of BH_4 in the presence of sepiapterin reductase and $NADP^+$ at pH 9.0. Reduction of this compound with $NaBD_4$ yielded monodeutero threo and erythro-BH_4, the deuterium was incorporated at the 2' position. This and the UV spectra were consistent with a 2'-oxo-tetrahydropterin structure. Dihydrofolate reductase (DHFR) catalyzed the reduction of BH_2 to BH_4 and was found to be specific for the pro-R-NADPH side. The sepiapterin reductase catalyzed the transfer of the pro-S hydrogen of NADPH during the reduction of sepiapterin to BH_2. In the presence of crude liver extracts the conversion of NH_2P_3 to BH_4 requires NADPH. Two deuterium atoms were incorporated from $(4S-^2H)NADHP$ in the 1' and 2' position of the BH_4 side chain. Incorporation of one hydrogen from the solvent was found at position C(6). These results are consistent with the occurrence of an intramolecular redox exchange between the pteridine nucleus and the side chain and formation of 6-pyruvoyl-5,6,7,8-tetrahydropterin(tetrahydro-1'-2'-dioxopterin) as intermediate.

Despite the numerous studies carried out on tetrahydrobiopterin (BH_4) biosynthesis in mammals, several controversial aspects still have to be clarified (Levine *et al.*, 1983a; Ghisla *et al.*, 1984). BH_4 is a cofactor for phenylalanine, tryptophan and tyrosine hydroxylases, and it has been suggested that it also plays an important role in the regulation of the synthesis of biogenic amine neurotransmitters (Levine *et al.*, 1983b). Errors in BH_4 biosynthesis and metabolism have been extensively studied in the rare childhood disease BH_4-deficient hyperphenylalaninaemia, alternatively referred to as atypical phenylketonuria (Niederwieser *et al.*, 1982), as well as in certain neurological and psychiatric disorders (Curtius *et al.*, 1982, 1983). The urinary excretion of neopterin (a metabolite of an intermediate in BH_4 biosynthesis) has been shown to be elevated in certain diseases where there is an alteration in the status of the immune system (Wachter *et al.*, 1983). A complete understanding of the enzymatic steps in the BH_4 biosynthesis in man is therefore of great importance.

The first reaction in mammalian BH_4 biosynthesis involves the conversion of GTP to dihydroneopterin triphosphate (NH_2P_3) by a single enzyme, GTP cyclohydrolase I. This has been reported in non-mammalians by Fan and Brown (1976) in *Drosophila* and by our group in humans (Blau and Niederwieser, 1983). We developed an enzyme assay for GTP cyclohydrolase I in human liver biopsies and lymphocytes and reported the first patient with GTP cyclohydrolase deficiency (Niederwieser *et al.*, 1984a). While the conversion of GTP to NH_2P_3 is catalyzed by a single enzyme in mammals, the further transformation of NH_2P_3 to BH_4 is likely to involve several enzymes. It should be pointed out that up to now in the biosynthesis

of BH_4, only the structures of GTP, NH_2P_3 and BH_4 have been established beyond doubt, as shown in Figure 1. Current discussions and controversies deal mainly with the steps leading from NH_2P_3 to BH_4.

Tanaka *et al.* (1981) reported that in chicken kidney, NH_2P_3 is converted through some intermediate "*x*" to L-sepiapterin by a heat stable, magnesium-dependent "fraction A_2". It was suggested that "*x*" was converted to

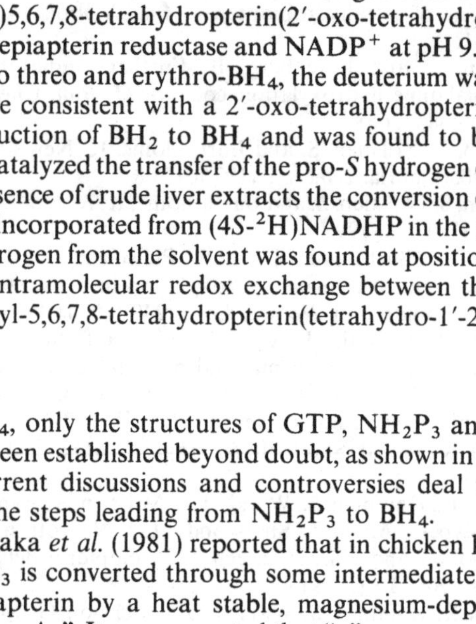

Figure 1 Biosynthesis of tetrahydrobiopterin from guanosine triphosphate. *Note* that only the structure of the molecules shown have been established beyond doubt. The parts of the molecules of NH_2P_3 which are subjected to reduction are denoted by squares, those which undergo inversion by circles

Journal of Inherited Metabolic Disease. ISSN 0141-8955. Copyright © SSIEM and MTP Press Limited, Queen Square, Lancaster, UK.

sepiapterin by the heat labile "fraction A_1" which was reported to be NADPH-dependent, and that "x" was a diketo-dihydropterin.

Regarding the potential of NADPH dependency of the sepiapterin formation from NH_2P_3, reported by some authors, it is puzzling that NADPH should be considered necessary since there is no net difference in the redox balance between NH_2P_3 and sepiapterin (Heintel *et al.*, 1984). Recently, however, we showed that NADPH is not necessary in human and vertebrates for sepiapterin formation. NH_2P_3 was shown to be converted to sepiapterin without addition of NADPH as well as under conditions that ensured the destruction of endogenous, free NADPH (Heintel *et al.*, 1984). Our results have also indicated that sepiapterin may not be an intermediate on the pathway leading to BH_4 biosynthesis under normal *in vivo* conditions.

Duch *et al.* (1983) demonstrated the formation of BH_4 in the presence of sufficient methotrexate to inhibit dihydrofolate reductase (DHFR) (EC 1.6.99.7) completely. This implied that sepiapterin is not on the biosynthetic pathway. This was also confirmed by Milstien and Kaufman (1983) and ourselves (Heintel *et al.*, 1984). Together with the groups of Kaufman, Nichol and Brown, we suggested the occurrence of internal oxidoreduction reactions leading to tetrahydropterins without the need of NADPH (Heintel *et al.*, 1984; Levine *et al.*, 1983a). This process appears to be thermodynamically feasible (Ghisla *et al.*, 1984).

A comparison of the chemical structures of NH_2P_3 and BH_4 reveals that three distinct chemical transformations are required for their interconversion (see Figure 1): (a) elimination, (b) inversion, (c) reduction.

(a) *Elimination*: The elimination of a leaving group such as (tri)phosphate is a facile chemical reaction requiring a base which catalyzes the abstraction of the C(2')-H as a proton. Several enzymes catalyzing phosphate elimination reactions are known, and the requirement for Mg^{2+} in reactions involving organic phosphates has been documented. During the reaction one proton from the solvent is introduced in the 3' position. However, a proton shift occurring at an active site shielded from H^+ exchange with solvent has also been proposed. This is shown in Figure 2. Whether, as in our case, such a shift occurs or not can be verified experimentally. Conservation of the 1' or of the 2' hydrogens in the 3'-CH_3 of BH_4 would be consistent with such hypothesis. Conversely, incorporation of (labeled) solvent hydrogen at C(3') would clearly exclude this type of mechanism. A possible enzyme catalyzing this conversion has been proposed by Tanaka *et al.* (1981), and is referred to as "fraction A_2" which has been shown to require Mg^{2+} for activity.

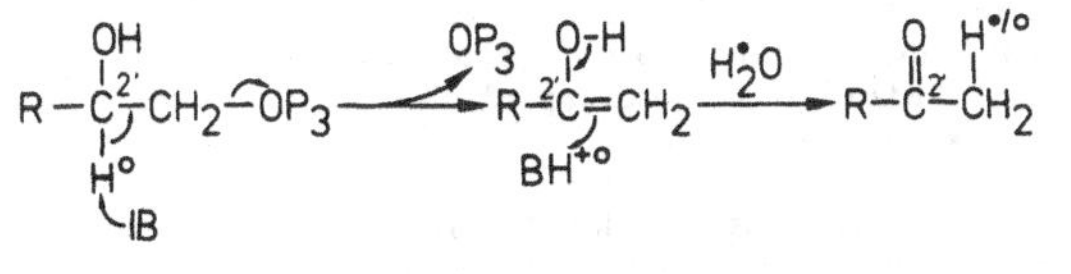

(b) *Inversion*: Two basically distinct types of biochemical inversions at chiral centers are known. One type of inversion can be induced directly by two enzyme active center bases and proceeds over a carbanionic transient. Alternatively, and as is likely to occur in our case, redox catalysis is involved and inversion could proceed via a planar sp^2 carbon center (Figure 3).

(c) *Reduction*: The difference in redox state between NH_2P_3 and BH_4 is $4e^-$. Reduction of the C(6)–N(5) imine might, at first sight, be considered a normal hydrogenation reaction, such as those catalyzed by pyridine nucleotide or flavin enzymes. In the case when an intramolecular rearrangement reaction takes place, a keto-group in the 1' position must be reduced (see Figure 10). The formal reduction at C(3'), on the other hand, might involve a more complicated set of events, i.e. triphosphate elimination to form an enol, ketonization of the latter and finally reduction of the 2'-keto group thus formed. The sequence of these events, elimination, intramolecular oxidoreduction reaction, inversion, and reduction of the keto-groups, is not established. Elimination can be an early event and has been proposed by Krivi and Brown (1979) to initiate the conversion. Milstien and Kaufman (1983), on the other hand, proposed that the sequence starts with the internal redox reaction.

Concerning biosynthesis, the following questions are still unclear:

(1) How is L-biopterin formed from D-neopterin with inversion of two chiral centers at 1' and 2'? (see Figure 1).

(2) Are quinonoid intermediates or dihydropteridine reductase (DHPR) involved in the biosynthesis?

(3) Is the tetrahydro form of the pterin nucleus formed by an intramolecular redox rearrangement?

(4) What is the mechanism of the reduction steps? Does direct transfer of NADPH hydride occur? If yes, from which (R or S) side?

(5) What is the role of sepiapterin reductase in the biosynthesis of BH_4. Can it be confirmed that folate reductase is not involved?

To clarify these questions we investigated the biosynthesis with stereospecific deuterium labeled pyridine nucleotides.

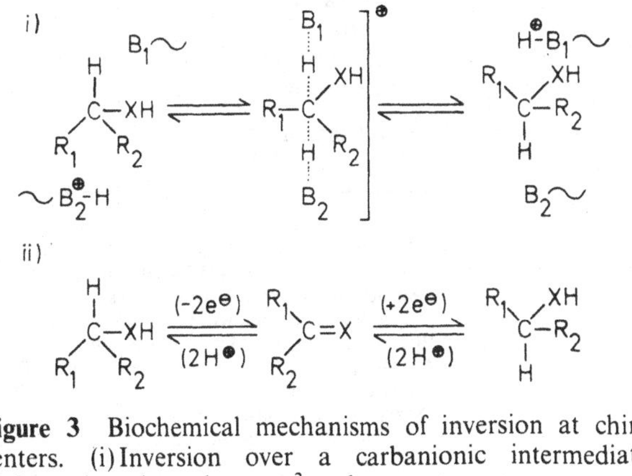

Figure 2. Elimination of triphosphate

Figure 3 Biochemical mechanisms of inversion at chiral centers. (i) Inversion over a carbanionic intermediate; (ii) inversion via a planar sp^2 carbon center

RESULTS AND DISCUSSION

(1) Isolation of "phosphate-eliminating enzyme"

We have isolated PEE from human liver by $(NH_4)_2SO_4$ fractionation and subsequent purification by several chromatographic columns. This enzyme was capable of synthesizing BH_4, in the presence of partially purified sepiapterin reductase, Mg^{2+} and NADPH. PEE is heat stable at 80 °C for 5 min and has a molecular weight of about 63 000 daltons, as determined by gel chromatography. The enzyme was purified ~750-fold. Our results are shown in Table 1.

In an experiment using labeled $[\alpha\text{-}^{32}P]GTP$, we could show that PEE eliminates the phosphates of NH_2P_3, and thus confirms the results of Tanaka *et al.* (1981) obtained with chicken kidney preparations. This suggests that the enzymes are similar in both cases. We succeeded in scaling down the assay of the PEE in order to carry out measurements with liver biopsy material. In controls from adult traffic accident victims we found an activity of the order of 1 nU mg protein^{-1}. In the liver biopsy of a patient with "BH_2-synthetase deficiency" no PEE activity could be detected (Niederwieser *et al.*, 1985).

These experiments allow us to conclude that $PEE + Mg^{2+}$ are necessary for the elimination and sepiapterin reductase + NADPH for the reduction processes. A third factor or enzyme might also be necessary for biosynthesis.

(2) Synthesis of 6-(1'-hydroxy-2'-oxopropyl)5,6,7,8-tetrahydropterin (2'-oxo-tetrahydropterin)

In the search for the intermediate in the biosynthetic pathway, many speculations have been published. Krivi and Brown (1979) proposed a dihydro-2'-keto compound; Suzuki and Goto (1973), and later on Tanaka *et al.* (1981) suggested a dihydro-diketo compound (compound *x*); our group (Heintel *et al.*, 1984), Smith and Nichol (1983), Milstien and Kaufman (1983), as well as Brown (Switchenko *et al.*, 1984) suggested a tetrahydromono or diketo pterin as intermediate. Recently, Smith and Nichol (1984) and Switchenko *et al.* (1984) published electrochemical data and a u.v. spectrum in favour of a tetrahydro compound without, however, proposing any chemical structure. They also claimed that there might be two NADPH-dependent reductases to reduce the keto compounds (Switchenko *et al.*, 1984; Smith and Nichol, 1984). In analogy with the oxidation of BH_2 to sepiapterin in the presence of NADP and sepiapterin reductase at pH 9.0, we attempted the dehydrogenation of BH_4 with sepiapterin reductase from human liver and rat erythrocytes as well as with crude homogenate from human liver (Figure 4). The formation of a new product was demonstrated by HPLC and with electrochemical detection (Figure 5). The u.v. spectrum of the corresponding HPLC fraction was in accordance with that of a tetrahydropterin. Upon reduction with sodium borohydride both erythro and threo BH_4 were formed. When sodium borodeuteride was used instead, a single deuterium was incorporated in the 2' position of the side chain of BH_4, as shown by GC–MS. These experiments prove the structure of the compound to be 2'-oxo-tetrahydropterin. The reactions of sepiapterin reductase are shown in Figure 6. The further oxidation of the 2'-oxo-tetrahydropterin by sepiapterin reductase and NADP to the postulated tetrahydro-diketo compound (6-pyruvoyl tetrahydropterin) has not yet been observed.

(3) Incubation studies with deuterated (R-or-S-^{2}H)-NADPH in H_2O and ^2H_2O

Recently, we studied the biosynthesis of tetrahydrobiopterin from either dihydroneopterin triphosphate,

Table 1 Yield of BH_4 after incubation of NH_2P_3 with PEE and sepiapterin reductase after various purification steps

	PEE, *human liver** (pmol BH_4 min^{-1})		
	Hydroxyapatite	*Gel filtration AcA 44*	*Heat treatment after AcA 44 (5 min, 80 °C)*
SR, human liver*			
Hydroxyapatite		68	112
Gel filtration AcA 44		58	88
Blue Sepharose CL-6B	148	‡	25
SR, rat erythrocytes†			
Matrex Red A		‡	15

The assay contained the following reaction components (final concentrations) in total volume of 125 μl: NH_2P_3 (0.02 mmol l^{-1}), $MgCl_2$ (8 mmol l^{-1}), NADPH (1 mmol l^{-1}), 10 μl sepiapterin reductase (in excess) and 20 μl PEE in 0.1 mol l^{-1} Tris–HCl pH 7.4. After incubation for 1 h at 37 °C the produced BH_4 was determined by HPLC and electrochemical detection (Niederwieser *et al.*, 1984b)
*Sepiapterin reductase was prepared as described by Sueoka and Katoh (1982). On the hydroxyapatite column, PEE could be separated from sepiapterin reductase. Both enzymes were further purified on 2.6 × 70 cm column of AcA 44 in 50 mmol l^{-1} potassium phosphate buffer, pH 6.0. Sepiapterin reductase was afterwards applied to a Blue Sepharose CL-6B column and eluted with NADPH (1 mmol l^{-1}) (Sueoka and Katoh, 1982)
†Sepiapterin reductase from rat erythrocytes was purified according to Sueoka and Katoh (1982)
‡BH_4 formation was ≤ the detection level. More recent experiments (Heintel and Curtius, unpublished) carried out under optimized conditions indicate substantial BH_4 production using highly purified PEE and sepiapterin reductase

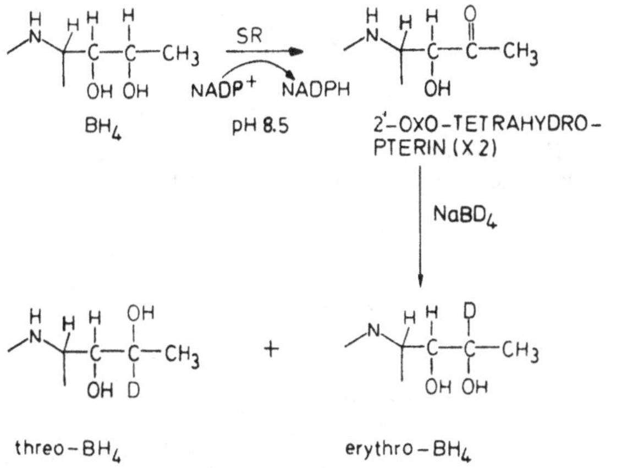

Figure 4 Reverse reaction of BH_4 to X2 with sepiapterin reductase. The reaction mixture contained (final concentrations) in a total volume of 2 ml, R-BH_4 (0.08 mmol l^{-1}), NADP$^+$ (0.4 mmol l^{-1}), 60 mU human sepiapterin reductase after purification on AcA 44 in 0.2 mol l^{-1} Tris–HCl pH 9.0. After 30 min at 25 °C, the mixture was acidified to pH 7.0 and the protein separated over Sephadex G 25. The column was equilibrated in degassed H_2O which contained DTE (1 mmol l^{-1}). The fractions which contained the BH_4 and X2 were lyophilized. Afterwards X2 was isolated by HPLC (system described by Niederwieser *et al.*, 1984b). Reduction of the isolated X2 was performed with NaB$^2H_4$ for 1 min at pH ~8.0 followed by adjustment to pH ~1 with HCl. The produced erythro-BH_4 was purified for GC–MS analysis

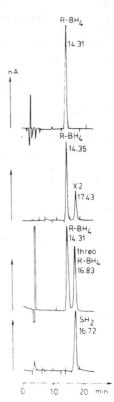

Figure 5 HPLC chromatography of tetrahydropterins with EC-detection. HPLC conditions as described elsewhere (Niederwieser *et al.*, 1984), except that the eluent contained 5% methanol

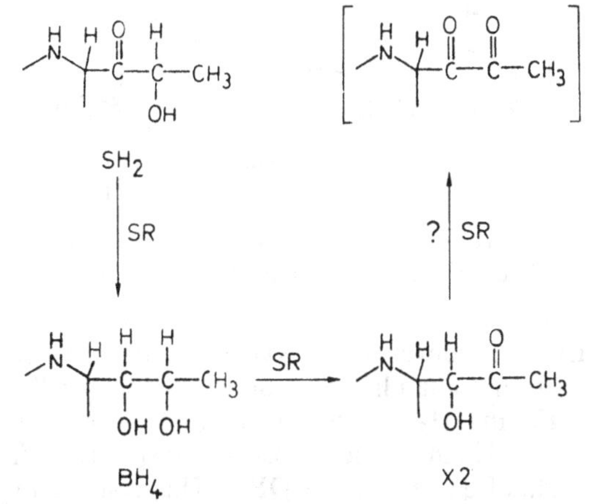

Figure 6 Reactions of sepiapterin reductase

sepiapterin or dihydrobiopterin using extracts from human liver, purified sepiapterin reductase from human liver, rat erythrocytes and dihydrofolate reductase (Curtius *et al.*, 1985). The incorporation of hydrogen in tetrahydrobiopterin was studied in either ^2H_2O or H_2O using deuterated (R- or S-^2H)NADH and deuterated (R- or S-^2H)NADPH. In NADPH-dependent enzyme reactions, the transfer of a hydride ion is stereospecific. Either the pro-R or pro-S hydride is transferred to the substrate (Figure 7).

Dihydrofolate reductase (DHFR)
In the formation of tetrahydrobiopterin from dihydrobiopterin in the presence of dihydrofolate reductase (DHFR), the pro-R hydrogen of NADPH was transferred to the C(6) position of the ring moiety of BH_4. Therefore DHFR is specific for the pro-R NADPH hydrogen (Figure 8).

Sepiapterin reductase
Sepiapterin reductase catalyzed the transfer of the pro-S hydrogen of NADPH during the reduction of sepiapterin at the side chain position C(1') to yield dihydrobiopterin (Figure 9).

Conversion of NH_2P_3 to BH_4
During the conversion of NH_2P_3 to BH_4 in the presence of human liver extract, arsenite to inhibit the H/D exchange of NADPH with solvent (see below), NADPH and ^2H_2O, one deuterium was incorporated in the 6-position of the ring. This is consistent with an intramolecular oxidoreduction reaction which is envisaged to occur via tautomerization in the C(6) position of the ring moiety and the C(1'), as shown in Figure 10.

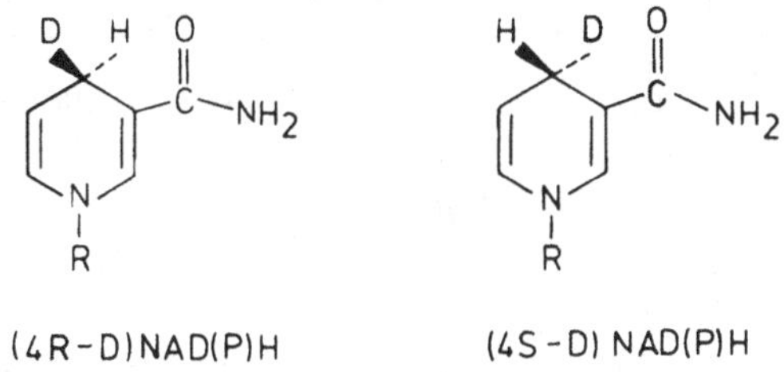

Figure 7 Transfer of either the pro-R or pro-S hydride in NADPH-dependent enzyme reactions

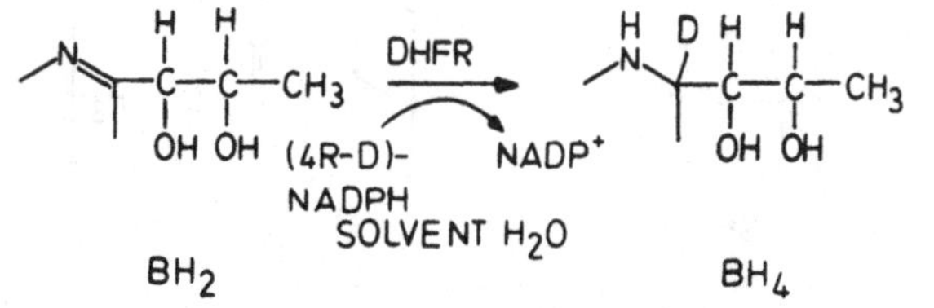

Figure 8 Hydrogen transfer from $(4R\text{-}^2H)$NADPH by dihydrofolate reductase (substrate BH_2, product BH_4)

During the conversion of NH_2P_3 to BH_4 with crude extract from human liver and deuterated $(R\text{-}$ or $S\text{-}^2H)$-NADPH in H_2O, two deuterium atoms were incorporated in the 1′ and 2′ positions, respectively, from the S side of deuterated NADPH. This could only be observed after inhibition of diaphorases which were present in the extract. The flavoprotein α-lipoyl dehydrogenase, a diaphorase present in liver tissue, can catalyze a hydrogen exchange between NADPH and H^+ of H_2O (Ernster *et al.*, 1965).

CONCLUSIONS

(1) DHFR has been shown to be specific for the pro-R NADPH side in the reduction of BH_2 to BH_4. During the conversion of NH_2P_3 to BH_4 with crude human liver extracts, no deuterium transfer to the ring moiety of BH_4 was found from either deuterated (S or R) NADPH. This indicates that DHFR is not involved in the biosynthesis of BH_4 from NH_2P_3 and that BH_2 is not an intermediate, which is in accordance with the conclusions of others (Duch *et al.*, 1983).

(2) Our finding of the incorporation of one deuterium from the solvent into position 6 is consistent with the occurrence of an intramolecular oxidoreduction (see Figure 10).

(3) Our results show that during the conversion of NH_2P_3 to BH_4 with deuterated $(S\text{-}^2H)$NADPH in H_2O, one deuterium atom is incorporated each at the 1′ and the 2′ position of the side chain. This requires that during biosynthesis, the intermediates must carry a diketo side chain at C(6).

(4) The dehydrogenation of BH_4 by sepiapterin reductase to form 2′-oxo-tetrahydropterin indicates that the reverse reaction can also be catalyzed by this enzyme and that sepiapterin reductase could indeed take place in the reduction of the 1′ and the 2′ keto functions.

(5) The PEE appears to be involved in the elimination of phosphate. The exact locus at which

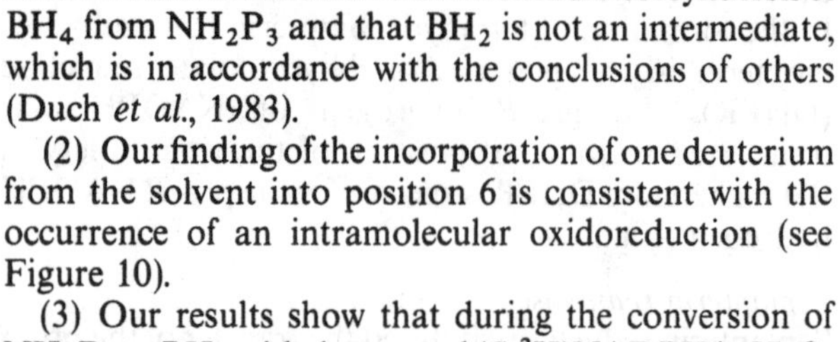

Figure 9 Hydrogen transfer from $(4S\text{-}^2H)$NADPH by sepiapterin reductase from rat erythrocytes (substrate sepiapterin, product BH_2)

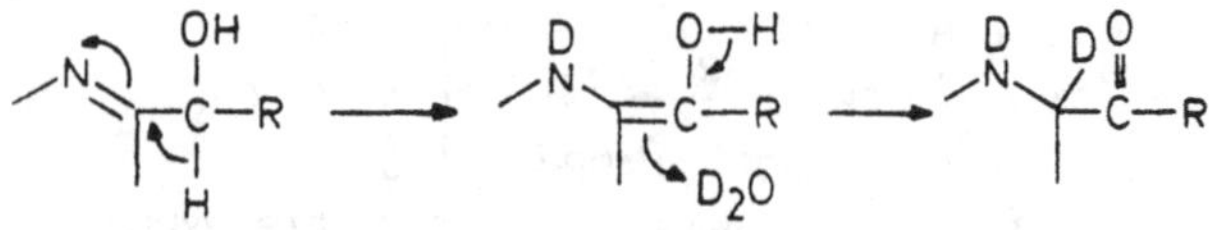

Figure 10 Intramolecular oxidoreduction reaction leading to tetrahydropterins without the need of NADPH

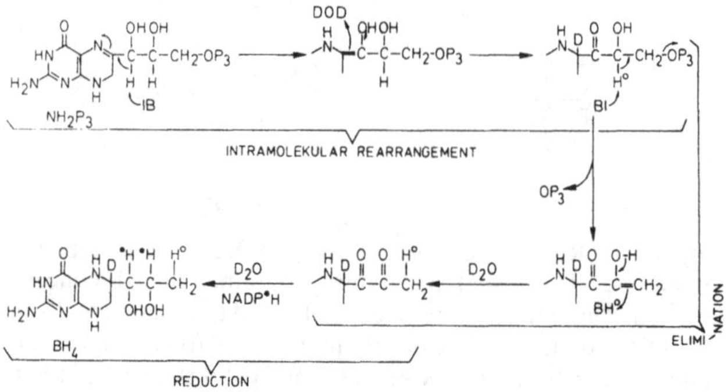

Figure 11 Possible pathway of BH_4 biosynthesis including recent GC–MS results of deuterated NADPH and D_2O studies

elimination occurs in the sequence in Figure 11 cannot be determined by the present experiments.

From these results it can be calculated that the metabolic scheme of Figure 11 may be the most likely.

We thank Mr U. Redweik, Mr W. Staudenmann and Ms M Sappelt for skilful technical assistance, and Dr B. Zagalak and Dr R. A. Levine (NIH, Bethesda, MD, USA) for valuable discussions. We thank Prof Dr H. Simon (Technical University of Munich, FRG) for a sample of $(4S\text{-}^2H)$NADH and for valuable discussions. This work was supported by the Swiss National Science Foundation, project no. 3′266-0.82.

References

Blau, N. and Niederwieser, A. Guanosine triphosphate cyclohydrolase I assay in human and rat liver using high-performance liquid chromatography of neopterin phosphates and guanine nucleotides. *Analyt. Biochem.* 128 (1983) 446–452

Curtius, H.-Ch., Müldner, H. and Niederwieser, A. Tetrahydrobiopterin: Efficacy in endogenous depression and Parkinson's disease. *J. Neural. Transmission* 55 (1982) 301–308

Curtius, H.-Ch., Niederwieser, A., Levine, R. A., Lovenberg, W., Woggon, B. and Angst, J. Successful treatment of depression with tetrahydrobiopterin. *Lancet* I (1983) 657–658

Curtius, H.-Ch., Heintel, D., Ghisla, S., Kuster, Th., Leimbacher, W. and Niederwieser, A. Tetrahydrobiopterin biosynthesis. Studies with specifically labelled (^2H)NAD(P)H and of enzymes involved. *Eur. J. Biochem.* 148 (1985) (in press)

Duch, D. S., Lee, C.-L., Edelstein, M. P. and Nichol, C. A. Biosynthesis of tetrahydrobiopterin in the presence of dihydrofolate reductase inhibitors. *Molec. Pharmacol.* 24 (1983) 103–108

Ernster, L., Hoberman, H. D., Howard, R. L., King, T. E., Lee, C.-P., Mackler, B. and Sottocasa, G. Stereospecificity of certain soluble and particulate preparations of mitochondrial reduced nicotinamide-adenine dinucleotide dehydrogenase from beef heart. *Nature, Lond.* 207 (1965) 940–941

Fan, C. L. and Brown, G. M. Partial purification and properties of guanosine triphosphate cyclohydrolase from *Drosophila melanogaster. Biochem. Genet.* 14 (1976) 259–270

Ghisla, S., Curtius, H.-Ch. and Levine, R. A. Chemical considerations on the biosynthesis of tetrahydrobiopterin. In Pfleiderer, W., Wachter, H. and Curtius, H.-Ch. (eds.) *Biochemical and Clinical Aspects of Pteridines,* Vol. 3, De Gruyter, Berlin, 1984, pp. 35–52

Heintel, D., Ghisla, S., Curtius, H.-Ch., Niederwieser, A. and Levine, R. A. Biosynthesis of tetrahydrobiopterin: Possible involvement of tetrahydrobiopterin intermediates. *Neurochem. Int.* 1 (1984) 141–155

Krivi, G. G. and Brown, G. M. Purification and properties of the enzymes from *Drosophila melanogaster* that catalyze the synthesis of sepiapterin from dihydroneopterin triphosphate. *Biochem. Genet.* 17 (1979) 371–390

Levine, R. A., Heintel, D., Leimbacher, W., Niederwieser, A., Curtius, H.-Ch. and Ghisla, S. Recent advances in tetrahydrobiopterin biosynthesis and the treatment of human disease. In Curtius, H.-Ch., Pfleiderer, W. and Wachter, H. (eds.) *Biochemical and Clinical Aspects of Pteridines,* Vol. 2, De Gruyter, Berlin, 1983a, pp. 325–337

Levine, R. A., Lovenberg, W., Curtius, H.-Ch. and Niederwieser, A. Speculation on the mechanism of therapeutic action of tetrahydrobiopterin in human disease. In Blair, J. A. (ed.) *Chemistry and Biology of Pteridines,* De Gruyter, Berlin, 1983b, pp. 833–837

Milstien, S. and Kaufman, S. Tetrahydro-sepiapterin is an intermediate in tetrahydrobiopterin biosynthesis. *Biochem. Biophys. Res. Commun.* 115 (1983) 888–893

Niederwieser, A., Blau, N., Wang, M., Joller, P., Atarés, M. and Cardesa-Garcia, J. GTP cyclohydrolase I deficiency, a new enzyme defect causing hyperphenylalaninemia with neopterin, biopterin, dopamine, and serotonin deficiencies and muscular hypotonia. *Eur. J. Pediatr.* 141 (1984a) 208–214

Niederwieser, A., Matasovic, A., Staudenmann, W., Wang, M. and Curtius, H.-Ch. Screening for tetrahydrobiopterin deficiency. In Wachter, H., Curtius, H.-Ch. and Pfleiderer, W. (eds.) *Biochemical and Clinical Aspects of Pteridines,* Vol. 1, De Gruyter, Berlin, 1982, pp. 293–306

Niederwieser, A., Staudenmann, W. and Wetzel, E. High-performance liquid chromatography with column switching for the analysis of biogenic amine metabolites and pterins. *J. Chromatogr.* 290 (1984b) 237–246

Niederwieser, A., Ponzone, A. and Curtius, H.-Ch. Differential diagnosis of tetrahydrobiopterin deficiency. *J. Inher. Metab. Dis.* 8 Suppl. 1 (1985) 34–38

Smith, G. K. and Nichol, C. A. Studies on the biosynthesis of tetrahydrobiopterin in bovine adrenal medulla preparations. In Curtius, H.-Ch., Pfleiderer, W. and Wachter, H. (eds.) *Biochemical and Clinical Aspects of Pteridines,* Vol. 2, De Gruyter, Berlin, 1983, pp. 123–131

Smith, G. K. and Nichol, C. A. Two new tetrahydropterin intermediates in the adrenal medullary *de novo* biosynthesis of tetrahydrobiopterin. *Biochem. Biophys. Res. Commun.* 120 (1984) 761–766

Sueoka, T. and Katoh, S. Purification and characterization of sepiapterin reductase from rat erythrocytes. *Biochim. Biophys. Acta* 717 (1982) 265–271

Suzuki, A. and Goto, M. Isolation of D-*erythro*-neopterin 2′:3′-cyclic phosphate from *Photobacterium phosphoreum. Biochim. Biophys. Acta* 304 (1973) 222–224

Switchenko, A. C., Primus, J. P. and Brown, G. M. Intermediates in the enzymic synthesis of tetrahydrobiopterin in *Drosophila melanogaster. Biochem. Biophys. Res. Commun.* 120 (1984) 754–760

Tanaka, K., Akino, M., Hagi, Y., Doi, M. and Shiota, T. The enzymatic synthesis of sepiapterin by chicken kidney preparations. *J. Biol. Chem.* 256 (1981) 2963–2972

Wachter, H. *et al.* In Curtius, H.-Ch., Pfleiderer, W. and Wachter, H. (eds.) *Biochemical and Clinical Aspects of Pteridines,* Vol. 2, De Gruyter, Berlin, 1983

J. Inher. Metab. Dis. 8 Suppl. 1 (1985) 34–38

Differential Diagnosis of Tetrahydrobiopterin Deficiency

A. Niederwieser[1], A. Ponzone[2] and H.-Ch. Curtius[1]

[1]*Department of Pediatrics, University of Zurich, Switzerland*
[2]*Department of Pediatrics, University of Torino, Italy*

Six hundred and seventy-three children (483 newborns and 190 older selected children) were screened for tetrahydrobiopterin (BH₄) deficiency by HPLC of urine pterins and BH₄ load test. One patient with GTP cyclohydrolase I deficiency, 36 patients with dihydrobiopterin synthetase (DHBS) deficiency (of which six were in the newborn and 30 in the older children) and 14 with dihydropteridine reductase deficiency (DHPR) were found. All 37 patients with defective BH₄ biosynthesis responded to a BH₄ load by lowering of the elevated serum phenylalanine concentration but four of 14 patients with DHPR deficiency did not. Measurement of DHPR activity in blood spots on Guthrie cards is recommended. Since subvariants of patients with BH₄ deficiency exist, homovanillic acid, 5-hydroxyindole acetic acid, pterins, phenylalanine, and tyrosine in cerebrospinal fluid should be measured for diagnosis and the control of therapy. The activity of the phosphate-eliminating enzyme (a key enzyme in BH₄ biosynthesis and part of "DHBS") was measured in human liver and activities of approx. 1 n U (mg protein)$^{-1}$ were found. In the liver biopsy of a patient with DHBS deficiency no activity (less than 3% of controls) was demonstrated.

Ten years ago the first patients with tetrahydrobiopterin (BH₄) deficiency were described independently by Bartholomé (1974) and Smith *et al.* (1974, 1975). At that time it became obvious that BH₄ was essential for human well-being and normal function of the central nervous system. Because tetrahydrobiopterin deficiency is a severe disease with progressive neurological symptoms (Danks *et al.*, 1978) and is treatable (Bartholomé and Byrd, 1975; Danks *et al.*, 1978), it became necessary to develop screening tests for the early detection of BH₄ deficiency in infancy. Every newborn with even only slight but persistent hyperphenylalaninaemia should be tested for BH₄ deficiency. Such tests have been introduced in many developed nations, but even today older children are detected because of the appearance of clinical symptoms, such as muscular hypotonia of the trunk, hypertonia of the extremities and often myoclonic epilepsy, which are unresponsive to a low phenylalanine diet.

Today we recognize four metabolic defects causing hyperphenylalaninaemia including the classical form with a defect in phenylalanine 4-hydroxylase (EC 1.4.16.1) (McKusick 26160) (Figure 1). The three variants are rare disorders, with an estimated incidence of 1% in newborns with hyperphenylalaninaemia, and lead to BH₄ deficiency either by a defect in regeneration of this cofactor or by one of two defects in biosynthesis. GTP cyclohydrolase I (EC 3.5.4.16) deficiency has been detected only recently (Niederwieser *et al.*, 1982c, 1984a) and four patients have been reported. This defect blocks BH₄ biosynthesis at the very first step of conversion of GTP to dihydroneopterin triphosphate and the patient is practically unable to form any pterins. Therefore, this disease may be a worthwhile model for investigating the potential involvement of pterins in other biological systems, in addition to the known cofactor role of BH₄ for phenylalanine, tyrosine, and tryptophan hydroxylases.

"Dihydrobiopterin synthetase" is a provisional name for an enzyme system described by Gál *et al.* (1978) converting dihydroneopterin triphosphate to BH₄. The system consists of two or three enzymes which have not yet been characterized in detail (Curtius, 1985). Most patients with BH₄ deficiency suffer from a defect in "dihydrobiopterin synthetase" (McKusick 26164, 26169). The first patient with this variant was described by Rey *et al.* (1977). The patients excrete huge amounts of dihydroneopterin and neopterin in urine (Niederwieser *et al.*, 1979; Kaufman *et al.*, 1979) as well as 3'-hydroxy-D-sepiapterin (Niederwieser *et al.*, 1980b) as degradation products of the accumulated dihydroneopterin triphosphate (Figure 1), and low concentrations only of biopterins.

Dihydropteridine reductase (DHPR) (EC 1.6.99.7) (McKusick 26163) deficiency was detected by Kaufman *et al.* (1975). Because of the absence of feedback inhibition of GTP cyclohydrolase I due to the lack of BH₄, biopterin biosynthesis is activated and leads to the

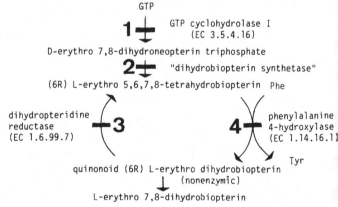

Figure 1 Possible metabolic defects in hyperphenylalaninaemia. BH₄ deficient variants: defects 1–3; classical phenylketonuria: defect 4

Journal of Inherited Metabolic Disease. ISSN 0141-8955. Copyright © SSIEM and MTP Press Limited, Queen Square, Lancaster, UK.

accumulation and excretion of the inactive 7,8-dihydrobiopterin and biopterin. The incidence is less than that of "dihydrobiopterin synthetase" deficiency and an increased frequency has been found in Sicily.

METHODS FOR DETECTION AND DIFFERENTIAL DIAGNOSIS OF BH₄ DEFICIENCY

A number of different methods are available. We use and recommend the following (Niederwieser *et al.*, 1982b): (1) Analysis of total pterins and creatinine in urine collected at elevated serum phenylalanine concentration (not on PKU diet). (2) Administration of a BH₄ load, 7.5 mg kg⁻¹ orally, and measurement of serum/plasma phenylalanine and tyrosine at zero, 4 and 8 h after the load. (3) DHPR activity should be measured in blood or dried blood spots (Guthrie cards) according to the method of Arai *et al.* (1982). In patients with BH₄ deficiency, we measure homovanillic acid and 5-hydroxyindole acetic acid in CSF by HPLC with electrochemical detection (Niederwieser *et al.*, 1984a), as well as pterins, phenylalanine, tyrosine, and tryptophan. Lumbar CSF should be taken between 10 and 12 a.m. (in newborns, discard the first 0.2 ml, collect the next 0.5–0.6 ml in an EDTA tube and freeze immediately).

For the analysis of pterins we have developed a routine method with a high degree of automation, selective for pterins and designed to detect other as yet unknown pterins which may differ widely in polarity (Niederwieser *et al.*, 1982d, 1984b). Other HPLC methods are available (Fukushima and Nixon, 1980; Lunte and Kissinger, 1983). BH₄ can be determined by differential oxidation in alkaline and acidic medium (Fukushima and Nixon, 1980) but can also be measured directly by HPLC with electrochemical detection (Niederwieser *et al.*, 1982d, 1984b; Lunte and Kissinger, 1983; Bräutigam *et al.*, 1984). Total biopterins can also be measured microbiologically in blood and urine (Leeming *et al.*, 1984).

Enzyme measurements are now possible for all three variants: GTP cyclohydrolase I in liver biopsies (Blau and Niederwieser, 1983: Niederwieser *et al.*, 1984a), DHPR in dried blood spots (Arai *et al.*, 1982) and the phosphate-eliminating enzyme (PEE) in liver biopsies from patients with "dihydrobiopterin synthetase" deficiency.

For measurement of the phosphate-eliminating enzyme activity, approx. 10 mg of liver tissue was homogenized in 100 µl of 10 mmol l⁻¹ potassium phosphate pH 6.8 and centrifuged at 12 000 g for 20 min. The supernatant was applied onto 500 µl of Sephadex G-25 in a Pasteur pipette and the brown zone eluted and collected. The volume and the protein concentration were determined; an aliquot of 150 µl was heated at 65 °C for 1 min and then centrifuged at 12 000 g for 20 min. Of the supernatant, 50 µl was incubated at 37 °C for 2 h at pH 7.4 in a total volume of 125 µl containing 24 mmol l⁻¹ Tris–HCl, 24 µmol l⁻¹ dihydroneopterin triphosphate, 8 mmol l⁻¹ magnesium chloride, 1 mmol l⁻¹ NADPH, 5 mmol l⁻¹ dithioerythritol, and approx. 1 mU of human liver sepiapterin reductase. The reaction was stopped by addition of 25 µl of 200 mmol l⁻¹ EDTA (final concentration 33 mmol l⁻¹), and the formation of BH₄ was measured immediately by HPLC with electrochemical detection (Niederwieser *et al.*, 1982, 1984b).

RESULTS AND DISCUSSION

Detection and differential diagnosis of BH₄ deficiency may often be possible directly from characteristic pattern of urinary pterins HPLC chromatograms (Niederwieser *et al.*, 1984a). In GTP cyclohydrolase deficiency only trace amounts of pterins are detected, while in "dihydrobiopterin synthetase" deficiency, the excessive concentrations of neopterin and monapterin, which is a neopterin isomer, are impressive. It should be emphasized, however, that small but significant peaks of biopterin can be detected, particularly in older children with this disease. We do not know the origin of this biopterin but it does not appear to result from a significant residual activity of biopterin biosynthesis in one of the children tested. A large peak of biopterin dominates the chromatograms from samples from patients with dihydropteridine reductase deficiency. Patients with classical PKU excrete increased amounts of pterins depending on the phenylalanine concentration in blood and tissue. On a low phenylalanine diet the excretion of pterins is nearly normal and, most important, patients with DHPR deficiency would not be diagnosed under such conditions. The differential diagnosis is straightforward when biopterin is expressed as a fraction of the sum of biopterin and neopterin (%B) and plotted versus the biopterin to creatinine ratio. The values then fall into characteristic areas for the different diseases and controls (Niederwieser *et al.*, 1980a, 1982a).

The results of our screening for BH₄ deficiency in children with hyperphenylalaninaemia is shown in Table 1. In a total of 673 cases (483 newborn, 190 older

Table 1 Results of screening children with hyperphenylalaninaemia for BH₄ deficiency caused by defects in GTP cyclohydrolase 1 (GTPCH), "dihydrobiopterin synthetase" (DHBS), or dihydropteridine reductase (DHPR)

Test used	Children investigated	Deficiencies found		
		GTPCH	*DHBS*	*DHPR*
HPLC of urinary pterins	483 newborns	0	6	0
	190 older, selected	1	30	14
	673 total	1	36	14
BH₄ test	total 440, responded:	1	36	10

selected cases) there was 1 patient with GTP cyclohydrolase I deficiency, 36 patients with "dihydro-biopterin synthetase" deficiency, and 14 patients with dihydropteridine reductase deficiency. In the 483 newborns we found six patients with BH_4 deficiency. The BH_4 loading test proposed originally by Danks *et al.* (1975) has been performed in a modified form (Niederwieser *et al.*, 1982a) in 440 children. A decrease of the serum phenylalanine after BH_4 indicates BH_4 deficiency. All of the patients with defects in biopterin biosynthesis showed a decrease; however, four of the 14 patients with dihydropteridine reductase did not respond to this test. Patients with classical PKU do not respond and in the nearly 400 cases investigated, no K_m mutant of phenylalanine-4-hydroxylase could be found.

Using this kind of screening, we did not identify a newborn with DHPR deficiency. Although there is no information that we have missed one, it is possible that this disease becomes manifest metabolically, later on. Therefore, measurement of DHPR activity in dried blood spots on Guthrie cards (Arai *et al.*, 1982) is recommended. The BH_4 test can be of advantage in the exclusion of BH_4 deficiency in children who show an abnormally high neopterin due to an infection. The increase in neopterin excretion in a number of diseases which are not related to hyperphenylalaninaemia has been reported by Wachter *et al.* (1983). Our own studies have shown that the neopterin increase is non-specific and is observed in various bacterial and viral infections (pneumonia, mumps, varicella, measles, influenza), and may become extreme in immune deficiencies, e.g. familial haemo-phagocytic lymphohistiocytosis and in severely ill patients with AIDS. A lack of decrease in serum phenylalanine in children with abnormally high neopterin will thus indicate the existence of an infection rather than a (partial) defect in biopterin biosynthesis. It should be noted here that neopterin and biopterin excretion are age-dependent (Niederwieser *et al.*, 1980a; Dhondt, 1981) and therefore, controls have to be age-matched.

Phenylalanine loading tests before and after administration of BH_4 can be used to detect a partial defect in biopterin biosynthesis. Güttler *et al.* (1984) reported a healthy 10-year-old girl with a partial deficiency of "dihydrobiopterin synthetase". With the exception of some unusual spikes in her EEG no clinical abnormality could be observed. On BH_4 treatment, her serum tyrosine concentration increased significantly after phenylalanine loading and the elevated neopterin in urine was nearly normalized. This patient shows that genetic heterogeneity, well known from PKU and other metabolic diseases, can also be observed in BH_4 deficiencies. There have been reports of patients where the defect seemed to be manifest only in the brain or only in the peripheral tissues (Hreidarsson *et al.*, 1982; Dhondt *et al.*, 1983) and transient defects have been observed (Rey *et al.*, 1980, 1983; Matalon, 1984). Direct measurement of the corresponding enzymes will be necessary to clarify such situations. Whereas measurement of dihydropteridine reductase can be performed in liver biopsies, fibroblast cultures and blood cells, measurement of GTP cyclohydrolase I activity has only

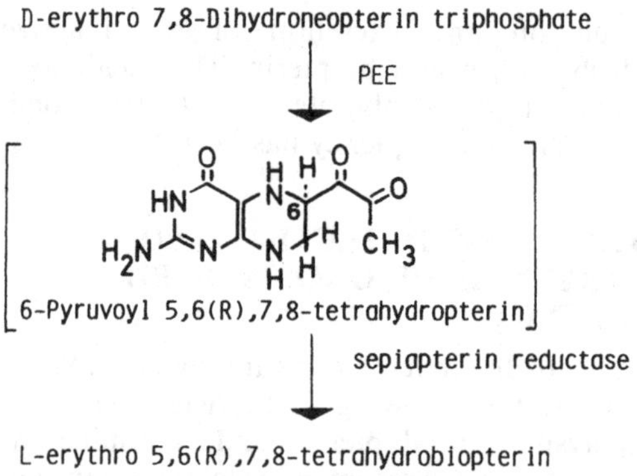

Figure 2 Postulated formation of BH_4 from D-erythro 7,8-dihydroneopterin triphosphate by "dihydrobiopterin synthetase", an enzyme system consisting of at least two enzymes: the phosphate-eliminating enzyme (PEE), which is defective in the patients, and sepiapterin reductase

recently been developed in liver biopsies (Blau and Niederwieser, 1983). Heterozygotes of GTP cyclohydrolase I defect may be recognized by measurement of the enzyme activity in stimulated mononuclear cells isolated from 20 ml of blood (Niederwieser *et al.*, 1984a; Blau *et al.*, 1985). Although the enzyme defective in "dihydro-biopterin synthetase" deficiency has not yet been characterized in detail (Curtius, 1985), we are now able to measure the corresponding PEE activity in liver biopsies. In the presence of sepiapterin reductase from human liver the hypothetical intermediate 6-pyruvoyl tetrahydropterin (Figure 2) is reduced to BH_4. No activity could be detected in the liver biopsy taken from a patient with "dihydrobiopterin synthetase" deficiency, whereas in a control sample of a child with thalassaemia, which was shipped concurrently, activity was present and four times higher than in the liver controls from adult traffic accident victims (Table 2). In trials to measure the defective biopterin biosynthesis in patients, other investigators have found activities as high as 50–60% of the controls (Yoshioka *et al.*, 1984). We assume that the "sepiapterin-synthesizing enzyme-1" activity measured via the determination of pterin formation by these investigators is only an indirect analysis.

An integral part of the diagnosis of BH_4 deficiency is the measurement of biogenic amine metabolites in CSF and it is of great importance to measure these

Table 2 Activity of phosphate-eliminating enzyme in human liver formation of BH_4 from 7,8-dihydroneopterin triphosphate in presence of human sepiapterin reductase

		nU (mg protein)$^{-1}$	%
Controls*	1	0.92	
	2	0.88	100
	3	1.22	
Child with thalassaemia age 6 years		3.99	396
Patient M.G. "dihydrobiopterin synthetase" deficiency		<0.03	<3

* Liver from traffic accident victims (adults)

metabolites before institution of the therapy. Only when baseline levels are known can the effect of therapy be followed. Because the blood–brain barrier is largely impermeable to BH_4 multicomponent therapy is necessary in most patients, consisting of L-DOPA, carbidopa, 5-hydroxytryptophan (Bartholomé and Byrd, 1975) and BH_4 instead of the low phenylalanine diet (Niederwieser *et al.*, 1979). In a few cases with "dihydrobiopterin synthetase" deficiency, monotherapy with BH_4 is possible (Leupold *et al.*, 1982; Niederwieser *et al.*, 1982a). 6-Methyltetrahydropterin (Kaufman *et al.*, 1983; McInnes *et al.*, 1984) cannot be recommended since therapeutic trials on three children have had to be interrupted because of the appearance of severe clinical symptoms (Leupold and Scheibenreiter, personal communication); in another case an increase of liver enzymes in serum in a patient given 6-methylpterin therapy was observed (Muenzer *et al.*, 1984). The institution and control of therapy is not easy and requires several weeks under careful clinical evaluation. For biochemical control we recommend measurement of the concentrations of homovanillic acid, 5-hydroxyindole acetic acid, phenylalanine, tyrosine, tryptophan and the pterins in cerebrospinal fluid (Table 3). All these measurements can be performed in 0.5–0.6 ml of CSF. In patients who can be treated with BH_4 monotherapy, homovanillic acid in CSF taken before institution of therapy was not as low as in those who required multicomponent therapy. This might indicate a different kind of defect. Neopterin concentration in CSF is extremely low in GTP cyclohydrolase I deficiency, and very high in "dihydrobiopterin synthetase" deficiency. Even on BH_4 therapy it remains elevated, indicating that dopaminergic or serotoninergic neurones are BH_4 deficient, in contrast to the peripheral tissues where neopterin concentration is nearly normalized.

In conclusion, BH_4 deficiency can be caused by three molecular defects which can be diagnosed by HPLC pterin analyses in the urine of children with hyperphenylalaninaemia. This test should be combined with the measurement of DHPR activity in dried blood spots on Guthrie cards. The two defects in biopterin biosynthesis can be proven now by measurement of enzyme activities in liver biopsies. A heterozygote test for GTP cyclohydrolase I deficiency is available but prenatal diagnosis is not yet possible.

The results could only be obtained due to extensive collaboration of many colleagues in pediatric hospitals of Europe and overseas. We thank Miss Dietlinde Gerloff, Mr W. Leimbacher, U. Redweik, and W. Staudenmann for skilful technical assistance. This work was also supported by the Swiss National Science Foundation, project No. 3.266-0.82.

References

Arai, N., Narisawa, K., Hayakawa, H. and Tada, K. Hyperphenylalaninaemia due to dihydropteridine reductase deficiency: Diagnosis by enzyme assay on dried blood spots. *Pediatrics* 98 (1982) 426–430

Bartholomé, K. A new molecular defect in phenylketonuria. *Lancet* II (1974) 1980

Bartholomé, K. and Byrd, D. J. L-Dopa and 5-hydroxytryptophan therapy in phenylketonuria with normal phenylalanine hydroxylase activity. *Lancet* II (1975) 1042

Blau, N., Joller, P., Atares, M., Cardesa-Garcia, J. and Niederwieser, A. Increase of GTP cyclohydrolase I activity in mononuclear blood cells by stimulation: Detection of heterozygotes of GTP cyclohydrolase I deficiency. *Clin. Chim. Acta* (In press) (1985)

Blau, N. and Niederwieser, A. GTP-cyclohydrolase I assay in human and rat liver using high-performance liquid chromatography of neopterin phosphates and guanine nucleotides. *Analyt. Biochem.* 128 (1983) 446–452

Bräutigam, M., Dreesen, R. and Herken, H. Tetrahydrobiopterin and total biopterin content of neuroblastoma (N1E-115, N2A) and pheochromocytoma (PC-12) clones and the dependence of catecholamine synthesis on tetrahydrobiopterin concentration in PC-12 cells. *J. Neurochem.* 42 (1984) 390–395

Table 3 Analysis of cerebrospinal fluid from patients with BH_4 deficiency for diagnosis and control of therapy

Deficiency	Patient	Age (years)	Hours after treatment	Treatment 1	2	3	4	HVA (nmol l^{-1})	5-HIAA	N (nmol l^{-1})	B	%B	Tyr (μmol l^{-1})	Phe
GTPCH	M.R.	5		—	—	—	—	37	50	1	2			
		5 11/12		5	—	—	—	48	95	1	5.2			
DHBS	M.G.	2		—	—	—	—	61	15	215	9.7	4.3	26	479
			49	20	—	—	—	137	51	187	12.5	6.3	26	35
				5	5	5	0.5	245	81	108	9.9	8.4	24	14.5
DHPR	R.A.	1		—	—	—	—	81	23	11	57	83	16	146
			8	7.5	—	—	—	104	24	24	199	89	28	49
				7.5	5	5	0.5	295	208	25	69	73	26	106
— Healthy controls		0.5–6		—	—	—	—	250–880	110–360	9–20	10–24	32–65	10–25	8–20

GTP cyclohydrolase I (GTPCH), "dihydrobiopterin synthetase" (DHBS), dihydropteridine reductase (DHPR); homovanillic acid (HVA), 5-hydroxyindole acetic acid (5-HIAA), neopterin (N), biopterin (B), %B = 100 B/(B + N), tyrosine (Tyr) and phenylalanine (Phe)

(1) BH_4, (2) DOPA, (3) 5-HTrp, (4) Carbidopa

Curtius, H.-Ch., Heintel, D., Ghisla, S., Kuster, Th., Leimbacher, W. and Niederwieser, A. Biosynthesis of tetrahydrobiopterin in man. *J. Inher. Metab. Dis.* 8 Suppl. 1 (1985) 28–33 .

Danks, D. M., Bartholomé, K., Clayton, B. E., Curtius, H.-Ch., Gröbe, H., Kaufman, S. *et al.* Malignant hyperphenylalaninaemia—Current status (June 1977). *J. Inher. Metab. Dis.* 1 (1978) 49–53

Danks, D. M., Cotton, R. G. and Schlesinger, P. Tetrahydro-biopterin treatment of variant forms of phenylketonuria. *Lancet* II (1975) 1043

Dhondt, J. L., Ardouin, P., Hayte, J.-M. and Farriaux, J.-P. Developmental aspects of pteridine metabolism and relationships with phenylalanine metabolism. *Clin. Chim. Acta* 116 (1981) 143–152.

Dhondt, J. L., Leroux, B., Farriaux, J. P., Largilliere, C. and Leeming, R. J. Dihydrobiopterin biosynthesis deficiency. *Eur. J. Pediatr.* 141 (1983) 92–95

Fukushima, T. and Nixon, J. C. Analysis of reduced forms of biopterin in biological tissues and fluids. *Analyt. Biochem.* 102 (1980) 176–188

Gál, E. M., Nelson, J. M. and Sherman, A. D. Biopterin III. Purification and characterization of enzymes involved in the cerebral synthesis of 7,8-dihydrobiopterin. *Neurochem. Res.* 3 (1978) 69–88

Güttler, F., Lou, H., Lykkelund, C. and Niederwieser, A. Combined tetrahydrobiopterin–phenylalanine loading test in the detection of partially defective biopterin biosynthesis. *Eur. J. Pediatr.* 142 (1984) 126–129

Hreidarsson, S., Valle, D., Kapatos, N. and Kaufman, S. A peripheral defect in biopterin synthesis: A new mutant? *Pediatr. Res.* 16 (1982) 192A

Kaufman, S. Biopterin and metabolic disease. In Kisliuk, R. L. and Brown, G. M. (eds.) *Chemistry and Biology of Pteridines*, Elsevier–North Holland, New York, 1979, pp. 117–124

Kaufman, S., Holtzman, N. A., Milstien, S., Butler, I. J. and Krumholz, A. Phenylketonuria due to a deficiency of dihydropteridine reductase. *N. Engl. J. Med.* 293 (1975) 785–790

Kaufman, S., Kapatos, G., Rizzo, W. B., Schulman, J. D., Tamarkin, L. and van Loon, G. R. Tetrahydropterin therapy for hyperphenylalaninaemia caused by defective synthesis of tetrahydrobiopterin. *Ann. Neurol.* 14 (1983) 308–315

Leeming, R. J., Barford, P. A., Blair, J. A. and Smith, I. Blood spots on Guthrie cards can be used for inherited tetrahydrobiopterin deficiency screening in hyperphenyl-alaninaemic infants. *Arch. Dis. Child.* 59 (1984) 58–61

Leupold, D., Wang, M. and Niederwieser, A. Tetrahydrobiopterin monotherapy in two siblings with dihydrobiopterin deficiency. In Wachter, H., Curtius, H.-Ch. and Pfleiderer, W. (eds.) *Biochemical and Clinical Aspects of Pteridines*, Vol. 1, De Gruyter, Berlin, 1982, pp. 307–317

Lunte, C. E., and Kissinger, P. T. The determination of pterins in biological samples by liquid-chromatography/electrochemistry. *Analyt. Biochem.* 129 (1983) 377–386

McInnes, R. R., Kaufman, S., Warsh, J. J., Van Loon, G. R., Milstien, S., Kapatos, G. *et al.* Biopterin synthesis defect. Treatment with L-Dopa and 5-hydroxytryptophan compared with therapy with a tetrahydropterin. *J. Clin. Invest.* 37 (1984) 458–469

Matalon, R. Current status of biopterin screening. *J. Pediatr.* 104 (1984) 579–580

Muenzer, J., Milstien, S., Sidbury, J., Berlow, S. and Kaufman, S. Treatment of phenylalaninaemia secondary to a deficiency of biopterin with reduced pterins. *Pediatr. Res.* 18 (1984) 297A

Niederwieser, A., Blau, N., Wang, M., Joller, P., Atarés, M. and

Cardesa-Garcia, J. GTP cyclohydrolase I deficiency, a new enzyme defect causing hyperphenylalaninaemia with neo-pterin, biopterin, dopamine, and serotonin deficiencies and muscular hypotonia. *Eur. J. Pediatr.* 141 (1984a) 208–214

Niederwieser, A., Curtius, H.-Ch., Bettoni, O., Bieri, J., Schircks, B., Viscontini, M. and Schaub, J. Atypical phenylketonuria caused by 7,8-dihydrobiopterin synthetase deficiency. *Lancet* I (1979) 131–133

Niederwieser, A., Curtius, H.-Ch., Gitzelmann, R., Otten, A., Baerlocher, K., Blehová, B. *et al.* Excretion of pterins in phenylketonuria and phenylketonuria variants. *Helv. Paediatr. Acta* 35 (1980a) 335–342

Niederwieser, A., Curtius, H.-Ch., Wang, M. and Leupold, D. Atypical phenylketonuria with defective biopterin meta-bolism. Monotherapy with tetrahydrobiopterin or sepia-pterin, screening and study of biosynthesis in man. *Eur. J. Pediatr.* 138 (1982a) 110–112

Niederwieser, A., Matasović, A., Curtius, H.-Ch., Endres, W. and Schaub, J. 3′-Hydroxysepiapterin in patients with dihydrobiopterin deficiency. *FEBS Lett.* 118 (1980b) 299–302

Niederwieser, A., Matasović, A., Staudenmann, W., Wang, M. and Curtius, H.-Ch. Screening for tetrahydrobiopterin deficiency. In Wachter, H., Curtius, H.-Ch. and Pfleiderer, W. (eds.) *Biochemical and Clinical Aspects of Pteridines*, Vol. 1, De Gruyter, Berlin, 1982b, pp. 293–306

Niederwieser, A., Staudenmann, W., Wang, M., Curtius, H.-Ch., Atares, M. and Cardesa-Garcia, J. Hyperphenyl-alaninaemia with neopterin deficiency. A new enzyme defect presumably of GTP cyclohydrolase. *Eur. J. Pediatr.* 138 (1982c) 97

Niederwieser, A., Staudenmann, W. and Wetzel, E. Automatic HPLC of pterins with or without column switching. In Wachter, H., Curtius, H.-Ch. and Pfleiderer, W. (eds.) *Biochemical and Clinical Aspects of Pteridines*, Vol. 1, De Gruyter, Berlin, 1982d, pp. 81–102

Niederwieser, A., Staudenmann, W. and Wetzel, E. High-performance liquid chromatography with column switching for the analysis of biogenic amine metabolites and pterins. *J. Chromatogr.* 290 (1984b) 237–246

Rey, F., Harpey, J. P. and Leeming, R. J. Les hyperphényl-alaninémies avec activité normale de la phenylalanine hydroxylase: Le déficit en tetrahydrobioptérine et la déficit en dihydropteridine reductase. *Arch. Fr. Pédiatr.* 34 (1977) 109–120

Rey, F., Leeming, R. J., Blair, J. A. and Rey, J. Biopterin defect in a normal appearing child affected by a transient phenylketonuria. *Arch. Dis. Child.* 55 (1980) 637–639

Rey, F., Saudubray, J. M., Leeming, R. J., Niederwieser, A., Curtius, H.-Ch. and Rey, J. Les déficits partiel en tétrahydrobioptérine. *Arch Fr. Pédiatr.* 40 (1983) 237–241

Smith, I. Atypical phenylketonuria accompanied by severe progressive neurological illness unresponsive to dietary treatment. *Arch. Dis. Child.* 49 (1974) 245

Smith, I., Clayton, B. E. and Wolff, O. H. New variant of phenylketonuria with progressive neurological illness unresponsive to phenylalanine restriction. *Lancet* 1 (1975) 1108

Wachter, H. *et al.* In Curtius, H.-Ch., Pfleiderer, W. and Wachter, H. (eds.) *Biochemical and Clinical Aspects of Pteridines*, Vols 2 and 3, De Gruyter, Berlin, 1983, 1984

Yoshioka, S., Masada, M., Yoshida, T., Mizokami, T., Akino, M. and Matsuo, N. Atypical phenylketonuria due to biopterin deficiency: Diagnosis by assay of an enzyme involved in the synthesis of sepiapterin from dihydro-neopterin triphosphate. *Zool. Sci.* 1 (1984) 74–81

J. Inher. Metab. Dis. 8 Suppl. 1 (1985) 39–45

Clinical Role of Pteridine Therapy in Tetrahydrobiopterin Deficiency

I. Smith, K. Hyland and B. Kendall
Departments of Child Health and Neuroradiology, Institute of Child Health, 30 Guilford Street, London WC1, UK

R. Leeming
Department of Haematology, The General Hospital, Birmingham, UK

In most patients with deficiency of tetrahydrobiopterin (BH_4) continuous administration of BH_4 or of a synthetic analogue such as 6-methyltetrahydropterin ($6\text{-}MPH_4$) lowers plasma phenylalanine concentrations to the therapeutic range. The effective dose of BH_4 varies from 1 to $2\,\text{mg}\,\text{kg}^{-1}$ daily in patients with defective biopterin synthesis, to $5\,\text{mg}\,\text{kg}^{-1}$ or more in patients with dihydropteridine reductase (DHPR) deficiency. The cost of $2\,\text{mg}\,\text{kg}^{-1}\,\text{day}^{-1}$ of BH_4 is comparable to the cost of a low phenylalanine diet.

Higher doses of pterins given orally ($20\,\text{mg}\,\text{kg}^{-1}$) raise the levels of tetrahydropterin in cerebrospinal fluid (CSF) to normal in patients with defective biopterin synthesis in whom initial concentration of biopterin species are low. In some, but not all, such patients pterin therapy also raises CSF amine metabolite concentrations and ameliorates symptoms. High dose therapy does not appear to be effective in raising CSF pterin levels in patients with DHPR deficiency who already accumulate dihydrobiopterin (BH_2) in CSF.

Central folate deficiency is an additional cause of neurological deterioration in patients with DHPR deficiency who require supplementation with folate as folinic acid. It is suggested that the accumulation of BH_2 in such patients competitively interferes with folate metabolism.

This paper discusses the role of pteridines (pterins and folates) in the clinical management of patients with inborn errors of biopterin metabolism, illustrating various points by reference to a patient (N.F.) with dihydropteridine reductase (DHPR) deficiency.

CASE REPORT

Patient N.F. was born at term weighing 3.8 kg. The perinatal period was uneventful. At 8 days of age plasma phenylalanine concentrations were moderately elevated ($540\,\mu\text{mol}\,\text{l}^{-1}$), then rose slowly to $1760\,\mu\text{mol}\,\text{l}^{-1}$ at 4 weeks when a low phenylalanine diet was introduced. Tolerance to dietary phenylalanine was noted to be higher than average. Routine testing for tetrahydrobiopterin (BH_4) deficiency (Smith *et al.*, 1982; Leeming *et al.*, 1984), using *Crithidia fasciculata* bioassay, showed persistently high values of plasma total biopterins ($21.6\,\text{ng}\,\text{ml}^{-1}$ pretreatment, $16\,\text{ng}\,\text{ml}^{-1}$ on diet, normal $1.8 \pm 1.1\,\text{ng}\,\text{ml}^{-1}$) suggesting a diagnosis of DHPR

deficiency confirmed by enzyme assay on a needle liver biopsy (Rey, unpublished results).

Minimal hypotonia and hypomobility were found on examination. EEG and CT scan were normal. Concentrations of homovanillic acid (HVA) and 5-hydroxyindoleacetic acid (5-HIAA), the major metabolites of dopamine and serotonin, respectively, were low in CSF (HVA 19.0; 5-HIAA $3.5\,\text{ng}\,\text{ml}^{-1}$) and serotonin was low in plasma ($25\,\text{ng}\,\text{ml}^{-1}$). Amine precursors consisting of L-dopa ($10\,\text{mg}\,\text{kg}^{-1}$) with carbidopa ($1\,\text{mg}\,\text{kg}^{-1}$) and 5-hydroxytryptophan ($10\,\text{mg}\,\text{kg}^{-1}$) were added to the diet at 3 months of age and adjusted to normalize CSF amine metabolite concentrations (Table 1). CSF, as well as plasma total biopterins, remained elevated. Symptoms disappeared, there were no problems in treatment, and development proceeded normally for the next 2 years. Continuous therapy with BH_4 in a dose of 50 mg daily replaced the diet from 10 months of age. Developmental quotients at 10 and 18 months were normal (86 and 84) and EEG at

Table 1 Response to therapy with amine precursors in a patient with dihydropteridine reductase (DHPR) deficiency

Age (months):	3.5	5	6	9	18	Normal values* Median (range)
CSF HVA ($\text{ng}\,\text{ml}^{-1}$)	40	51	91	102	84	104 (66–174)
5-HIAA ($\text{ng}\,\text{ml}^{-1}$)	48	31	33	38	28	90 (48–104)
TB ($\text{ng}\,\text{ml}^{-1}$)			11	9	7	3.9 (2.4–5.1)
Blood 5-HT ($\text{ng}\,\text{ml}^{-1}$)	568	522	524	372		† (100–150)

Homovanillic acid (HVA), 5-hydroxyindoleacetic acid (5-HIAA), and total biopterin (TB) in CSF and serotonin (5-HT) in whole blood
*15 children under 2 years of age with severe neurological disease but without movement disorder
†Adult range

Journal of Inherited Metabolic Disease. ISSN 0141-8955. Copyright © SSIEM and MTP Press Limited, Queen Square, Lancaster, UK.

10, 18 and 24 months and CT scan at 18 months were also normal. After the second birthday, progress slowed down and from 29 to 33 months the patient suffered a period of frank neurological deterioration due to folate deficiency.

THERAPY WITH PTERINS

Plasma phenylalanine fall in response to BH_4

Danks *et al.* (1975) first showed that intravenous (i.v.) administration of BH_4 lowered plasma phenylalanine concentrations in a patient with defective biopterin metabolism due to DHPR deficiency and the response to a standardized oral load ($7.5\,mg\,kg^{-1}$) has been widely used as a test for BH_4 deficiency (Niederwieser *et al.*, 1982). In patients with defective synthesis of biopterins there is a brisk fall in phenylalanine to normal (Niederwieser *et al.*, 1982, 1984). The positive but rather modest response in patient N.F. (Figure 1) is typical of DHPR deficiency. Patients with phenylalanine hydroxylase deficiency show no response to BH_4. Some patients with DHPR deficiency also show no fall in phenylalanine and might therefore be missed if diagnosis depended solely on this test. Intravenous loading as first proposed (Danks *et al.*, 1975), or subcutaneous injection, may be more reliable in this respect.

Continuous oral administration of BH_4 instead of a diet has been used successfully to control phenylalanine accumulation in several patients with defective biopterin synthesis (Curtius *et al.*, 1979; Niederwieser *et al.*, 1982; Enders *et al.*, 1982). One, who was treated with a combination of BH_4 ($2.5\,mg\,kg^{-1}$) and amine precursors from early infancy, was, however, mentally retarded at 2 years of age, raising the question of the safety and/or effectiveness of such therapy (Enders *et al.*, 1982). No data concerning CSF amine metabolite concentrations are available for these cases.

N.F. started therapy with BH_4 in a dose of $50\,mg\,day^{-1}$ at the age of 10 months. Amine precursor therapy was continued and the diet was stopped. Control of blood phenylalanine concentrations was as good or better than on diet (Table 2) until dosage fell (with growth) to below $3\,mg\,kg^{-1}$ at around 3 years of age. The cost of therapy was £6.5 per day compared with the cost of diet at 2 years of around £3 per day. In patients with defective biopterin synthesis the requirements of BH_4 are lower so that the relative cost of continuous therapy compares favourably with the cost of dietary treatment.

Physical health and developmental progress were good for over 1 year of BH_4 therapy in patient N.F. and

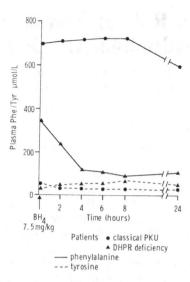

Figure 1 Response of plasma phenylalanine and tyrosine to oral administration of BH_4 ($7.5\,mg\,kg^{-1}$) in patient with DHPR deficiency and a patient with PH deficiency

no toxic effects were observed. Neurological deterioration occurred after the second birthday, although for the reasons discussed it is unlikely that this was caused by BH_4 therapy.

Entry of BH_4 into peripheral tissues

In patients with defective synthesis of biopterin total biopterin concentrations in plasma and urine (Rey *et al.*, 1977; Niederwieser *et al.*, 1982, 1984; Kaufman *et al.*, 1983) are low and rise on oral administration of BH_4. An increase in intracellular hepatic BH_4 levels in the presence of normal DHPR activity can explain the phenylalanine response. 7,8-Dihydrobiopterin (BH_2) and sepiapterin, which is converted to BH_2, are at least as effective as BH_4 in lowering plasma phenylalanine. BH_2 is converted to BH_4 *in vivo*, a step probably requiring dihydrofolate reductase (DHFR) (Hausermann *et al.*, 1981) since DHPR will only accept quinonoid-dihydrobiopterin (q-BH_2) as substrate (Kaufman, 1971).

As Kaufman (1975) has emphasized, in patients with DHPR deficiency BH_4 should be required in a roughly 1:1 molar ratio with phenylalanine intake (approximately $100\,mg\,day^{-1}$) to prevent phenylalanine accumulation. In N.F. far less BH_4 than this lowered plasma phenylalanine concentrations, suggesting that there is an alternative mechanism for reduction of q-BH_2. 5,10-Methylenetetrahydrofolate reductase (5,10-CH_2THFR) will accept q-BH_2 as substrate *in vitro*

Table 2 Phenylalanine concentrations in patient N.F. on low phenylalanine (Phe) diet and whilst receiving normal diet and BH_4

	Low Phe diet	BH_4 ($50\,mg\,day^{-1}$) normal diet		
Age (months)	1–9	10–24	25–33	34–39
Median (range) ($\mu mol\,l^{-1}$)	360 (60–720)	240 (60–720)	300 (60–600)	420 (180–600)

(Matthews and Kaufman, 1980), and might therefore serve to maintain biopterin in the tetrahydro form *in vivo*. Since patient N.F. accumulates biopterins mainly as BH_2 (unpublished observations) the combined action of DHFR and $5,10\text{-}CH_2THFR$ can perhaps explain the rather modest phenylalanine accumulation. The possible consequences for folate metabolism of these folate enzymes acting on biopterin turnover are discussed in the second half of this paper.

Entry of BH_4 into CNS

In rats BH_4, given intramuscularly at a dose of $20\,mg\,kg^{-1}$, raised levels of tetrahydropterin in brain tissue by a factor of two (Kapatos and Kaufman, 1981). In human subjects with defective biopterin synthesis comparable oral doses increased plasma total biopterins from around $1\,ng\,ml^{-1}$ to over $100\,ng\,ml^{-1}$, at the same time increasing CSF total biopterin by a factor of 20 (Kaufman *et al.*, 1983). Smaller doses of BH_4 ($5\,mg\,kg^{-1}$) raised CSF biopterin to a lesser degree in a patient with GTP cyclochydrolase deficiency (Niederwieser *et al.*, 1984), but $2.5\,mg\,l^{-1}$ was ineffective in a patient with defective conversion of dihydroneopterin triphosphate to BH_4 (Kaufman *et al.*, 1983). Subcutaneous or i.v. administration of pterins have not been explored sufficiently but are likely to be effective at much smaller doses than oral administration. 6-Methyltetrahydropterin ($6\text{-}MPH_4$), a synthetic pterin which is more lipid-soluble than BH_4 and has high cofactor activity *in vitro*, enters plasma as effectively as BH_4 and produces even higher CSF tetrahydropterin levels (Kaufman *et al.*, 1983; Kapatos and Kaufman, 1981).

Less information is available concerning the entry of BH_4 into the CNS in patients with DHPR deficiency. In patient N.F., who was given $20\,mg\,kg^{-1}$ BH_4 daily for 30 days, plasma total biopterin (*Crithidia fasciculata* assay) rose from 11 to $73\,ng\,ml^{-1}$ whereas CSF biopterin remained elevated but unchanged, at around $10\,ng\,ml^{-1}$ (Figure 2).

Effects of BH_4 on amine metabolism

One of the most important questions concerning the clinical role of administered BH_4 is whether or not it increases amine synthesis in the CNS and could therefore be used as a complete therapy for patients with BH_4 deficiency. In patients with defective biopterin synthesis doses of between 5 and $20\,mg\,kg^{-1}$ BH_4 may

improve or abolish neurological symptoms and increase concentrations of amine metabolites in urine and CSF and of amines in plasma (Niederwieser *et al.*, 1982, 1984; Kaufman *et al.*, 1983). $6\text{-}MPH_4$ appears to be equally effective. The responses are, however, variable, as well as being dose-dependent and some patients show no central response of amine metabolism or symptoms, despite good entry of pterin into CSF (McInnes *et al.*, 1984).

The amine response to BH_4 in DHPR deficiency has not been reported previously. In patient N.F. a single dose of $7.5\,mg\,kg^{-1}$ BH_4 at 3 months of age failed to raise CSF amine metabolites or increase blood serotonin (Table 3). At 10 months $20\,mg\,kg^{-1}$ daily combined with a reducing dose of amine precursors led initially to a rise in CSF HVA and, to a lesser extent, 5-HIAA and in blood serotonin (Figure 3). When amine precursors were omitted, however, hypotonia and oculogyric crisis occurred after 8 days and CSF amine metabolites fell to below normal even before symptoms appeared. Blood serotonin also fell but only from high values to the normal range. Reintroduction of amine precursors led to disappearance of symptoms within hours.

The data suggest that in DHPR deficiency BH_4 in a dose of $20\,mg\,kg^{-1}$ increases peripheral amine synthesis and, in the presence of amine precursor therapy including a decarboxylase inhibitor, also increases central amine turnover. The central effects may, however, have been mediated through increased peripheral synthesis of dopa and 5-hydroxytryptophan which, in the presence of a

Table 3 Amine response to oral administration of a single dose of BH_4 ($7.5\,mg\,kg^{-1}$)

		Baseline	6 h
CSF	HVA ($ng\,ml^{-1}$)	17	16
	5-HIAA ($ng\,ml^{-1}$)	5	5
Blood	5-HT ($ng\,ml^{-1}$)	26	24

See Figure 1 for phenylalanine response

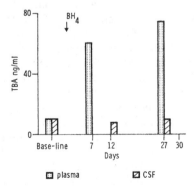

Figure 2 Plasma and CSF total biopterin (TBA) concentrations during 30-day trial of BH_4 ($20\,mg\,kg^{-1}$ orally)

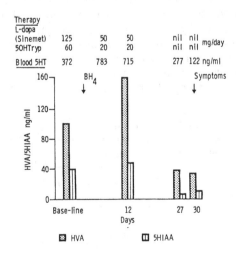

Figure 3 CSF HVA, 5-HIAA and blood serotonin (5 HT) with BH_4 administration ($20\,mg\,kg^{-1}$)

decarboxylase inhibitor, would lead to a rise in the plasma concentrations of these two compounds. Both cross the blood–brain barrier and could cause a rise in central amine synthesis. This explanation is consistent with the absence of any detectable rise in CSF biopterins and the reversal of the rise in HVA and 5-HIAA when the decarboxylase inhibitor was withdrawn. A similar peripheral effect of BH_4 on plasma concentrations of L-dopa and 5-hydroxytryptophan, combined with more effective control of plasma phenylalanine concentrations, could also explain how low doses of BH_4 (which probably do not cause a rise of cofactor levels in the CNS) in some patients with defective biopterin synthesis reduce the requirement of amine precursors and may even abolish symptoms in the absence of precursor therapy (Niederwieser *et al.*, 1982; Curtius *et al.*, 1979).

THERAPY WITH FOLATES

Clinical response to folate therapy

Tetrahydrofolate has some hydroxylase cofactor activity *in vitro* (Kaufman, 1971). In a patient with defective biopterin synthesis folic acid administration led to a fall in plasma phenylalanine, a rise in tyrosine and a rise in blood serotonin (Hase *et al.*, 1982). If confirmed, these findings suggest that folates may have cofactor activity *in vivo* as well as *in vitro*.

In patients with DHFR deficiency folates have a different and essential role in therapy. Several reports have documented low levels of total folate in serum, red cells, CSF and brain in such patients (Butler *et al.*, 1978; Pollock and Kaufman, 1978; Tada *et al.*, 1980; Harpey, 1983). Despite the low tissue levels of folate there were no haematological abnormalities, but in Harpey's (1983) patients neurological deterioration appeared to be due to the lack of folate. Folinic acid (but not folic acid) therapy produced dramatic clinical improvement.

Character of folate disturbance in DHPR deficiency

During the first year of life, whilst receiving a diet which contained 0.75 mg folic acid per day, N.F. was not deficient in folate (Table 4). By 33 months of age, coincident with neurologic deterioration, total folates were profoundly reduced. In retrospect it appeared that CSF folate was low at 29 months of age when deterioration had become evident but not in the first year of life when he was making good progress. There was no evidence of anaemia, macrocytosis, megalo-

blastic change, growth impairment or other of the usual signs of peripheral folate deficiency despite erythrocyte folate concentration of only $60 \, ng \, ml^{-1}$ (normal $>150 \, ng \, ml^{-1}$). Mean cell volumes which were examined at regular intervals throughout follow-up were normal (81–84 fl). This unusual picture is characteristically seen in patients with deficiency of $5,10\text{-}CH_2THFR$ (Niederwieser, 1979; Rowe, 1983), which causes defective synthesis of 5-methyltetrahydrofolate (5-CH_3THF) and severe neurological damage.

Neurological symptoms associated with lack of folate

Neurological deterioration in N.F. began a few months after the second birthday with slowing in the rate of development, occasional minor and later major convulsions, appearance of an intention tremor and increasingly erratic control of CSF HVA and 5-HIAA. At first symptoms were relatively minor and were attributed to inadequate amine precursor therapy since HVA and 5-HIAA in CSF were low (HVA $33 \, ng \, ml^{-1}$; 5-HIAA $11 \, ng \, ml^{-1}$ at 27 months), but as time passed it became clear that low CSF amine metabolite levels, and later symptoms attributable to amine deficiency, were not explained by inadequate precursor therapy. Despite raising CSF metabolites for a period to supranormal levels (HVA $225 \, ng \, ml^{-1}$; 5-HIAA $84 \, ng \, ml^{-1}$) symptoms progressed with hypotonia and pin-point pupils, especially in the early morning, intermittent peripheral cyanosis due to venous stasis, drooling, hyperpyrexia without infection, irritability and hypomobility, ataxia, loss of balance when stationary, deterioration of speech, abnormally brisk tendon jerks, increased limb-tone, and finally extensor plantar responses with loss of ankle jerks. The neurological picture indicated amine lack, long tract degeneration and cerebral damage and was similar to that described previously by Harpey (1983) in another patient with DHPR deficiency who was also folate-deficient. The clinical diagnosis was subacute combined degeneration of the cord, with cerebral involvement due to folate deficiency. Serum B_{12} was normal ($360 \, ng \, ml^{-1}$).

Folate therapy in DHPR deficiency

In N.F. therapy was started at 33 months with $2.5 \, mg \, day^{-1}$ of folic acid. Symptoms worsened over 10 days culminating in persistent hyperpyrexia, hypotonia and a series of grand-mal convulsions. CSF amine metabolites fell to low levels and, despite a rise in RBC and serum folate concentrations, total folate in CSF was even lower than before (Table 5). During infancy comparable amounts of folic acid were given without harm and probably prevented development of folate deficiency. Most folate normally present in plasma is 5-CH_3THF but folic acid administration leads to a rise of non-methyl derivatives (Ratanasthien *et al.*, 1977) which could compete with the natural compound for transport into the CNS (Rowe, 1983). This may explain how folic acid therapy appeared to worsen an already critical CNS folate deficiency. The response to folic acid is reminiscent of the clinical effects of folate therapy in patients with subacute combined degeneration due to B_{12} deficiency.

Table 4 Total folate (*Lactobacillus casei* assay) in red cells (RBC), serum and CSF before (3 and 9 months) and after (29 and 33 months), neurological deterioration

Age (months)	Total folate ($ng \, ml^{-1}$) 3	9	29	33	Normal values
RBC	1210	920		61	150–800
Serum	34	26		2.5	10–25
CSF	36*	25*	5.9*	4.2	15–50

*Assay on stored specimens

Table 5 Effects of folic acid administration on serum, RBC and CSF total folates and CSF amine metabolites

	Folic acid therapy (2.5 mg day^{-1} for 10 days)	
	Day 0	Day 10
Total folate (ng ml^{-1})		
RBC	61	134
Serum	2.5	13
CSF	4.2	3.3
Amine metabolites in CSF (ng ml^{-1})		
HVA	116	19.5
5-HIAA	60	11.5

At the height of the neurological problems following folic acid therapy 15 mg folinic acid was given intramuscularly. There was an immediate and dramatic clinical improvement. Folinic acid was continued orally (3 mg day^{-1}). From that time to the present (8 months follow-up) the patient had made steady progress. There has been no further hypotonia, pin-point pupils, peripheral cyanosis, drooling or hyperpyrexia. Within 3 weeks the parents were convinced that speech, gait and tremor were also improving. Four months after the start of folinic acid therapy CSF folate concentration (26 ng ml^{-1}) and amine metabolites (HVA 110 ng ml^{-1}; 5-HIAA 28 ng ml^{-1}) were normal and there have been no further difficulties with treatment. Upper motor neurone signs persist, balance is still somewhat impaired, gait is wide-based and a developmental quotient is 64. Unfortunately permanent damage to the CNS appears to have been sustained.

A CT scan showed multiple areas of low density in the cerebral white matter with calcification (indicative of necrosis) in the basal ganglia radiating out into the white matter (Figure 4). The appearances were in striking contrast to the normal scan at 18 months of age. The scan appearances are almost identical to those in the cases of Harpey (1983) and of Tada *et al.* (1980), to the appearance in children with congenital folate malabsorption (Niederwieser, 1979; Rowe, 1983) and in those with methotrexate toxicity (Kendall, personal communication).

Speculation on the mechanism and effects of folate disturbance in DHPR deficiency

It is suggested that in patients with DHPR deficiency 5,10-CH$_2$THFR maintains a minimum turnover of q-BH$_2$ and BH$_4$, thus accounting for the incomplete block in phenylalanine metabolism. Conversion of 5,10-CH$_2$THF to 5-CH$_3$THF is then competitively inhibited by a rise of intracellular q-BH$_2$ so that, as in patients with an inherited defect of 5,10-CH$_2$THFR, normal folate intake, whilst sufficient to maintain adequate levels of the folate cofactors (5,10-CH$_2$THF and 10-formylTHF) peripherally, is insufficient to sustain adequate concentrations of 5-CH$_3$THF in plasma for entry of folate into the CNS. Folic acid administration is harmful once CNS folate deficiency supervenes, due to a rise of non-methylfolate in plasma and further inhibition of 5-CH$_3$THF uptake into the CNS, whereas folinic acid, by providing increased amounts of natural substrate for 5,10-CH$_2$THFR, corrects the peripheral and central deficiency of 5-CH$_3$THF.

Pollock and Kaufman (1978) have suggested that

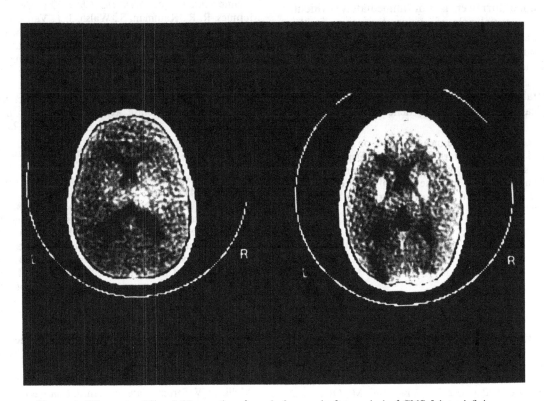

Figure 4 CT scan at 18 and 35 months of age before and after period of CNS folate deficiency

DHPR is required in the CNS to maintain folates in the tetrahydro form since DHFR activity is low in brain tissue. If this is correct then patients with DHPR deficiency would be particularly susceptible to the damaging effects of folate deficiency and, indeed, the calcification present on the CT scan suggests that necrosis had occurred. Alternatively biopterins may competitively inhibit DHFR as well as $5,10\text{-}CH_2THFR$, thus exacerbating the effects of folate deficiency in the CNS. The similarity between the scan appearances in N.F. and the appearances seen in children with methotrexate toxicity supports the latter explanation.

The association of folate deficiency with disturbance in amine metabolism has been reported previously (Harpey, 1983). In both cases symptoms of amine disturbance occurred in the face of an exogenous supply of L-dopa and 5-hydroxytryptophan indicating that the disturbance is probably due to defective control of amine release rather than impaired synthesis. Recent unpublished studies in a patient with $5,10\text{-}CH_2THFR$ deficiency who, like patient N.F., exhibited symptoms of amine deficiency as well as signs of long tract degeneration and cerebral involvement, showed profoundly reduced amine metabolites and total biopterins in CSF although plasma and urine biopterins were normal. At postmortem this patient showed the classical appearances of subacute combined degeneration (Harding, personal communication). It is logical that deficiency of $5\text{-}CH_3THF$ should lead to similar neurological damage as deficiency of B_{12} since the latter functions to transfer the methyl group from $5\text{-}CH_3THF$ to homocysteine to form methionine and tetrahydrofolate.

How folate deficiency causes severe impairment of central amine turnover is not immediately evident. Given the essential role of purine derivatives in the control of amine release, however, the requirement for folate in purine synthesis is perhaps the site of folate metabolism most likely to be involved. If these speculations are correct then disturbance of central amine metabolism is also to be expected in patients with neurological disease due to B_{12} deficiency.

The initial amine metabolite measurements on patient N.F. were carried out by Dr Mark Tricklebank, Department of Neurochemistry, Institute of Neurology, London. I.S. is in receipt of financial support from the Medical Research Council and K.H. is in receipt of a Fellowship from the McAlpine Foundation.

References

Butler, I. J., Koslow, S. H., Krumholz, A., Holtzman, N. A. and Kaufman, S. A disorder of biogenic amines in dihydropteridine reductase deficiency. *Ann. Neurol.* 3 (1978) 224–230

Curtius, H.-Ch., Niederwieser, A., Viscontini, M., Otten, A., Schaub, J., Scheibenreiter, S. and Schmidt, H. Atypical phenylketonuria due to tetrahydrobiopterin deficiency. Diagnosis and treatment with tetrahydrobiopterin, dihydrobiopterin and sepiapterin. *Clin. Chim. Acta* 93 (1979) 251–262

Danks, D. M., Cotton, R. G. H. and Schlesinger, B. Tetrahydrobiopterin treatment of variant form of phenylketonuria. *Lancet* 11 (1975) 1043 (letter)

Enders, W., Niederwieser, A., Curtius, H.-Ch., Wang, M., Ohrt, B. and Schaub, J. Atypical phenylketonuria due to biopterin deficiency. Early treatment with tetrahydrobiopterin and neurotransmitter precursors, trials of tetrahydrobiopterin monotherapy. *Helv. Paediatr. Acta* 37 (1982) 489–498

Harpey, J.-P. Les défauts de synthèse des bioptérines. Les déficits complets (réductase et synthétase). *Arch. Fr. Pédiatr. Suppl. 1* 40 (1983) 231–235

Hase, Y., Shintaku, H., Turuhara, T., Oura, T., Kobashi, M. and Iwai, K. A case of tetrahydrobiopterin deficiency due to a defective synthesis of dihydrobiopterin. *J. Inher. Metab. Dis.* 5 (1982) 81–82

Hausermann, M., Ghisla, S., Niederwieser, A. and Curtius, H.-Ch. New aspects of biopterin biosynthesis in man. *FEBS Lett.* 131 (1981) 275–278

Kapatos, G. and Kaufman, S. Peripherally administered reduced pterins do enter the brain. *Science* 212 (1981) 955–956

Kaufman, S. The phenylalanine hydroxylating system from mammalian liver. *Adv. Enzymol.* 35 (1971) 245–319

Kaufman, S. Pterin administration as a therapy for PKU due to dihydropteridine reductase deficiency. *Lancet* 2 (1975) 767 (letter)

Kaufman, S., Kapatos, G., Rizzo, W. B., Schulman, J. D., Tamarkin, L. and Van Loon, G. R. Tetrahydrobiopterin therapy of hyperphenylalaninaemia due to defective synthesis of tetrahydrobiopterin. *Ann. Neurol.* 14 (1983) 308–315

Leeming, R. J., Barford, P. A., Blair, J. A. and Smith, I. Blood spots on Guthrie cards can be used for inherited tetrahydrobiopterin deficiency screening in hyperphenylalaninaemic infants. *Arch. Dis. Child.* 59 (1984) 58–61

McInnes, R. R., Kaufman, S., Walsh, J. J., Van Loon, G. R., Milstien, S., Kapatos, G., Soldin, S., Walsh, P., MacGregor, D. and Hanley, W. H. Biopterin synthesis defect. Treatment with L-dopa and 5-hydroxytryptophan compared with therapy with tetrahydropterin. *J. Clin. Invest.* 73 (1984) 458–469

Matthews, R. G. and Kaufman, S. Characterization of dihydropterin reductase activity of pig liver methylene tetrahydrofolate reductase. *J. Biol. Chem.* 255 (1980) 6014–6017

Niederwieser, A. Inborn errors of pterin metabolism. In Botez, M. I. and Reynolds, E. H. (eds.) *Folic Acid in Neurology, Psychiatry and Internal Medicine*, Raven Press, New York, 1979, pp. 349–384

Niederwieser, A., Blau, N., Wang, M., Joller, P., Atarés, M. and Cardesa-Garcia, J. GTP cyclohydrase deficiency; a new enzyme defect causing hyperphenylalaninaemia with neopterin, biopterin, dopamine and serotonin deficiencies and muscular hypotonia. *Eur. J. Pediatr.* 141 (1984) 208–214

Niederwieser, A., Curtius, H.-Ch., Wang, M. and Leupold, D. Atypical phenylketonuria with defective biopterin metabolism. Monotherapy with tetrahydrobiopterin or sepiapterin. Screening and a study of biosynthesis in man. *Eur. J. Pediatr.* 138 (1982) 110–112

Pollock, R. J. and Kaufman, S. Dihydropteridine reductase may function in tetrahydrofolate metabolism. *J. Neurochem.* 31 (1978) 115–123

Ratanasthien, K., Blair, J. A., Leeming, R. J., Cooke, W. T. and Melikian, V. Serum folates in man. *J. Clin. Pathol.* 30 (1977) 438–448

Rey, F., Harpey, J.-P., Leeming, R. J., Blair, J. A., Aicardi, J. and Rey, J. Les hyperphénylalaninémies avec activité normal de la phénylalanine hydroxylase: Le déficit en tetrahydro-biopterine et le déficit en dihydropteridine reductase. *Arch. Fr. Pédiatr.* 34 (1977) 109–120

Rowe, P. B. Inherited disorders of folate metabolism. In Stanbury, J. B., Wyngaarden, J. B., Fredrickson, D. S., Goldstein, J. and Brown, M. S. (eds.) *The Metabolic Basis of Inherited Disease*, McGraw-Hill, New York, 1983

Smith, I., Leeming, R. J. and Wolff, O. H. Screening for tetrahydrobiopterin deficiency among newborns with phenylketonuria. *Arch. Dis. Child.* 57 (1982) 799 (Abstr.)

Tada, K., Narisawa, K., Arai, N., Ogesawa, Y. and Ishizawa, S. A sibling case of hyperphenylalaninaemia due to deficiency of dihydropteridine reductase. Biochemical and pathological findings. *Tohoku J. Exp. Med.* 132 (1980) 123–131

J. Inher. Metab. Dis. 8 Suppl. 1 (1985) 46–52

Enzyme Studies in Biotin-responsive Disorders

K. Bartlett, H. K. Ghneim, H.-J. Stirk and H. Wastell

Departments of Child Health and Clinical Biochemistry, Medical School, University of Newcastle-upon-Tyne, Newcastle-upon-Tyne NE2 4HH, UK

There appear to be at least two underlying aetiologies for combined carboxylase deficiency; firstly, a failure of biotinylation of apocarboxylases due to a mutation of holocarboxylase synthetase (EC 6.3.4.10) which results in an enzyme with a high K_m with respect to biotin and secondly, a failure of biotinylation due to a lowered availability of biotin due to biotinidase deficiency (EC 3.5.1.12). In both these disorders secondary defects of all four biotin-dependent carboxylases result which in turn causes the excretion of the metabolites characteristic of the isolated carboxylase deficiencies. In addition, both disorders respond biochemically and clinically to the administration of large amounts of biotin.

There are four biotin-dependent carboxylases in mammalian tissues, their place in intermediary metabolism is shown in Figure 1. Pyruvate carboxylase (EC 6.4.1.1) and acetyl-CoA carboxylase (EC 6.4.1.2) are key regulatory enzymes. Propionyl-CoA carboxylase (EC 6.4.1.3) is involved in the oxidation of a number of substrates including valine, isoleucine and methionine, and 3-methylcrotonyl-CoA carboxylase (EC 6.4.1.4) is part of the degradative pathway of leucine. Each enzyme is an ATP-dependent CO_2 fixation reaction and biotin functions as a CO_2 carrier on the surface of the enzyme. All bar acetyl-CoA carboxylase are located in the mitochondrial subcellular compartment.

Biotin is covalently linked to the apocarboxylases via the epsilon amino group of a lysine residue (Moss and Lane, 1971) and the biotinylated site is highly conserved with respect to species and enzyme (Maloy *et al.*, 1978). Biotinylation of apocarboxylases involves the intermediacy of biotinyl adenylate followed by the transfer of biotin to the apocarboxylase to yield holocarboxylase (Siegel *et al.*, 1965a). These steps are catalysed by a single enzyme—holocarboxylase synthetase, although the enzyme has never been purified to homogeneity.

Figure 2 shows a general scheme for the metabolism of a vitamin. However, knowledge of the gut uptake, possible processing within the enterocyte, plasma transport and cellular uptake of biotin is scarce. The degradation of biotin-dependent enzymes results in the formation of biocytin, that is the lysyl derivative of biotin, rather than free biotin (Thoma and Petersen, 1954). The free vitamin can then be regenerated by the action of biotinidase (Wright *et al.*, 1954). The degree to which biotin is recycled and contributes to the overall requirement is uncertain.

Isolated defects of the three mitochondrial carboxylases have been documented. Propionyl-CoA carboxylase deficiency (McCusick 23200) is characterised by the excretion of propionic acid, 3-hydroxypropionate, methylcitrate, tiglylglycine and a number of other compounds characteristic of ketosis (Duran *et al.*, 1978). Eldjarn *et al.* (1970) were the first to describe a condition characterised by the excretion of 3-hydroxyisovalerate, 3-methylcrotonate and 3-methylcrotonylglycine and presumed a deficiency of 3-methylcrotonyl-CoA carboxylase. Some of the cases originally designated 3-methylcrontonyl-CoA carboxylase deficiency were

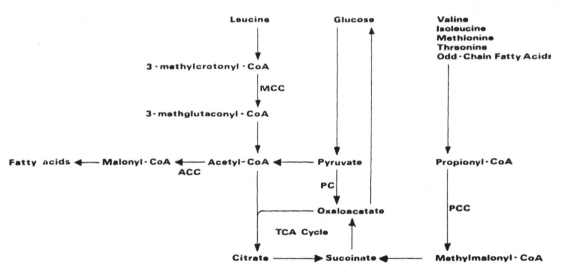

Figure 1 The role of biotin-dependent enzymes in intermediary metabolism. MCC, 3-methylcrontonyl-CoA carboxylase deficiency; PCC, propionyl-CoA carboxylase; PC, pyruvate carboxylase; AC, acetyl-CoA carboxylase

Journal of Inherited Metabolic Disease. ISSN 0141-8955. Copyright © SSIEM and MTP Press Limited, Queen Square, Lancaster, UK.

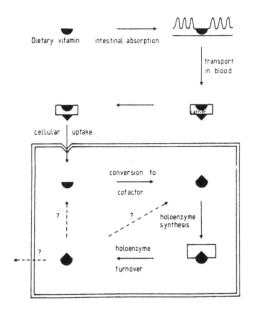

Figure 2 A general scheme for the metabolism of a vitamin

probably combined defects of all carboxylases (see below). However, proven isolated 3-methylcrotonyl-CoA carboxylase deficiency has been documented (Beemer *et al.*, 1982; Bartlett *et al.*, 1984a; McKusick 21020). Pyruvate carboxylase deficiency was first reported by Hommes *et al.* and is characterised by lacticacidaemia, pyruvicacidaemia and hyperketonaemia (Hommes *et al.*, 1968; McKusick 26615).

In addition to the isolated defects there are also a heterogeneous group of disorders which have two major characteristics in common; firstly, a range of abnormal metabolites are excreted which include those characteristic of deficiencies of all three mitochondrial carboxylases, and secondly, there is a marked and dramatic clinical and biochemical response to large doses of biotin (about 1000-fold the normal daily intake). It is with this group of multiple or combined carboxylase deficiencies that this review is concerned.

A clear and dramatic clinical and biochemical response to biotin was first reported by Gompertz *et al.* (1971) in an infant with protein intolerance, severe acidosis and who excreted large amounts of 3-methylcrotonylglycine, characteristic of 3-methylcrotonyl-CoA carboxylase deficiency, and tiglylglycine, characteristic of propionyl-CoA carboxylase deficiency (Duran *et al.*, 1978). The administration of biotin resulted in the correction of the acid–base disturbance, the abnormal metabolites disappeared and dietary protein could be reintroduced. A combined defect of propionyl-CoA carboxylase and 3-methylcrotonyl-CoA carboxylase was demonstrated in cultured cells (Bartlett and Gompertz, 1976; Weyler *et al.*, 1977) which was reversed by culture in the presence of high concentrations of biotin (Figure 3(A)). This response was shown to be independent of *de novo* protein synthesis and suggested that the underlying defect was of holocarboxylase synthetase or cellular biotin transport (Bartlett and Gompertz, 1978).

Following these early studies of combined defect of all

three mitochondrial carboxylases was shown in a patient who presented at 14 months with an episode of ketosis and acidosis (Bartlett *et al.*, 1980b). The major abnormal urinary metabolites were characteristic of 3-methylcrotonyl-CoA carboxylase deficiency, with smaller amounts of 3-hydroxypropionate and methylcitrate characteristic of propionyl-CoA carboxylase deficiency. Treatment with biotin resulted in complete normalisation of urinary organic acids and there have been no further episodes of ketoacidosis since treatment commenced. There was deficiency of all three mitochondrial carboxylases in fibroblasts cultured in minimum essential medium but normalisation of activity in cells grown in the presence of high concentrations of biotin (Figure 3(B)). Acetyl-CoA carboxylase and citrate synthase remained constant. Acetyl-CoA carboxylase deficiency has been reported in cultured cells from a similar patient (Feldman and Wolf, 1981), although we were not able to demonstrate this presumably because the biotin concentration was not low enough.

A third, previously unpublished patient who presented at 7 months of age but with the same abnormal urinary metabolites, also responded well to biotin and cultured cells again demonstrated an *in vitro* response (Figure 3(C)).

HOLOCARBOXYLASE SYNTHETASE DEFICIENCY

One explanation for these findings and other similar patients reported in the literature (Roth *et al.*, 1976; Lehnert *et al.*, 1980; Packman *et al.*, 1981a; Munnich *et al.*, 1981b; Saunders *et al.*, 1982), is a failure of biotinylation of apocarboxylases, that is a deficiency of the holocarboxylase synthetase. Since large amounts of biotin, both *in vitro* and *in vivo*, reversed the deficiencies we presumed this to be a K_m defect and devised an assay of holocarboxylase synthetase using cultured cells. The method is in three stages and is summarised in Table 1. In stage 1 fibroblast or fibroblast mitochondrial homogenate from cells which had been passaged three times in biotin-depleted medium (Ghneim *et al.*, 1981), was incubated with biotin, ATP and buffer. In stages 2 and 3 the resultant holopropionyl-CoA carboxylase was measured by the $^{14}CO_2$ fixation method. We thus utilised the endogenous apopropionyl-CoA carboxylase to assay holocarboxylase synthetase. We were unable to use either apopyruvate carboxylase or apo-3-methylcrotonyl-CoA carboxylase because biotin-deficiency appeared to switch off the synthesis of these apocarboxylases (Bartlett *et al.*, 1985).

The assay was linear with respect to protein and to time to about 3 h. The K_m with respect to ATP was $3–5 \mu mol \, l^{-1}$, in good agreement with the literature (Siegel *et al.*, 1965b). The K_m with respect to biotin was $0.2 \mu mol \, l^{-1}$ which is 10–40-fold higher than reported in the literature (Siegel *et al.*, 1965b). Presumably this is a second substrate effect since previous studies have utilised large amounts of exogenous apocarboxylase. However, it could be argued that Michaelis–Menten kinetics should not be used in this system since one of the

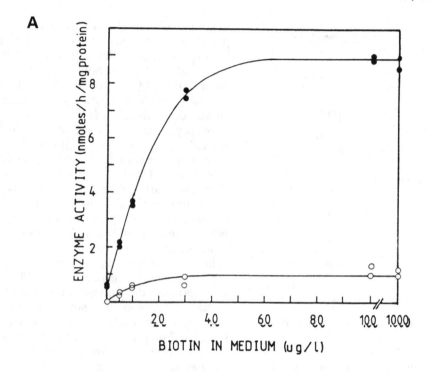

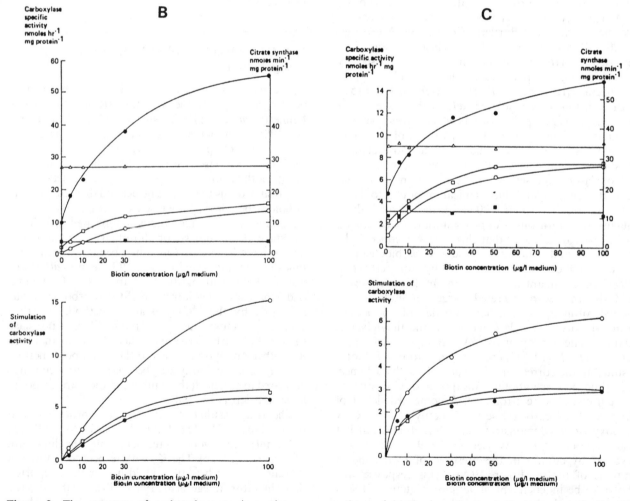

Figure 3 The response of carboxylases to increasing concentrations of biotin in cultures derived from patients with holocarboxylase synthetase deficiency. (A) Patient 1 (Gompertz *et al.*, 1971); (B) patient 2 (Bartlett *et al.*, 1980); (C) patient 3 (unpublished). ●, propionyl-CoA carboxylase; ○, 3-methylcrotonyl-CoA carboxylase; ■, pyruvate carboxylase; □, acetyl-CoA carboxylase; △, citrate synthase

Table 1 Assay of holocarboxylase synthetase

Biotin-deficient fibroblasts or mitochondria prepared from them by differential centrifugation were sonicated in 0.2–1.0 ml 50 mmol l^{-1} potassium phosphate (pH = 7.0) containing 0.1 % bovine serum albumin.

FIRST STAGE—biotinylation of apoenzyme

Potassium phosphate	100 mmol l^{-1} (pH = 6.5)
Potassium chloride	140 mmol l^{-1}
Magnesium chloride	6.3 mmol l^{-1}
Dithiothreitol	0.5 mmol l^{-1}
Biotin	0.06–25 µmol l^{-1} (normal enzyme)
	10–500 µmol l^{-1} (mutant enzyme)
ATP	20 µmol l^{-1}
Apopropionyl-CoA carboxylase (cell or mitochondrial homogenate)	
Total volume	400 µl

Incubate at 37 °C for 1.5 h

SECOND STAGE—assay of generated holopropionyl-CoA carboxylase

Tris (pH = 8.6) to give final pH = 7.7	
Propionyl-CoA	0.75 mmol l^{-1}
ATP	3 mmol l^{-1}
NaH^{14}CO$_3$	40 µCi (1.9×10^4 dpm nmol^{-1})
Final volume	800 µl

Incubate at 30 °C for 0.5 h

THIRD STAGE—determination of fixed ^{14}CO$_2$

Addition of 50 µl perchloric acid (5 mol l^{-1}) was followed by centrifugation. Aliquots (100 µl) were applied to filter paper, dried overnight to allow unfixed ^{14}CO$_2$ to exchange, and radioactivity determined by the external standard channels ratio method.

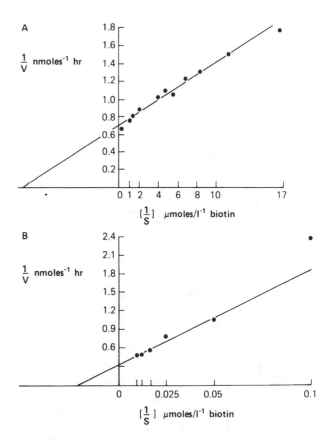

Figure 4 Kinetic properties of fibroblast mitochondrial holocarboxylase synthetase from (A) control, (B) patient 2 (Bartlett *et al.*, 1980)

assumptions in the derivation of the rate equations is that the substrate (apocarboxylase) should be present at concentrations much greater than the enzyme (holocarboxylase synthetase) (Dixon *et al.*, 1979).

The same procedure, that is utilising mitochondrial homogenates from biotin-deficient fibroblasts, was carried out on cells from patient 2 with combined carboxylase deficiency. The K_m with respect to ATP was normal (5.3 µmol l^{-1}). Whereas the K_m with respect to biotin was grossly elevated (54 nmol l^{-1}), that is about 500 times higher than controls (Figure 4, Ghneim and Bartlett, 1982). The same conclusion was reached by Burri and coworkers who measured holocarboxylase synthetase by measuring the biotinylation of exogenous apopropionyl-CoA carboxylase (Burri *et al.*, 1981).

Holocarboxylase synthetase has also been measured by following the activation of biotin to biotinyl-AMP (Zamboni *et al.*, 1982). These workers were unable to detect deficiency in any of their patients with combined carboxylase deficiency. Some of their patients have subsequently been shown to have biotinidase deficiency (see below) and it is not surprising that these patients had normal activity. They suggest that it is the second step of the overall biotinylation reaction which is defective: i.e. biotinyl-AMP + apocarboxylase → holocarboxylase.

BIOTINIDASE DEFICIENCY

The clinical, biochemical and genetic heterogeneity of patients with combined carboxylase deficiency has been noted by a number of groups (Sweetman, 1981; Packman *et al.*, 1981b; Saunders *et al.*, 1979). We have investigated a number of children who presented with the same general picture of abnormal urinary organic acids and a variety of other clinical features usually including alopecia and skin rash, all of which were corrected by the administration of large doses of biotin. In all these patients the plasma biotin concentrations were normal or low–normal, as measured by our avidin competitive-binding assay. The activities of the four biotin-dependent carboxylases in leukocytes are shown in Table 2 in a typical example. All four enzymes return to normal with biotin treatment, in fact supranormal activities were observed with prolonged biotin treatment, an effect which we and others have observed in normal subjects (Hsai *et al.*, 1977; Bartlett *et al.*, 1980a; Stirk *et al.*, 1983).

However, no matter what the biotin concentration of the culture medium, we were unable to demonstrate any deficiency in cultured cells (Bartlett *et al.*, 1984b). Cells were made biotin-deficient and then subcultured in media of increasing biotin concentration; the profiles of reactivation were identical to those obtained with normal cells. Thus, although combined carboxylase deficiency could be demonstrated in leukocytes prior to

Table 2   Specific activities of carboxylases and citrate synthase in leukocytes and plasma biotin concentrations from case 4 before and after biotin administration (10 mg daily)

Enzyme	Prebiotin	Postbiotin		Normal range
Propionyl-CoA carboxylase*	0.4	1.70	6.20	1.64–4.69
3-Methylcrotonyl-CoA carboxylase*	0.004	0.90	4.50	0.18–1.76
Pyruvate carboxylase*	0	0.20	0.62	0.11–0.53
Acetyl-CoA carboxylase*	0	0.04	0.33	0.08–0.26
Citrate synthase†	7.3	5.9	10.4	5.48–17.25
Plasma biotin‡	0.3	113		0.25–1.14
Date	1.4.80	2.7.80	4.5.81	

* nmol h^{-1} mg protein^{-1}
† nmol min^{-1} mg protein^{-1}
‡ nmol l^{-1}

biotin therapy, no such deficiency could be shown in cultured cells. These studies also excluded a defect in biotin cellular or mitochondrial transport. This paradox has been resolved by the studies of Wolf and colleagues, who were the first to demonstrate biotinidase deficiency in these patients (Wolf *et al.*, 1983a,c, 1984, 1985). Biotinidase catalyses the hydrolysis of biotinyllysine (biocytin) derived from the turnover of biotin-dependent enzymes. One might expect that such individuals would become biotin-deficient. Indeed the characteristic alopecia and skin rash of dietary biotin deficiency are features of biotinidase deficiency. However, the plasma biotin concentrations reported were either normal or only just below the normal range (Packman *et al.*, 1981b; Munnich *et al.*, 1981a; Thoene *et al.*, 1981; Table 2, present study). This seeming paradox is a consequence of the methods used to measure biotin. Most biotin assays are based on the essentially irreversible binding of biotin by avidin (Horsborough and Gompertz, 1978; Yankovsky *et al.*, 1981), or on bioassay using biotin auxotrophs (Baker *et al.*, 1962). However, these methods do not distinguish biotin and biocytin and it is therefore not surprising that biotin deficiency could not be convincingly demonstrated in patients with biotinidase deficiency. This problem and the related observation of impaired renal reabsorption of biotin in these patients has been studied by Baumgartner *et al.* (1982, 1984, 1985). This group has demonstrated that there is a renal loss of biotin and biocytin which were distinguished by chromatography and specific bioassay. The plasma concentrations of biotin in biotinidase-deficient patients are low when measured by these methods (Bonjour *et al.*, 1984; Baumgartner *et al.*, 1985).

Impaired intestinal absorption of biotin has been claimed by two groups (Munnich *et al.*, 1981a; Thoene *et al.*, 1983). These were studies in which the biotin concentrations in plasma were measured following small incremental oral doses of the vitamin prior to full biotin therapy. However, it has been suggested that the effects observed were due to tissue depletion of the vitamin rather than in inherited defect of intestinal transport (Thoene and Wolf, 1983).

We measured biotinidase activity in the plasma and cultured cells from patient 4 (Table 2) and demonstrated a complete deficiency. This child was thus functionally

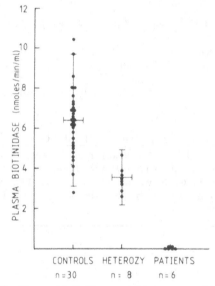

Figure 5   Plasma biotinidase activities measured fluorimetrically (Wastell *et al.*, 1984) in controls, patients and heterozygotes

biotin-deficient due to an inability to either recycle endogenous biotin from the turnover of biotin-dependent enzymes or to utilise dietary protein-bound biotin. We have now detected a total of seven patients with biotinidase deficiency (Figure 5). The late presentation of some of these children (Sweetman, 1981; Wolf *et al.*, 1983b), which is presumably due to the slow development of biotin deficiency following birth, since there is a transplacental gradient in favour of the fetus with respect to biotin, is not necessarily a good discriminant between biotinidase deficiency and holocarboxylase synthetase deficiency. Patients 2 and 3, with proven holocarboxylase synthetase deficiency, presented at 7 and 18 months of age, respectively.

Biocytin is the presumed natural substrate of biotinidase (Wright *et al.*, 1954), although other biotinyl peptides are also substrates (Craft *et al.*, 1985) and it is probable that biotinidase deficiency results in the excretion of such compounds in addition to biocytin. The enzyme is generally measured by a colourimetric end-point assay using biotinyl-4-aminobenzoate (Figure 6) as a model substrate (Knappe *et al.*, 1963). We have devised a simple fluorimetric rate assay which

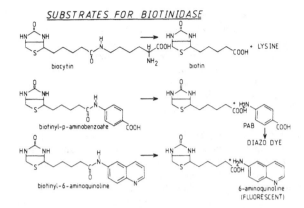

SUBSTRATES FOR BIOTINIDASE

Figure 6 Natural and synthetic substrates for biotinidase

utilises biotinyl-6-aminoquinoline (Figure 6; Wastell *et al.*, 1984). This assay is of sufficient sensitivity to measure biotinidase activity in fibroblasts, leukocytes, and subcellular fractions (unpublished observations).

References

Baker, H., Frank, O., Matovitch, V., Pasher, I., Aaronson, S., Hunter, S. and Sabotka, H. A new assay method for biotin in blood, serum, urine and tissue. *Analyt. Biochem.* 3 (1962) 31–39

Bartlett, K., Bennett, M. J., Hill, R. P., Lashford, L. S., Pollitt, R. J. and Worth, H. G. J. Isolated biotin-resistant 3-methylcrotonyl-CoA carboxylase deficiency presenting with life-threatening hypoglycaemia. *J. Inher. Metab. Dis.* 7 (1984a) 184

Bartlett, K., Ghneim, H. K., Stirk, J.-H., Dale, G. and Alberti, K. G. M. M. Pyruvate carboxylase deficiency. *J. Inher. Metab. Dis.* 7, Suppl. 1 (1984b) 74–78

Bartlett, K., Ghneim, H. K., Stirk, J.-H., Wastell, H. J., Sherratt, H. S. A. and Leonard, J. V. Enzyme studies in combined carboxylase deficiency. *Proc. Natl. Acad. Sci. USA* (In press) (1985)

Bartlett, K. and Gompertz, D. Combined carboxylase defects: biotin-responsiveness in cultured fibroblasts. *Lancet* 2 (1976) 803

Bartlett, K. and Gompertz, D. Biotin activation of carboxylase activity in cultured cells from a child with a combined carboxylase defect. *Clin. Chim. Acta* 84 (1978) 399–401

Bartlett, K., Horsborough, T. and Gompertz, D. The relationship between plasma biotin concentration and circulating leucocyte 3-methylcrotonyl-CoA carboxylase and propionyl-CoA carboxylase. *Clin. Sci.* 58 (1980a) 111–114

Bartlett, K., Ng, H. and Leonard, J. V. A combined defect of three mitochondrial carboxylases presenting as biotin responsive 3-methylcrotonylglycinuria and 3-hydroxy-isovaleric aciduria. *Clin. Chim. Acta* 100 (1980b) 183–186

Baumgartner, E. R., Suomala, T. and Wick, H. Biotin-responsive multiple carboxylase deficiency (MCD): deficient biotinidase activity associated with renal loss of biotin. *J. Inher. Metab. Dis.* 7, Suppl. 2 (1984) 501–503

Baumgartner, E. R., Suomala, T. and Wick, H. Biotinidase deficiency: factors responsible for the increased biotin requirement. *J. Inher. Metab. Dis.* 8 (1985) 00–00

Baumgartner, E. R., Suomala, T., Wick, H., Geisert, J. and Lehnert, W. Infantile multiple carboxylase deficiency: evidence for normal intestinal absorption but renal loss of biotin. *Helv. Paediatr. Acta* 37 (1982) 499–502

Beemer, F. A., Bartlett, K., Duran, M., Ghneim, H. K., Wadman, S. K., Bruinvis, L. and Ketting, D. Isolated biotin-resistant 3-methylcrotonyl-CoA carboxylase deficiency in two sibs. *Eur. J. Pediatr.* 138 (1982) 351–354

Bonjour, J. P., Bausch, J., Suomala, T. and Baumgartner, E. R. Detection of biocytin in urine of children with congenital biotinidase deficiency. *Int. J. Vit. Nutr. Res.* 54 (1984) 223–231

Burri, B. J., Sweetman, L. and Nyhan, W. L. Mutant holocarboxylase synthetase: evidence for the enzyme defect in early infantile biotin-responsive multiple carboxylase deficiency. *J. Clin. Invest.* 68 (1981) 1491–1495

Craft, D. V., Goss, N. H., Chandramouli, N. and Wood, H. G. Purification of biotinidase from human serum and its activity on biotinyl peptides. *Proc. Natl. Acad. Sci. USA* (In press) (1985)

Dixon, M., Webb, E. C., Thorne, C. J. R. and Tipton, K. F. *Enzymes*, Longman, London, 1979

Duran, M., Gompertz, D., Bruinvis, L., Ketting, D. and Wadman, S. K. The variability of metabolite excretion in propionic acidaemia. *Clin. Chim. Acta* 82 (1978) 93–99

Eldjarn, L., Jellum, E., Stokke, O., Pande, H. and Waaler, P. E. 3-Hydroxyisovaleric aciduria and 3-methylcrotonyl-glycinuria. A new inborn error of metabolism. *Lancet* 2 (1970) 521–522

Feldman, G. L. and Wolf, B. Deficient acetyl-CoA carboxylase activity in multiple carboxylase deficiency. *Clin. Chim. Acta* 111 (1981) 147–151

Ghneim, H. K. and Bartlett, K. Mechanism of biotin-responsive combined carboxylase deficiency. *Lancet* 1 (1982) 1187–1188

Ghneim, H. K., Noy, G. and Bartlett, K. Biotin-dependent carboxylases and cultured human fibroblasts. *Biochem. Soc. Trans.* 9 (1981) 405–406

Gompertz, D., Draffan, G. H., Watts, J. L. and Hull, D. Biotin-responsive 3-methylcrotonylglycinuria. *Lancet* 2 (1971) 22–24

Hommes, F. A., Polman, H. A. and Reerink, J. D. Leigh's encephalopathy: an inborn error of gluconeogenesis. *Arch. Dis. Child.* 43 (1968) 423–426

Horsborough, T. and Gompertz, D. A protein binding assay for measurement of biotin in physiological fluids. *Clin. Chim. Acta* 82 (1978) 215–223

Hsai, Y. E., Rosenberg, L. E. and Wolf, B. Stimulation of propionyl-CoA carboxylase and 3-methylcrotonyl-CoA carboxylase activity following high dose biotin administration in man. *Am. J. Hum. Genet.* 29 (1977) 116A

Knappe, J., Brunner, W. and Biederbick, K. Reinigung und Eigenschaften der biotinidase aus Schweinenieren und lactobacillus casei. *Biochem. Z.* 338 (1963) 599–613

Lehnert, W., Niederhoff, H. and Saule, H. Convulsions in an infant with biotin-dependent 3-methylcrotonylglycinuria. *Monatsschr. Kinderheilkd.* 128 (1980) 380–381

Maloy, W. L., Bowier, B. U., Zwolinski, G. K., Kumar, K. G., Wood, H. G., Ericsson, L. H. and Walsh, K. A. Amino acid sequence of the biotinyl subunit from transcarboxylase. *J. Biol. Chem.* 254 (1979) 11612–11622

Moss, J. and Lane, M. D. The biotin-dependent enzymes. *Adv. Enzymol.* 35 (1971) 321–441

Munnich, A., Saudubray, J. M., Carré, G., Goode, F. X., Ogier, H., Charpentier, C. and Frézal, J. Defective biotin absorption in multiple carboxylase deficiency. *Lancet* 2 (1981a) 263

Munnich, A., Saudubray, J. M., Cotisson, A., Coudé, F.-X.,

Ogier, H., Charpentier, C., Marsac, C., Carré, G., Bourgeay-Causse, M. and Frézal, J. Biotin-dependent multiple carboxylase deficiency presenting as congenital lactic acidosis. *Eur. J. Pediatr.* 137 (1981b) 203–206

Packman, S., Sweetman, L., Baker, H. and Wall, S. The neonatal form of biotin-responsive multiple carboxylase deficiency. *J. Pediatr.* 99 (1981a) 418–420

Packman, S., Sweetman, L., Yoshino, M., Baker, H. and Cowan, M. Biotin-responsive carboxylase deficiency of infantile onset. *J. Pediatr.* 99 (1981b) 421–423

Roth, K., Yandrasitz, J., Preti, G., Dodd, P. and Segal, S. Beta-methylcrotonic aciduria associated with lactic acidosis. *J. Pediatr.* 88 (1976) 229–235

Saunders, M. E., Sherwood, W. G., Duthie, M. and Gravel, R. A. Evidence for a defect of holocarboxylase synthetase activity in cultured lymphocytes from a patient with biotin-responsive multiple carboxylase. *Am. J. Hum. Genet.* 34 (1982) 590–601

Saunders, M., Sweetman, L., Robinson, B., Roth, K., Cohn, R. and Gravel, R. A. Biotin-responsive organicaciduria. Multiple carboxylase defects and complementation studies with propionicacidemia in cultured fibroblasts. *J. Clin. Invest.* 64 (1979) 1695–1702

Siegel, L., Foote, J. L., Christener, J. E. and Coon, M. J. Propionyl-CoA holocarboxylase synthesis from biotinyl adenylate and the apocarboxylase in the presence of an activating enzyme. *Biochem. Biophys. Res. Commun.* 13 (1965a) 307–312

Siegel, L., Foote, J. L. and Coon, M. J. The enzymatic synthesis of propionyl-CoA carboxylase from *d*-biotinyl-5′-adenylate and the apocarboxylase. *J. Biol. Chem.* 240 (1965b) 1025–1031

Stirk, J.-H., Alberti, K. G. M. M. and Bartlett, K. The effects of large doses of biotin on leucocyte carboxylases in humans. *Biochem. Soc. Trans.* 11 (1983) 185–186

Sweetman, L. Two forms of biotin-responsive multiple carboxylase deficiency. *J. Inher. Metab. Dis.* 4 (1981) 43–54

Thoene, J., Baker, H., Yoshino, M. and Sweetman, L. Biotin-responsive carboxylase deficiency associated with sub-normal plasma and urinary biotin. *N. Engl. J. Med.* 304 (1981) 817–820

Thoene, J. G., Lemons, R. M. and Baker, H. Impaired intestinal absorption of biotin in juvenile multiple carboxylase deficiency. *N. Engl. J. Med.* 308 (1983) 639–642

Thoene, J. G. and Wolf, B. Biotinidase deficiency in juvenile multiple carboxylase deficiency. *Lancet* 2 (1983) 398

Thoma, R. W. and Petersen, W. H. The enzymatic degradation of soluble bound biotin. *J. Biol. Chem.* 210 (1954) 569–579

Wastell, H., Dale, G. and Bartlett, K. A sensitive fluorimetric assay for biotinidase using a new derivative of biotin, biotinyl-6-aminoquinoline. *Analyt. Biochem.* 140 (1984) 69–73

Weyler, W., Sweetman, L., Maggio, D. C. and Nyhan, W. L. Deficiency of propionyl-CoA carboxylase and 3-methyl-crotonyl-CoA carboxylase in a patient with methylcrotonyl-glycinuria. *Clin. Chim. Acta* 76 (1977) 321–328

Wolf, B., Grier, R. E., Allen, R. J., Goodman, S. I. and Kien, C. L. Biotinidase deficiency: the enzymatic defect in late-onset multiple carboxylase deficiency. *Clin. Chim. Acta* 131 (1983a) 273–281

Wolf, B., Grier, R. E., Allen, R. J., Goodman, S. I., Kien, G. L., Parker, W. D., Howell, D. M. and Hunt, D. L. Phenotypic variation in biotinidase deficiency. *J. Pediatr.* 103 (1983b) 233–235

Wolf, B., Grier, R. E., Parker, W. D., Goodman, S. I. and Allen, R. J. Deficient biotinidase activity in late-onset multiple carboxylase deficiency. *N. Engl. J. Med.* 308 (1983c) 161

Wolf, B., Grier, R. E., McVoy, J. S. and Heard, H. S. Biotinidase deficiency: a novel vitamin recycling defect. *J. Inher. Metab. Dis.* 8 Suppl. 1 (1985) 53–58

Wolf, B., Heard, G. S., McVoy, J. S. and Raetz, H. M. Biotinidase deficiency: the possible role of biotinidase in the processing of dietary protein-bound biotin. *J. Inher. Metab. Dis.* 7, Suppl. 2 (1984)

Wright, L. D., Driscoll, C. A. and Boger, W. P. Biocytinase, an enzyme concerned with the hydrolytic cleavage of biocytin. *Proc. Soc. Exp. Biol. Med.* 86 (1954) 335–337

Yankofsky, S. A., Gurevitch, R., Niv, A., Cohen, G. and Goldstein, L. Solid-phase assay for biotin on avidin-cellulose disks. *Analyt. Biochem.* 118 (1981) 307–314

Zamboni, M., Gauday, M., Marquet, A., Munnich, A., Saudubray, J. M. and Marsac, C. Search for the biochemical basis of biotin-dependent multiple carboxylase deficiencies: determination of biotin activation in cultured fibroblasts. *Clin. Chim. Acta* 122 (1982) 241–248

J. Inher. Metab. Dis. 8 Suppl. 1 (1985) 53–58

Biotinidase Deficiency: A Novel Vitamin Recycling Defect

B. WOLF, R. E. GRIER, J. R. SECOR MCVOY and G. S. HEARD
Departments of Human Genetics and Pediatrics, Medical College of Virginia, Richmond, VA 23298-0001, USA

The recent finding that biotinidase deficiency is the primary biochemical defect in late-onset multiple carboxylase deficiency has stimulated new interest in the inherited disorders of biotin-dependent carboxylases. The clinical and biochemical features of biotinidase deficiency are discussed. We also speculate about two exciting areas currently being investigated: the localization of action of biotinidase, and the possible role of the enzyme as a binding or carrier protein for biotin.

Multiple carboxylase deficiency (MCD) (McKusick 25327) describes a group of inherited metabolic disorders which are characterized by deficient activities of the biotin-dependent carboxylases (Sweetman, 1981; Wolf and Feldman, 1982). Based on differences in clinical features and the times of their appearance, MCD has been catagorized into two major forms. Most children with the first form, neonatal or early-onset MCD, have been shown to have a primary enzyme deficiency in the activity of biotin holocarboxylase synthetase, the enzyme that attaches biotin covalently to the various apocarboxylases forming holoenzyme (Burri *et al.*, 1981; Saunders *et al.*, 1982). We have recently demonstrated that most individuals with the second form, juvenile or late-onset MCD, are deficient in the activity of biotinidase [EC 3.5.1.12] (Wolf *et al.*, 1983a,b). This enzyme catalyzes the cleavage of biotin from biocytin (ε-*N*-biotinyl-L-lysine) or biotinyl-peptides (Craft, 1984), the products of carboxylase degradation (Wright *et al.*, 1954; Thoma and Peterson, 1954). Biotinidase is not only important for the recycling of endogenous biotin but it appears to play an integral role in the processing of dietary, protein-bound biotin. This disorder is unique among the inherited vitamin-responsive metabolic diseases for two reasons. First, all children with biotinidase deficiency have improved clinically following the administration of oral biotin and treatment initiated early has been essentially "curative". Second, we now have evidence that biotinidase deficiency can be successfully treated with daily doses of biotin in the physiologic range rather than with pharmacologic doses.

THE ENZYME DEFECT

Biotinidase activity has been determined by measuring the release of biotin from biocytin, using several microbiological assays (Wright *et al.*, 1954; Koivusalo and Pispa, 1963) and by the release of chromophoric amino compounds from biotinylated substrates (Knappe *et al.*, 1963; Pispa, 1965). We determined enzyme activity using a modification of the method of Knappe *et al.* (1963), in which *p*-aminobenzoate (PABA) is released from the substrate, *N*-biotinyl-*p*-amino-benzoate.

The biotinidase activity in the serum of 18 healthy, fasting, normal children and adults was 5.80 ± 0.89 nmol min^{-1} ml^{-1} (Table 1). Biotinidase activity in the serum of children with the clinical features of late-onset MCD was deficient with a mean of 3.4% of mean normal activity. No increase in activity was found after increasing the concentration of substrate in the assay to 60 mmol^{-1} (an 800-fold increase). The activities in the serum of parents who were available for study were intermediate between those of the affected children and normal controls with a mean of 57% of mean control activity. Biotinidase activity in serum from one patient with biotin holocarboxylase synthetase deficiency was normal (Sweetman and Burri, 1981). We demonstrated that the deficient activity in the serum of affected children was not due to the presence of inhibitors, including biotin at concentrations usually attained after treatment with pharmacologic doses of the vitamin.

Very little biotinidase activity was detectable in concentrated extracts of fibroblasts from normal individuals using the colorimetric assay (Wolf *et al.*, 1983a). Therefore we developed a sensitive radioassay based on the liberation of [^{14}C-carboxyl]-*p*-amino-benzoate from *N*-biotinyl-[^{14}C-carboxyl]-*p*-amino-benzoate (Wolf and Secor McVoy, 1984). This assay is approximately 100 times more sensitive than the colorimetric method.

Using the radioassay we found biotinidase activity in extracts of peripheral blood leukocytes and fibroblasts of normal individuals but essentially no detectable activity in the serum of individuals who were shown previously to be biotinidase-deficient using the colorimetric assay (Wolf *et al.*, 1983a). Activities in the extracts of peripheral blood leukocytes and fibroblasts of patients with biotinidase-deficient serum were found to be less than 1% of mean normal activities. The specific activities in normal leukocytes and fibroblasts are similar to those reported in other mammalian tissues (Koivusalo and Pispa, 1963; Pispa, 1965). These studies and a report of deficient activity in the liver of an affected child (Gaudry *et al.*, 1983) also demonstrate that the deficiency of biotinidase activity in affected patients is not confined to serum and substantiate further that biotinidase deficiency is the primary defect in most patients with late-onset MCD.

Journal of Inherited Metabolic Disease. ISSN 0141–8955. Copyright © SSIEM and MTP Press Limited, Queen Square, Lancaster, UK.

Table 1   Biotinidase activity in the sera of affected children and their parents

Group	Number of samples	Biotinidase activity in serum (nmol PABA min^{-1} ml^{-1}) Mean*	Range
Normal individuals	18	5.80 ± 0.89	4.30–7.54
Affected children	15	0.20	0–0.90
Parents	18	3.29 ± 0.60	2.40–4.50

* Duplicate determinations were performed on each sample. Values are means $\pm$ 1 SD

CLINICAL AND BIOCHEMICAL FEATURES

Fifteen children with biotinidase deficiency have been diagnosed by our laboratory. The clinical features of these and five other patients with biotinidase deficiency (Charles *et al.*, 1979; Leonard *et al.*, 1981, case 4; Munnich *et al.*, 1981b; Gaudry *et al.*, 1983) are summarized in Table 2. There are 12 females and eight males from 16 families; consanguinity of the parents was reported in four families. This, together with the finding of about half-normal activity in the parents, indicates that biotinidase deficiency is inherited as an autosomal recessive trait. All of the children exhibited some or all of the symptoms usually seen in patients with late-onset MCD (Sweetman, 1981; Bonjour, 1981; Wolf and Feldman, 1982). The age of onset of symptoms varied from 3 weeks to 2 years of age (median age is 3 months, mean age is 6.3 months). The disorder was usually suspected when the children exhibited alopecia, skin rash and seizures, with the seizures frequently being the initial symptom. Fourteen of the patients were diagnosed because they had organic aciduria in addition to those neurologic and cutaneous features characteristic of the late-onset disorder. Of the remaining patients some had either the neurologic features or the cutaneous features characteristic of MCD; some had both but did not exhibit metabolic acidosis or organic aciduria. There is clinical variability among affected individuals from different families and, as demonstrated by siblings with

the disorder, there is also considerable variability in expression of the disorder among affected family members (Wolf *et al.*, 1983b).

In previously reported cases the diagnosis of the late-onset disease depended in part on the presence of demonstrable organic aciduria. Failure to detect this finding would have excluded about one-third of our cases of biotinidase deficiency. Although the biochemical abnormalities attributed to biotinidase deficiency are often life-threatening, they appear to represent relatively late effects of the disorder. The cutaneous symptoms and some of the neurologic signs are similar to those seen in biotin deficiency states (Sweetman *et al.*, 1981; Mock *et al.*, 1981; McClain *et al.*, 1982) and they usually occur early in the course of the disease. Biotin deficiency does not alter biotinidase activity. The enzyme activity in the sera of several patients who became biotin-deficient while receiving parenteral hyperalimentation was normal (Kien *et al.*, 1981) and biotin-deficient rats have similar biotinidase activities to rats receiving adequate dietary biotin (Suchy *et al.*, 1984). It seems likely that the cutaneous and neurologic symptoms of biotinidase deficiency result from a mild to moderate depletion of biotin when the residual carboxylase activities are still adequate to maintain normal metabolic balance. Only after protracted biotin deficiency do ketoacidosis and organic aciduria appear.

Hearing loss, which in several children was attributable to neurosensory impairment, has been diagnosed in about half the children with biotinidase deficiency (Taitz *et al.*, 1983; Wolf *et al.*, 1983c). Patients usually exhibited hearing loss before the initiation of biotin treatment but the deficit did not appear to improve after biotin therapy. It is possible that the hearing loss is caused by the accumulation of organic acids or by the accumulation of biocytin or larger biotinyl-peptides which, in the biotin-deficient state, may alter the metabolic pathways involved in the development and/or function of the auditory system (Taitz *et al.*, 1983). Although these metabolites should continue to accumulate after biotin treatment is begun, further hearing loss may be prevented in the presence of adequate biotin.

Immunoregulatory dysfunction has been reported in several children with biotinidase deficiency (Cowan *et al.*, 1979; Fischer *et al.*, 1982). However, too few patients have undergone immunological evaluation to enable a clear description of either the specific immunological abnormalities in biotinidase deficiency, or their clinical significance.

Table 2   Clinical and biochemical features of biotinidase deficiency

Feature	Frequency
Alopecia	17/20
Skin rash	15/20
Seizures	14/20
Ataxia	9/20
Conjunctivitis	9/20
Hypotonia	9/20
Hearing loss	8/16
Developmental delay	10/18
Fungal infections	6/20
Metabolic acidosis	14/19
Lactic acidosis	13/18
Hyperammonaemia	6/13
Organic acidaemia	14/18

Because of their inability to recycle biotin, biotinidase-deficient children are dependent upon exogenous biotin to prevent the clinical and biochemical features of biotin deficiency. Previous reports have described 'impaired' intestinal absorption of biotin in two patients with MCD (Munnich *et al.*, 1981a; Thoene *et al.*, 1983). However, both patients have since been shown to be biotinidase-deficient (Thoene and Wolf, 1983; J.M. Saudubray, personal communication). It has been shown in one of these patients that the response to oral biotin is normal if the loading test is conducted when the tissues are not depleted of biotin (Thoene and Wolf, 1983). Loading tests, performed on patients whose tissues are severely biotin-depleted, apparently result in the rapid entry of the vitamin into these tissues and in plasma concentrations of biotin which are misleadingly low. We would expect that the second patient would respond similarly if the appropriate loading study was performed.

Humans cannot synthesize biotin and therefore must derive the vitamin from the turnover of biotin-containing enzymes and from the absorption of biotin from dietary and/or microbial origin. The concentrations of free and protein-bound biotin in foods are variable but most of the biotin in foods such as meats and cereals is protein-bound (György, 1939; Thompson *et al.*, 1941). Therefore biotinidase may also play a critical role in the processing of dietary, protein-bound biotin. We have shown that although intestinal mucosa has biotinidase activity, the activity is not enriched in intestinal brush-border membranes (Wolf *et al.*, 1984). Biotinidase may be secreted by the columnar or specialized glandular cells. We found no activity in bile but considerable activity in pancreatic juice. The combined action of secreted gastrointestinal proteases and those associated with brush-border membranes on dietary, biotin-containing proteins may result in the liberation of biocytin or biotinyl-peptides. These compounds may then either be absorbed and hydrolyzed in the mucosa or be hydrolyzed in the intestinal lumen by biotinidase which originates from bacteria, pancreatic juice, the intestinal mucosa or all of these sources. Furthermore, if biotinidase production by intestinal flora is quantitatively unimportant, then patients with biotinidase deficiency would lack a mechanism for liberating protein-bound biotin from food and, if the contribution of the microflora to the free biotin pool is small or negligible, then these patients would depend entirely on dietary free biotin to meet their requirements for the vitamin.

Children with biotinidase deficiency have been treated successfully with pharmacologic doses of biotin, 10–20 mg day^{-1}, an empirically determined dose rate. Patients with holocarboxylase synthetase deficiency must be treated with pharmacologic doses of biotin and some are unable to normalize their carboxylase activities even with biotin dosages as high as 80 mg day^{-1}. This phenomenon is attributable to an extremely high K_m for biotin in these patients (Sweetman and Burri, 1981). In contrast, all patients with biotinidase deficiency have improved following treatment with pharmacologic doses of biotin. It has been suspected that these doses

supply more biotin than is actually required to meet the metabolic needs of these patients. One patient who was brought to our attention recently has been asymptomatic for eight years on a daily dose of biotin of about 150 µg day^{-1} (Diamantopoulos *et al.*, 1985). An important modifying factor in the treatment of this disorder may be the amount of free biotin in the diet; thus individuals consuming diets containing predominantly free biotin may require less supplemental biotin that those whose diet consists mostly of biotin in the bound form.

PRENATAL DIAGNOSIS AND NEONATAL SCREENING OF BIOTINIDASE DEFICIENCY

Using the radioassay we have found that biotinidase activity is also measurable in both amniotic fluid and cultured amniotic cells of normal pregnancies obtained by amniocentesis (Secor McVoy *et al.*, 1985). Since enzymes in amniotic fluid may be of maternal or fetal origin, the definitive diagnosis of biotinidase deficiency in the fetus depends on the determination of enzyme activity in extracts of amniotic fluid cells.

Although the tissues of heterozygous mothers have half-normal biotinidase activity, affected neonates are asymptomatic. This indicates that these mothers can supply the developing infant with adequate free biotin. However, the prenatal diagnosis of biotinidase deficiency may indicate whether prenatal treatment with biotin is warranted.

We have also developed a method of neonatal screening for biotinidase deficiency which involves the qualitative colorimetric assessment of biotinidase activity in the same samples of whole blood spotted on filter paper used in phenylketonuria screening (Heard *et al.*, 1984a). Samples with biotinidase activity show a characteristic purple color after incubation with *N*-biotinyl-*p*-aminobenzoate, whereas those with little or no activity remain straw-colored. Positive screening tests can be confirmed by a quantitative assay of enzyme activity using additional samples of dried blood or fresh serum. A pilot study, using samples obtained by the Commonwealth of Virginia for phenylketonuria testing, is currently being conducted to estimate the incidence of the disorder.

This technique also offers a simple, rapid method for the physician to obtain specimens from patients suspected of having biotinidase deficiency. Since the enzyme activity in the blood spots is stable for up to 18 months the cards may be sent to an appropriate reference laboratory.

SPECULATION

There are several major questions about the function of biotinidase that remain unanswered. First, where does the enzyme primarily function? Our preliminary studies have shown that serum biotinidase activity correlates positively with the concentration of serum albumin. The concentrations of albumin and the activities of biotinidase in sera of patients with cirrhosis were lowered (Weiner *et al.*, 1983), indicating that in the human as well as in the rat (Pispa, 1965) serum biotinidase originates principally from the liver. Given that the pH optimum for biotinidase activity is pH 5–7.5 (Pispa, 1965, Wolf *et al.*, 1983a) and that there is evidence that at least pyruvate carboxylase is degraded in lysosomes (Chandler and Ballard, 1983) it is attractive to assume that biotinidase is localized in the lysosome where it can readily hydrolyze biotinyl-substrates. However, subcellular fractionation studies show that biotinidase activity is enriched in the microsomal fraction (Pispa, 1965; Heard *et al.*, 1985), and not enriched in the lysosomal fraction. The enzyme, which migrates in the α_1-region on serum electrophoresis, is sialylated in serum and is asialylated in tissues (Heard *et al.*, 1985). In addition, biotinidase activity is readily determined in various tissues with secretory function, such as liver, fibroblasts, leukocytes and pancreas (Pispa, 1965; Wolf and Secor McVoy, 1984), as well as in pancreatic juice and isolated zymogen granules (Heard *et al.*, 1984b). These results are compatable with a model in which biotinidase is a secretory enzyme that hydrolyzes the products of carboxylase degradation that reach the blood. Finding a relatively greater specific activity of biotinidase in the serum (about 120 pmol min^{-1} mg protein^{-1}) than in the tissues (10–50 pmol min^{-1} mg protein^{-1}) could be explained if the enzyme primarily functioned in the serum. In fact, there is evidence that biotin originating from degraded carboxylases is not recycled in the cells, but in the extracellular compartment (Chandler and Ballard, 1983; Freytag and Utter, 1983).

Second, is biotinidase a binding or carrier protein for biotin in serum? The specificity of biotinidase resides in the biotinyl moiety of its substrate. If few molecules of biocytin or biotinyl-peptide are available to interact with biotinidase in the serum at any instant, then biotin which is a known competitive inhibitor of biocytin for biotinidase should be in equilibrium with the enzyme. Biotinidase has been purified 5000-fold to homogeneity from serum and has a molecular weight of approximately 76 000 daltons (Craft and Goss, 1982). Therefore, we would expect there to be about 200 pmol enzyme ml serum^{-1} and, if a typical serum biotin concentration of 2 pmol ml^{-1} is assumed, then the ratio of enzyme to biotin would be 100:1. Baumgartner *et al.* (1982) attributed abnormally high urinary output of biotin by a biotinidase-deficient patient to defective tubular reabsorption but also suggested that it could be due to the absence of or to a functionally deficient plasma biotin-binding protein. Biotinidase activity is present in the kidney but it is not enriched in the renal brush border membrane (Wolf *et al.*, 1984) and probably does not play a role in biotin recycling in the kidney.

If biotinidase is a biotin-binding protein in serum and is absent from the sera of biotinidase-deficient patients or so altered structurally as to be unable to interact with biotin, then the increased excretion of biotin in these patients can easily be explained. Assuming that in the biotin-replete state normal individuals and biotinidase-deficient patients have similar concentrations of biotin in their sera, then the gradient between the serum and the lumen of renal tubules for free biotin would be greater in the patients and, hence, they would excrete more biotin. Figure 1 summarizes schematically the various possible mechanisms of biotinidase function. Answers to these important questions are currently being actively pursued in our laboratory.

CONCLUSION

Biotinidase is necessary for the normal recycling of biotin that has been incorporated into the carboxylases. The presence of biotinidase activity in normal individuals confers some independence from exogenous biotin. In patients with biotinidase deficiency, the biotin salvage pathway is blocked and sufficient biotin must be ingested to prevent the development of symptoms of biotin deficiency from occurring. The potential exists for prenatal and neonatal diagnosis of the disorder, and we have initiated a pilot neonatal screening program to estimate its incidence. Daily physiologic doses, rather than pharmacologic doses, of biotin are likely to be sufficient to alleviate the symptoms of biotin deficiency, and biotinidase deficiency thus joins pyridoxine-responsive seizures as a specific and treatable form of infantile seizures. Elucidation of biotinidase deficiency as the primary defect in late-onset MCD has not only furthered interest in the inherited disorders of biotin-dependent carboxylases, but has led to new approaches for understanding the basic metabolism of biotin and its role in nutrition.

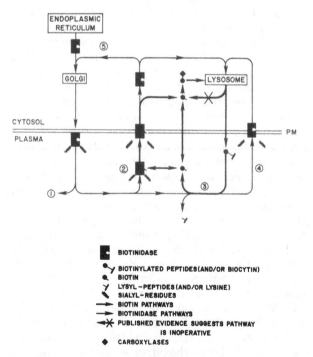

Figure 1 A schematic model for the recycling of biotin and biotinidase. The pathways labeled in the diagram represent the following processes: (1) transfer of biotinidase to tissues other than the sites of production; (2) binding of biotin to biotinidase (or another biotin-binding protein) and transport of this bound biotin into cells; (3) cleavage of biotinylated peptides or biocytin; (4) desialylation and re-entry of biotinidase into cells which may be followed by degradation; or (5) recycling of the enzyme.

We thank Drs R. J. Allen, M. Batshaw, C. Bachmann, D. Crisp, S. I. Goodman, D. M. Howell, D. L. Hurst, C. L. Kien, R. Matalon, S. Packman, M. Painter, W. D. Parker, M. Smith-Wright, J. Thoene and J. Thompson for providing fibroblasts and/or blood from patients, and Rosa M. Vaughan for her excellent secretarial assistance. This work was supported by grants from The National Institutes of Health (AM 25675 and AM 33022) and from the National Foundation-March of Dimes (6-342). This is paper number 247 from the Department of Human Genetics of The Medical College of Virginia.

References

Baumgartner, R., Suormala, T., Wick, H., Geisert, J. and Lehnert, W. Infantile multiple carboxylase deficiency: evidence for normal intestinal absorption but renal loss of biotin. *Helv. Paediatr. Acta* 37 (1982) 499–502

Bonjour, J. P. Biotin-dependent enzymes in inborn errors of metabolism in humans. *Wld Rev. Nutr. Diet.* 38 (1981) 1–88

Burri, B. J., Sweetman, L. and Nyhan, W. L. Mutant holocarboxylase synthetase: Evidence for the enzyme defect in early infantile biotin-responsive multiple carboxylase deficiency. *J. Clin. Invest.* 68 (1981) 1491–1495

Chandler, C. S. and Ballard, F. J. Inhibition of pyruvate carboxylase degradation and total protein breakdown by lyposomotropic agents in 3T3-L1 cells. *Biochem. J.* 210 (1983) 845–853

Charles, B., Hosking, G., Green, A., Pollit, R., Bartlett, K. and Taitz, L. S. Biotin-responsive alopecia and developmental regression. *Lancet* 2 (1979) 118–120

Cowan, M. J., Wana, D. W., Packman, S., Ammann, A. J., Yoshino, M., Sweetman, L. and Nyhan, W. Multiple biotin-dependent carboxylase deficiencies associated with defects in T-cell and B-cell immunity. *Lancet* 2 (1979) 115–118

Craft, D. V. Studies of biotinidase and biotin holoenzyme synthetase. Master's degree thesis, Case Western Reserve University, Cleveland, Ohio, 1984, pp. 126–130

Craft, D. V. and Goss, N. H. Enzymatic degradation of protein bound biotin by biotinidase. *Fed. Proc.* 41 (1982) 2753

Diamantopoulos, N., Painter, M. J., Wolf, B., Heard, G. S. and Roe, C. Preferential involvement of the CNS in biotinidase deficiency. *Ann. Neurol.* 16 (1985) 385

Fischer, A., Munnich, A., Saudubray, J. M., Mamas, S., Coudé, F. X., Charpentier, C., Dray, F., Frézal, J. and Griscelli, C. Biotin responsive immunoregulatory dysfunction in multiple carboxylase deficiency. *J. Clin. Immunol.* 2 (1982) 35–38

Freytag, S. O. and Utter, M. F. Regulation of the synthesis and degradation of pyruvate carboxylase in 3T3-L1 cells. *J. Biol. Chem.* 258 (1983) 6307–6312

Gaudry, M., Munnich, A., Ogier, H., Marsac, C., Marquet, A., Saudubray, J. M., Mitchell, G., Causse, M. and Frézal, J. Deficient liver biotinidase activity in multiple carboxylase deficiency. *Lancet* 2 (1983) 397

György, P. The curative factor (vitamin H) for egg white injury, with particular reference to its presence in different foodstuffs and in yeast. *J. Biol. Chem.* 131 (1939) 733–744

Heard, G. S., Grier, R. E., Weiner, D. L., Secor McVoy, J. R. and Wolf, B. Biotinidase—a possible mechanism for the recycling of biotin. *Ann. N.Y. Acad. Sci.* (in press) (1985)

Heard, G. S., Secor McVoy, J. R. and Wolf, B. A screening method for biotinidase deficiency in newborns. *Clin. Chem.* 30 (1984a) 125–127

Heard, G. S., Wolf, B. and Reddy, J. K. Pancreatic biotinidase activity: The potential for intestinal processing of dietary protein-bound biotin. *Pediatr. Res.* 18 (1984b) 198A

Kien, C. L., Kohler, E., Goodman, S. I., Berlow, S., Hong, R., Horowitz, S. P., and Baker, H. Biotin responsive *in vivo*

carboxylase deficiency in two siblings with secretory diarrhea receiving total parenteral nutrition. *J. Pediatr.* 99 (1981) 546–550

Knappe, J., Brommer, W. and Brederbick, K. Reinigung und Eigenschaften der Biotinidase aus Schweinenieren und *Lactobacillus casei*. *Biochem. Z.* 338 (1963) 599–613

Koivusalo, M. and Pispa, J. Biotinidase activity in animal tissue. *Acta Physiol. Scand.* 58 (1963) 13–19

Leonard, J. V., Seakins, J. W. T., Bartlett, K., Hyde, J., Wilson, J. and Clayton, B. Inherited disorders of 3-methylcrotonyl CoA carboxylation. *Arch. Dis. Child.* 56 (1981) 53–59

McClain, C. J., Baker, H. and Onstad, G. R. Biotin deficiency in an adult during home parenteral nutrition. *J. Am. Med. Assoc.* 247 (1982) 3116–3117

Mock, D. M., Delorimer, A. A., Liebman, W. M., Sweetman, L. and Baker, H. Biotin-responsive *in vivo* carboxylase deficiency in two siblings with secretory diarrhea receiving total parenteral nutrition. *N. Engl. J. Med.* 304 (1981) 820–823

Munnich, A., Saudubray, J. M., Carre, G., Goode, F. X., Ogier, H., Charpentier, C. and Frézal,. J. Defective biotin absorption in multiple carboxylase deficiency. *Lancet* 2 (1981a) 263

Munnich, A., Saudubray, J. M., Ogier, H., Coudé, F-X., Marsac, C., Roccichioli, F., Labarthe, J. C., Cuznave, C., Laugier, J., Charpentier, C. and Frézal, J. Déficit multiple des carboxylases. *Arch. Fr. Pediatr.* 38 (1981b) 83–90

Pispa, J. Animal biotinidase. *Ann. Med. Exp. Biol. Fenn.* 43, Suppl. 5 (1965) 5–39

Saunders, M. E., Sherwood, W. G., Duthie, M., Surh, L. and Gravel, R. A. Evidence for a defect of holocarboxylase synthetase activity in cultured lymphoblasts from a patient with biotin-responsive multiple carboxylase deficiency. *Am. J. Hum. Genet.* 34 (1982) 590–601

Secor McVoy, J. R., Heard, G. S. and Wolf, B. The potential for the prenatal diagnosis of biotinidase deficiency. *Prenatal Diagn.* (in press) (1985)

Suchy, S. F., Rizzo, W. B. and Wolf, B. Fatty acids in biotin deficiency. *Ann. NY Acad. Sci.* (in press) (1985)

Sweetman, L. Two forms of biotin responsive multiple carboxylase deficiency. *J. Inher. Metab. Dis.* 4 (1981) 53–54

Sweetman, L. and Burri, B. Abnormal holocarboxylase synthetases with elevated K_m values for biotin as the cause of one form of the inherited human disorder, biotin-responsive multiple carboxylase deficiency. *Int. Symp. Biotin-Dependent Enzymes*, Glenelg, Australia, 1981

Sweetman, L., Surh, L., Baker, H., Peterson, R. M. and Nyhan, W. L. Clinical and metabolic abnormalities in a boy with dietary deficiency of biotin. *Pediatrics* 68 (1981) 553–558

Taitz, L. S., Green, A., Strachan, I., Bartlett, K. and Bennet, M. Biotinidase deficiency and the eye and ear. *Lancet* 2 (1983) 918

Thoene, J. G., Lemons, R. M. and Baker, H. Impaired intestinal absorption of biotin in juvenile multiple carboxylase deficiency. *N. Engl. J. Med.* 308 (1983) 639–642

Thoene, J. and Wolf, B. Biotinidase deficiency in juvenile multiple carboxylase deficiency. *Lancet* 2 (1983) 398

Thoma, R. W. and Peterson, W. H. The enzymatic degradation of soluble bound biotin. *J. Biol. Chem.* 210 (1954) 569–579

Thompson, R. C., Eakin, R. E. and Williams, R. J. The extraction of biotin from tissues. *Science* 94 (1941) 589–590

Weiner, D. L., Grier, R. E., Watkins, P., Heard, G. S. and Wolf, B. Tissue origin of serum biotinidase; Implication in biotinidase deficiency. *Am. J. Hum. Genet.* 34 (1983) 56A

Wolf, B. and Feldman, G. L. The biotin-dependent carboxylase deficiencies. *Am. J. Hum. Genet.* 34 (1982) 699–716

Wolf, B., Grier, R. E., Allen, R. J., Goodman, S. I. and Kien, C.

L. Biotinidase deficiency: the enzymatic defect in late-onset multiple carboxylase deficiency. *Clin. Chim. Acta* 131 (1983a) 272–281

Wolf, B., Grier, R. E., Allen, R. J., Goodman, S. I., Kien, C. L., Parker, W. D., Howell, D. M. and Hurst, D. L. Phenotypic variation in biotinidase deficiency. *J. Pediatr.* 103 (1983b) 233–237

Wolf, B., Grier, R. E. and Heard, G. S. Hearing loss in biotinidase deficiency. *Lancet* 2 (1983c) 1365–1366

Wolf, B., Heard, G. S., McVoy, J. S. and Raetz, H. M. Biotinidase deficiency: The possible role of biotinidase in the processing of dietary protein-bound biotin. *J. Inher. Metab. Dis.* 7, Suppl. 2 (1984) 121–122

Wolf, B. and Secor McVoy, J. R. A sensitive radioassay for biotinidase activity: Deficient activity in tissues of serum biotinidase-deficient individuals. *Clin. Chim. Acta* 135 (1984) 275–281

Wright, L. D., Driscoll, C. A. and Boger, W. P. Biocytinase, an enzyme concerned with hydrolytic cleavage of biocytin. *Proc. Soc. Exp. Biol. Med.* 86 (1954) 335–337

J. Inher. Metab. Dis. 8 Suppl. 1 (1985) 59–64

Biotinidase Deficiency: Factors Responsible for the Increased Biotin Requirement

E. R. Baumgartner, T. Suormala and H. Wick
University Children's Hospital, Römergasse 8, CH-4005 Basel, Switzerland

J. Bausch and J.-P. Bonjour
Department of Vitamin and Nutrition Research, F. Hoffmann-La Roche & Co. Ltd, Basel, Switzerland

Inability to recycle biotin from endogenous biocytin in congenital biotinidase deficiency is associated with increased requirement of exogenous free biotin. We have observed that severe biotin depletion with clinical and biochemial consequences occurs within 12 days after birth in a newborn patient and within 15–20 days after withdrawal of biotin supplementation in four other patients. Our studies have shown that:

(1) Urinary loss of biotin and biocytin are major causes for this rapid biotin depletion.

(2) Intestinal absorption of biotin seems to be normal at least at the loading dose of $1.5\,\mu g/kg$.

(3) At normal or subnormal plasma biotin concentrations biocytin is found in low concentrations (below $1\,\text{nmol}\,l^{-1}$) in plasma of patients but at much higher concentrations in urine ($100–600\,\text{nmol}\,l^{-1}$).

(4) An oral load of biocytin results in patients in unchanged biotin levels but in a marked rise of biocytin in plasma followed by rapid renal excretion of biocytin whereas in controls biotin levels in plasma increase rapidly and biocytin remains below detection levels.

It is now widely recognized that biotinidase deficiency, first described in 1983 by Wolf *et al.* (1983d) is the primary enzyme defect in "late-onset" multiple carboxylase deficiency (MCD). Patients with this autosomal recessive disorder usually present during the first postnatal months with neurological symptoms (seizures, ataxia, developmental delay), muscular hypotonia, skin rash, alopecia and metabolic acidosis. There is, however, a considerable variability in clinical symptoms and time of onset (Wolf *et al.*, 1983b). The biochemical key feature is an abnormal urinary organic acid profile characteristic of deficient activity of the three mitochondrial biotin-dependent enzymes: propionyl-CoA carboxylase (PCC, EC 6.4.1.3), 3-methylcrotonyl-CoA carboxylase (MCC, EC 6.4.1.4) and pyruvate carboxylase (PC, EC 6.4.1.1). In contrast to holocarboxylase synthetase deficiency, the other known defect in biotin metabolism, which causes the "neonatal" form of MCD (Burri *et al.*, 1981; Ghneim and Bartlett, 1982), patients with biotinidase deficiency have subnormal levels of biotin in plasma (if measured specifically) while carboxylase activities in their cultured skin fibroblasts are indistinguishable from normal. Most of the clinical and biochemical abnormalities rapidly disappear with pharmacological doses of biotin.

Biotinidase (EC 3.5.1.12) cleaves biotin from its covalent linkage to the ε-aminolysyl residue of carboxylases after they have been metabolically degraded to biocytin (ε-*N*-biotinyllysine) or short biotinyl peptides (Craft *et al.*, 1984). The study of patients with congenital biotinidase deficiency has clearly demonstrated that biotinidase plays an important role in the recycling of endogenous biotin (Wolf *et al.*, 1983a). Biotin stores are rapidly depleted as soon as biotin therapy is discontinued. As a consequence carboxylase activities decline and clinical symptoms

appear (Baumgartner *et al.*, 1985).

The present report is concerned with studies aimed at elucidating how biotinidase deficiency leads to the rapid biotin depletion and hence increased biotin requirement observed in patients with biotinidase deficiency. We further present some data on the handling of biocytin by these patients.

PATIENTS

The five patients studied stem from four unrelated families. Biotinidase activity in plasma was severely decreased (1.4–4% of control values; Baumgartner *et al.*, 1985). The time of onset of clinical symptoms varied from age 7 weeks up to 2 years in the four index cases. Neurological abnormalities were always present and in most cases were the initial symptoms. Notably in a younger sibling (C.K.) of an index case (C.G) minor seizures were noticed as early as 7 days of age and EEG changes (temporal spikes during sleep) at 10 days. Her mother had not received biotin supplementation. In the four index patients organic aciduria was the key finding in establishing the diagnosis of MCD. Short case histories have been reported elsewhere (Baumgartner *et al.*, 1985).

METHODS

Biotin was routinely measured in plasma and urine samples by a microbiological assay method using *Lactobacillus plantarum* (ATCC 8014) (Frigg and Brubacher, 1976). This method is specific for biotin, i.e. it does not measure biocytin or other biotin metabolites, with the exception of biotin sulphoxide. In contrast, the widely used competitive binding assays based on avidin

Journal of Inherited Metabolic Disease. ISSN 0141-8955. Copyright © SSIEM and MTP Press Limited, Queen Square, Lancaster, UK.

and ^{3}H-biotin measure any biotin-containing compound in which the ureido ring of the biotin moiety is intact and accessible to avidin. This latter method with avidin–Sepharose as binder was used for selected urine samples (Bausch and Rettenmaier, unpublished results).

Biocytin in urine and plasma samples was estimated by two different methods:

(1) Separation by TLC (ethanol/water 4:1) followed by assaying the resulting fractions using the avidin–Sepharose method as described (Bonjour *et al.*, 1984).

(2) Normal plasma was used as source of biotinidase to cleave the biocytin (and possibly short biotinyl peptides) present in urine and plasma of the patients. The samples were assayed by the microbiological method before and after incubation with control plasma (1 ml urine + 120 µl control plasma, 2 ml plasma + 50 µl control plasma for 1 h at 37 °C). The difference of the results before and after such incubation is indicated as "liberated" biotin and corresponds to biocytin and probably also to short biotinyl peptides. Details of the method have been described (Bonjour *et al.*, 1984).

Carboxylase activities (PCC, MCC and PC) were assayed in lymphocytes as described (Suormala *et al.*, 1985a).

RESULTS

Course of biotin depletion

The two index patients (S.V. and C.G.), who could be evaluated in detail before biotin treatment was initiated, had subnormal biotin levels in plasma and urine and decreased carboxylase activities in lymphocytes (Table 1). With oral biotin treatment (2×5 mg day^{-1}) plasma biotin levels in patients rose to approximately 50–100 times normal and carboxylase activities in lymphocytes rose to supranormal values as observed by us and other authors (Wolf and Rosenberg, 1979; Stirk *et al.*, 1983) in normal controls under prolonged biotin treatment (Table 1). However, when biotin supplementation was withheld, plasma biotin fell at a much faster rate in the patients than in controls, reaching the normal range within 86 h and subnormal concentrations within less

than 5 days; later, between 6 and 10 days, it was below the detection limit (0.4 nmol l^{-1}) in all patients tested (Figure 1). Similarly, the decrease in urinary biotin concentration was much faster in patients than in controls. The rapid fall of plasma biotin was followed by a progressive decrease in carboxylase activities in lymphocytes resulting in about 25 % of control values 20 days after cessation of biotin therapy (Baumgartner *et al.*, 1985).

We were able to follow the natural course of biotin depletion in a newborn, C.K., younger sibling of C.G., whose mother had not received biotin supplementation during pregnancy. Plasma biotin and carboxylase activities in lymphocytes of cord blood were at the lower limit of the normal range. However, by age 10 days when EEG changes were already present, abnormal urinary metabolites were clearly increased, plasma biotin was subnormal (0.84 nmol l^{-1}) and carboxylase activities were decreased to 30 % of normal mean values (Figure 2).

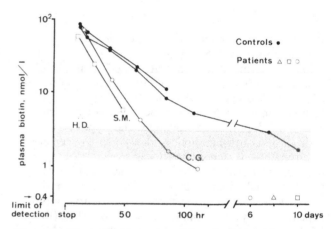

Figure 1 Plasma biotin concentrations in three patients and two adult controls after cessation of biotin supplementation (2×5 mg daily, except H.D. 2×1.25 mg daily). The normal range is indicated by the shaded area. Reprinted with permission of the authors and publishers of Baumgartner *et al.* (1985)

Table 1 Plasma biotin and propionyl-CoA carboxylase (PCC) and 3-methylcrotonyl-CoA carboxylase (MCC) activities in lymphocytes of patients and controls with and without biotin supplementation

Subject (age)	Biotin supplementation	Plasma biotin (nmol l^{-1})	Carboxylase activities in lymphocytes (pmol mg protein^{-1} min^{-1}) PCC		MCC	
			− biotin	+ biotin	− biotin	+ biotin
Patient C.G. (3 months)	Before supplementation	0.89	148		132	
	2×5 mg day^{-1} for several months		62‡		939	896
Patient S.V. (2 1/4 yrs)	Before supplementation	<0.4*	13		8	
	2×5 mg day^{-1} for 5 days		167†		576	538
Controls ($n = 5$)	0	1.58 ± 0.56	684 ± 84		472 ± 76	
	2×10 mg day^{-1} for 7–14 days		160 ± 48†		938 ± 85	696 ± 139

* Detection limit: 0.4 nmol l^{-1}
† 12 h after last biotin dose
‡ Exact time of last biotin dose not known
For controls, the data are given as mean values ± SD

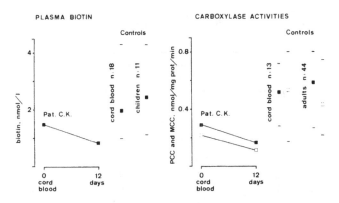

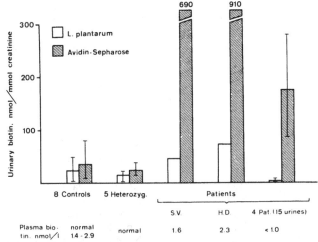

Figure 2 Plasma biotin concentrations and carboxylase (PCC = closed squares, MCC = open squares) activities in lymphocytes of patient C.K. at birth (cord blood) and at 12 days of age. Reference values (median value and range) are indicated by the shaded bars

Figure 3 Urinary biotin concentrations in patients, five heterozygotes and controls measured microbiologically and by the avidin-binding assay. Biotin supplementation had been discontinued in patients until their biotin plasma concentration had reached the normal (patients S.V. and H.D.) or subnormal (S.V., H.D., C.K. and C.G.) range

Renal excretion of biotin and biocytin

Urinary excretion of biotin was measured in patients and controls after prolonged biotin supplementation had been discontinued. At that time biotin plasma concentrations were similarly elevated in patients and controls. During the first hours after biotin supplementation had been stopped, urinary biotin concentrations in the patients were about one order of magnitude higher than in controls. In patients, urinary biotin levels remained higher than in controls at comparable plasma biotin concentrations (e.g. 775 and 669 nmol biotin (mmol creatinine)$^{-1}$ at plasma biotin concentrations of 15 and 22 nmol l^{-1} in two patients, compared to 213 $\pm$ 83 nmol (mmol creatinine)$^{-1}$ at plasma biotin concentrations of 20.7 $\pm$ 5.4 nmol l^{-1} in eight controls) until their plasma biotin became grossly subnormal. This stage was usually reached at 6–7 days after biotin withdrawal.

Biotin clearance studies confirmed the observation of renal loss of biotin in the patients. To compare biotin clearance in patients and controls, biotin supplementation in patients was withheld until their plasma biotin had reached the normal range. Under these conditions, biotin clearance in the patients was equal to or slightly higher than the creatinine clearance (clearance in ml min^{-1} 1.73 m^{-2}: biotin 118–158, creatinine 97–134) resulting in a ratio (biotin/creatinine) of 1.0–1.3. In control children and adults, biotin clearance was much lower than the creatinine clearance with a mean ratio of 0.41 in adults and 0.44 in children (Baumgartner *et al.*, 1985).

All these results were obtained by the microbiological assay which measures biotin only, not biocytin or other biotin metabolites. Analysis of urine samples by the avidin–Sepharose assay yielded values approximately 1.5 times those obtained with the microbiological assay in the urine of normal and heterozygous subjects. However, in the urine of patients this difference was much greater: 10–190 times more avidin-combinable material than "true" biotin was found (at normal and subnormal biotin plasma levels) (Figure 3).

Analysis of urine samples of the patients by TLC revealed the presence of a component with the R_f of

authentic biocytin, in addition to a component with the R_f of biotin (Figure 4). Incubation of the urine with control plasma as a source of biotinidase resulted in disappearance of the biocytin peak and a corresponding increase of the biotin peak (Figure 4). This confirmed the presence of biocytin in the patients' urine. In control urine no biocytin could be detected.

The amount of biocytin (possibly including short biotinyl peptides) excreted in urine of the patients (after withdrawal of biotin supplementation, at normal or subnormal plasma biotin levels) ranged from 22 to 100 nmol (mmol creatinine)$^{-1}$, as estimated by the microbiological assay before and after incubation of the urine sample with plasma-biotinidase (Table 2). Comparison with control values shows that during this period the biotin excretion of the patients was subnormal (except in S.V.), whereas biocytin excretion

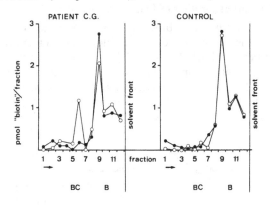

Figure 4 Thin-layer chromatograms of urine samples (corresponding to 80 nmol creatinine) of patient C.G. (20 days after cessation of biotin supplementation) and of a healthy control (without biotin supplementation). Before (open circles) and after (closed circles) incubation with normal plasma as source of biotinidase. The individual fractions were analysed for avidin-combinable material by the avidin–Sepharose method as described by Bonjour *et al.* (1984). Biotin (B) and biocytin (BC) were applied as reference substances

Table 2 Biotin concentration in urine of patients and controls after withdrawal of biotin supplementation and the effect of a biocytin load

Subjects	Biotin supplementation	Urinary biotin* (nmol (mmol creatinine)$^{-1}$)		
		− plasma†	+ plasma†	"Liberated biotin" $\approx$ biocytin
Patients				
S.M.	None for 3 days	1.7	63.6	61.9
S.M.	None for 7 days	1.2	78.3	77.1
S.V.	None for 3 days	18.3	56.6	38.3
H.D.	None for 3 days	1.7	28.5	26.8
H.D.	None for 7 days	2.3	29.8	27.5
H.D.	None for 20 days	0.8	22.6	21.8
C.G.	None for 20 days	0.6	51.7	51.1
C.K.	None for 5 days, before biocytin load	2.2	84.8	82.6
	4.8 h after biocytin load‡	38.3	404.8	366.5
Controls				
Children, n = 8§	None	33 ± 15	31 ± 13	0
(1.5–6 years)		(14–50)	(13–50)	
1 Adult	None, before biocytin load	9	9	0
	4.5 h after biocytin load‡	809	812	3

* Microbiological assay (*L. plantarum*) before and after incubation of the urine samples with normal plasma as source of biotinidase†
† For details see Methods
‡ Biocytin was given as a single oral dose of 0.4 μmol kg body weight^{-1}
§ Control values are given as $\bar{x} \pm$ SD and (range)

in most instances was considerably higher than the biotin excretion of controls. The amount of biocytin determined by this method did not fully account for the difference found between the avidin and microbiological assay, due to the additional excretion of biotin-metabolites which we have not yet identified.

Using the microbiological assay without and with plasma-biotinidase pretreatment, 0.65 to 0.96 nmol biocytin l^{-1} was found in the patients' plasma while their "true" biotin was subnormal (C.K. and C.G.) and in the normal range (S.V.) (Table 3).

Intestinal absorption of biotin and biocytin

Oral biotin and biocytin absorption tests were performed in the patients after biotin supplementation had been withheld for several days. At this time plasma biotin levels in one patient (C.G.) were at the lower normal limit and carboxylase activities were within the normal range, while in the two other patients plasma biotin and carboxylase activities were subnormal.

Table 3 Plasma biotin (nmol l^{-1}; *L. plantarum*) in patients after withdrawal of biotin supplementation

Patients	− plasma	+ plasma	"Liberated biotin" $\approx$ biocytin
C.K.	0.67	1.38	0.71
C.G.	0.57	1.16	0.59
S.V.	1.71	2.67	0.96
S.V.	1.51	2.16	0.65

Effect of incubation with normal plasma as source of biotinidase

Ingestion of a very small, almost physiological dose of biotin (1.5 μg (kg body weight)$^{-1}$) caused a similar increase of plasma biotin concentrations in patients and controls, with a peak after 45–60 min (Figure 5) (Suormala *et al.*, 1985b; Baumgartner *et al.*, 1982). These results disagree with the biotin absorption studies of Munnich *et al.* (1983) and Thoene *et al.* (1983a). Their patients were probably so severely biotin-depleted that a large proportion of the ingested biotin was rapidly incorporated into tissue carboxylases resulting in a flat absorption curve due to a high apparent distribution volume. A second study by Thoene and Wolf (1983b) using different experimental conditions is in agreement with our results.

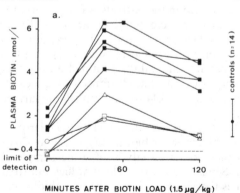

Figure 5 Response of plasma biotin concentrations to a single oral biotin load of 1.5 μg kg^{-1} in patients S.M. (△), C.G. (○) and H.D. (□), and healthy adult controls (■). The vertical bar indicates reference values (mean value and range) of biotin plasma concentrations in adult controls not on supplemental biotin. Reprinted with permission of the authors and publishers of Suormala *et al.* (1985b)

Absorption tests with a higher dose of biotin ($100 \mu g \, kg^{-1} \approx 0.4 \mu mol \, kg^{-1}$) resulted in biotin plasma peak values approximately 100 times normal in both patients and controls; initially decreased carboxylase activities in patients became normal within 2 h (Baumgartner *et al.*, 1981; Suormala *et al.*, 1985b).

However, after an equimolar oral dose of biocytin ($0.4 \mu mol \, kg^{-1}$), plasma biotin concentrations did not rise in the patients and the decreased carboxylase activities remained unchanged. Preliminary results have shown that in the patients biocytin is absorbed uncleaved giving rise to plasma biocytin levels of $7-16 \, nmol \, l^{-1}$ within 2–4 h, followed by rapid excretion of biocytin in the urine (Figure 6, Table 2). In contrast, in controls given the same biocytin load, biotin plasma levels rose to approximately $60 \, nmol \, l^{-1}$ within 2–3 h and urinary biotin concentrations increased approximately 10-fold (Table 2) whereas no biocytin could be detected. These findings indicate that the biocytin administered to controls is rapidly cleaved to biotin and lysine in the intestinal cells or in plasma as already observed previously (Wright *et al.*, 1954).

CONCLUSIONS

Patients with biotinidase deficiency suffer rapid depletion of biotin stores after birth, as illustrated by our patient C.K. The mechanisms for this rapid biotin depletion are not fully understood. The relationship between biotinidase deficiency and biotin depletion—hence increased biotin requirement—remains to be solved. Since patients with biotinidase deficiency are unable to cleave biocytin to biotin, biocytin itself might interfere with biotin handling processes such as intestinal absorption, cellular transport or holocarboxylase synthesis as suggested by Wolf *et al.* (1983a).

In our studies we have demonstrated that:

(1) After withdrawal of biotin supplementation, biocytin (and possibly biotinyl peptides) are indeed present in the patients' plasma and urine; at low concentrations (below $1 \, nmol \, l^{-1}$) in plasma but at much higher concentrations in urine ($20-100 \, nmol \, (mmol \, creatinine)^{-1}$ corresponding to $100-600 \, nmol \, l^{-1}$).

(2) In addition, the patients excrete about 10 times more biotin in urine than controls at similar biotin plasma concentrations. This is of course only true as long as the patients are not biotin-depleted. The renal loss of biotin is best documented by the elevated renal biotin clearance of the patients. Specific estimation of biotin concentrations (using the microbiological assay with *L. plantarum* rather than one of the less specific avidin-binding assays) is a prerequisite for such investigations.

(3) In contrast to some earlier reports in the literature, we could show that intestinal absorption of free biotin was not impaired in our patients.

(4) In patients, but not in controls, orally administered biocytin appears uncleaved in plasma and cannot be utilized as cofactor for the carboxylases. It is rapidly excreted by the kidney and does not accumulate significantly in plasma of the patients.

It is conceivable that the relatively high concentrations of biocytin in the urine of patients impair the renal handling of biotin. At the concentrations observed biocytin could interfere with tubular reabsorption or—rather unlikely—with binding of biotin to an as yet hypothetical biotin-binding protein in plasma (Baumgartner *et al.*, 1985). Further investigations are needed to clarify these questions.

The considerable loss of biocytin and biotin through the kidney is certainly a major factor leading to the increased biotin requirement. A further factor might be the patients' inability to utilize dietary biotinyl compounds arising during digestive degradation of proteins which are probably a major source of dietary biotin under normal conditions (Wolf *et al.*, 1984).

An important question for further investigations is whether biocytin plays a role in the hearing loss and optic nerve atrophy observed in an increasing number of these patients (Taitz *et al.*, 1983; Wolf *et al.*, 1983c). If so, it would be important to know whether biotin therapy increases biocytin levels in plasma and tissues significantly by inducing a more rapid turnover of carboxylases. Careful observations of patients who have been treated with biotin from birth will add to our knowledge in this respect.

We are indebted to our colleagues for their excellent collaboration in the clinical studies: Drs U. Caflisch, K. H. Jaggi, R. Clauss, H.-P. Haastert, E. Harms and A. J. Geisert. We would like to thank Ms J. Engler and her group (Department of Vitamin and Nutrition Research, F. Hoffmann-La Roche & Co. Ltd, Basel) for the microbiological biotin determinations.

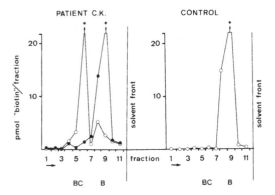

Figure 6 Thin layer chromatograms of urine samples (corresponding to 80 nmol creatinine) 4.8 h after a single oral biocytin load ($0.4 \mu mol \, kg^{-1}$) in patient C.K. and a healthy control. Details of the method and symbols as in Figure 4. *More than 30 pmol biotin per fraction

References

Baumgartner, E. R., Suormala, T., Wick, H. and Bonjour, J. P. Biotin-responsive multiple carboxylase deficiency (MCD): deficient biotinidase activity associated with renal loss of biotin. *J. Inher. Metab. Dis.* 7, Suppl. 2 (1984) 123–125

Baumgartner, E. R., Suormala, T., Wick, H., Geisert, J. and Lehnert, W. Infantile multiple carboxylase deficiency: evidence for normal intestinal absorption but renal loss of biotin. *Helv. Paediatr. Acta* 37 (1982) 499–502

Baumgartner, E. R., Suormala, T., Wick, H., Bausch, J. and Bonjour, J. P. Biotinidase deficiency associated with renal loss of biocytin and biotin. *Ann. N.Y. Acad. Sci.* (In press) (1985)

Baumgartner, E. R., Suormala, T., Wick, H., Bachmann, C. and Jaggi, K. H. Biotin dependency causing multiple carboxylase deficiency *in vivo. Pediatr. Res.* 15 (1981) 1189

Bonjour, J. P., Bausch, J., Suormala, T. and Baumgartner, E. R. Detection of biocytin in urine of children with congenital biotinidase deficiency. *Int. J. Vit. Nutr. Res.* 54 (1984) 223–231

Burri, B. J., Sweetman, L. and Nyhan, W. L. Mutant holocarboxylase synthetase. Evidence for the enzyme defect in early infantile biotin-responsive multiple carboxylase deficiency. *J. Clin. Invest.* 68 (1981) 1491–1495

Craft, D. V., Goss, N. H., Chandramouli, N. and Wood, H. G. Purification of biotinidase from human serum and its activity on biotinyl peptides. *Biochemistry* (In press) (1984)

Frigg, M. and Brubacher, G. Biotin deficiency in chicks fed a wheat-based diet. *Int. J. Vit. Nutr. Res.* 46 (1976) 314–321

Ghneim, H. K. and Bartlett, K. Mechanism of biotin-responsive combined carboxylase deficiency. *Lancet* i (1982) 1187–1188

Munnich, A., Saudubray, J. M., Carré, G., Coudé, F. X., Ogier, H., Charpentier, C. and Frézal, J. Defective biotin absorption in multiple carboxylase deficiency. *Lancet* ii (1983) 263

Stirk, J. H., George, K., Alberti, M. M. and Bartlett, K. The effect of large dose of biotin on leukocyte carboxylases in humans. *Biochem. Soc. Trans.* 11 (1983) 185–186

Suormala, T., Wick, H., Bonjour, J. P. and Baumgartner, E. R. Rapid differential diagnosis of carboxylase deficiencies and evaluation for biotin-responsiveness in a single blood sample, *Clin. Chim. Acta* 145 (1985a) 151–162

Suormala, T., Wick, H., Bonjour, J. P. and Baumgartner, E. R. Intestinal absorption and renal excretion of biotin in patients with biotinidase deficiency. *Eur. J. Pediatr.* (In press) (1985b)

Taitz, L. S., Green, A., Strachan, I., Bartlett, K. and Bennet, M. Biotinidase deficiency and the eye and ear. *Lancet* ii (1983) 918

Thoene, J., Lemons, R. and Baker, H. Impaired intestinal absorption of biotin in juvenile multiple carboxylase deficiency, *N. Engl. J. Med.* 308 (1983a) 639–642

Thoene, J. and Wolf, B. Biotinidase deficiency in juvenile multiple carboxylase deficiency. *Lancet* ii (1983b) 398

Wolf, B., Grier, R. E., Allen, R. J., Goodman, S. I. and Kien, C.L. Biotinidase deficiency: the enzymatic defect in late-onset multiple carboxylase deficiency. *Clin. Chim. Acta* 131 (1983a) 273–281

Wolf, B., Grier, R. E., Allen, R. J., Goodman, S. I., Kien, G. L. Parker, W. D., Howell, D. M. and Hurst, D. L. Phenotypic variation in biotinidase deficiency. *J. Pediatr.* 103 (1983b) 233

Wolf, B., Grier, R. E. and Heard, G. S. Hearing loss in biotinidase deficiency. *Lancet* ii (1983c) 1365–1366

Wolf, B., Grier, R. E., Parker, W. D., Goodman, S. I. and Allen, R. J. Deficient biotinidase activity in late-onset multiple carboxylase deficiency. *N. Engl. J. Med.* 308 (1983d) 161

Wolf, B., Heard, G. S., Secor McVoy, J. R. and Raetz, H. M. Biotinidase deficiency: the possible role of biotinidase in the processing of dietary protein-bound biotin. *J. Inher. Metab. Dis.* 7, Suppl. 2 (1984) 121–122

Wolf, B. and Rosenberg, L. E. Stimulation of propionyl-CoA and beta-methylcrotonyl-CoA carboxylase activities in human leukocytes and cultured fibroblasts by biotin. *Pediatr. Res.* 13 (1979) 1275–1279

Wright, L. D., Driscoll, C. A. and Boger, W. P. Biocytinase, an enzyme concerned with hydrolytic cleavage of biocytin. *Proc. Soc. Exp. Biol. Med.* 86 (1954) 335–337

J. Inher. Metab. Dis. 8 Suppl. 1 (1985) 65–69

Riboflavin-responsive Defects of β-Oxidation

N. GREGERSEN

Research Laboratory for Metabolic Disorders, University Department of Clinical Chemistry, Aarhus kommunehospital, DK-8000 Aarhus C, Denmark

The key reaction in the β-oxidation of fatty acids is the acyl-CoA dehydrogenation, catalyzed by short chain, medium chain, and long chain acyl-CoA dehydrogenases. Acyl-CoA dehydrogenation reactions are also involved in the metabolism of the branched chain amino acids, where isovaleryl-CoA and 2-methylbutyryl-CoA dehydrogenases are involved and in the metabolism of lysine, 5-hydroxylysine and tryptophan, where glutaryl-CoA dehydrogenase functions. In all of these dehydrogenation systems reducing equivalents are transported to the main respiratory chain by electron transfer flavoprotein (ETF) and electron transfer flavoprotein dehydrogenase (ETFDH), which are common to all the dehydrogenation systems. The acyl-CoA dehydrogenation enzymes are dependent on flavin adenine dinucleotide (FAD) as coenzyme, for which riboflavin is the precursor. Patients with multiple acyl-CoA dehydrogenation deficiencies have been found in whom the defect has been located to ETF and/or ETFDH. A few patients with multiple acyl-CoA dehydrogenation deficiencies have been described, in whom no defects in acyl-CoA dehydrogenases, ETF or ETFDH have been found but who respond clinically and biochemically to pharmacological doses of riboflavin. This indicates a defect related to the metabolism of FAD. An uptake defect of riboflavin or a synthesis defect of FAD from riboflavin have been excluded by *in vivo* and *in vitro* studies. A mitochondrial transport defect of FAD or a defect in the binding FAD to ETF and/or ETFDH remains possible.

Multiple acyl-CoA dehydrogenation deficiency is the functional term for a group of human metabolic diseases characterised by defects in the oxidation of acyl-CoA esters in the fatty acid, branched chain amino acid, lysine, 5-hydroxylysine and tryptophan metabolism. The clinical picture can vary considerably from that reported in the first severe cases of the neonatal form (neonatal glutaric aciduria type II) (McKusick 23168), who exhibit serious metabolic disturbances (hypoglycaemia, metabolic acidosis, coma) leading to early death (Przyrembel *et al.*, 1976; Gregersen *et al.*, 1980; Goodman *et al.*, 1980; Sweetman *et al.*, 1980), to that in the later reported milder forms, from which the patients recover following symptomatic treatment (Mantagos *et al.*, 1979; Dusheiko *et al.*, 1979; Gregersen *et al.*, 1982) after attacks of drowsiness (coma) accompanied by hypoglycaemia and acidosis.

Biochemically these diseases are characterised by the excretion of metabolites derived from accumulated acyl-CoA esters, i.e. C_6–C_{10}-dicarboxylic and hydroxy-monocarboxylic acids, ethylmalonic and methylsuccinic acids, free and glycine conjugated isobutyric, 2-methylbutyric, isovaleric, butyric, hexanoic and glutaric acids. Despite the qualitative similarity in the metabolic profiles, the quantitative pattern of metabolites is quite variable. In neonatal glutaric aciduria type II, the glutaric acid dominates the urinary metabolites, whereas the fatty acid derived metabolites dominate in some of the milder forms (Mantagos *et al.*, 1979; Gregersen *et al.*, 1982).

Most certainly these differences in excretion pattern reflect the different molecular forms of the acyl-CoA dehydrogenation deficiencies, but it is also probable that they reflect an individual's ability to utilize alternative metabolic pathways for acyl-CoA esters (Gregersen *et al.*, 1982; Gregersen, 1984).

THE ACYL-CoA DEHYDROGENATION COMPLEX

Acyl-CoA dehydrogenation is shown in Figure 1, where the dehydrogenation of hexanoyl-CoA is depicted as an example. The first enzyme involved is an acyl-CoA dehydrogenase, of which there are six. Two branched chain acyl-CoA dehydrogenases have been isolated

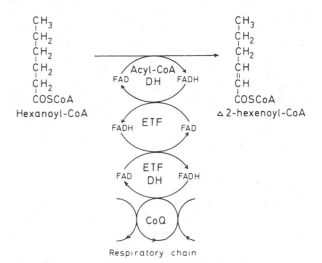

Figure 1 The acyl-CoA dehydrogenation system. The enzymes of the system are: acyl-CoA dehydrogenase (acyl-CoA DH), electron transfer flavoprotein (ETF) and electron transfer flavoprotein dehydrogenase (ETFDH), which all require flavin adenine dinucleotide (FAD) as coenzyme

Journal of Inherited Metabolic Disease. ISSN 0141-8955. Copyright © SSIEM and MTP Press Limited, Queen Square, Lancaster, UK.

(Noda *et al.*, 1980; Ikeda and Tanaka, 1982, 1983; Ikeda *et al.*, 1983), and in the fatty acid β-oxidation pathway there are three different enzymes with overlapping chain length specificity (Furuta *et al.*, 1981; Ikeda *et al.*, 1983; Dommes and Kunau, 1984). Finally, glutaryl-CoA dehydrogenase is unique because, in addition to dehydrogenation, the enzyme also catalyzes the subsequent decarboxylation to crotonyl-CoA or the two enzymes' activities are closely integrated (Besrat *et al.*, 1969; Noda *et al.*, 1980).

The two other components of the dehydrogenation system, which transport the reducing equivalents to coenzyme Q in the respiratory chain (Figure 1), are electron transfer flavoprotein (ETF) and ETF dehydrogenase (ETFDH) (Hall and Kamin, 1975; Ruzicka and Beinert, 1977). ETF and ETFDH are common to all the dehydrogenation processes.

The acyl-CoA dehydrogenases, ETF and ETFDH, all require FAD as coenzyme. FAD is tightly bound in a non-covalent way to the apoenzymes. The K_m values of rat liver acyl-CoA dehydrogenases for FAD are in the micromolar range (Ikeda *et al.*, 1983) and the K_m of human glutaryl-CoA dehydrogenase for FAD is approximately $5 \mu mol \, l^{-1}$ (Christensen and Brandt, 1978). The binding of FAD to ETF and ETFDH has not been measured experimentally, but it must be tight since FAD is not lost from ETF during purification procedures (Hall and Kamin, 1975; Ikeda and Tanaka, 1983), and the fact that ETF is not effected in riboflavin-deficient rats whereas the acyl-CoA dehydrogenase is decreased (Sakurai *et al.*, 1982) indicates that FAD is more tightly bound to ETF than to the acyl-CoA dehydrogenases. As FAD remains bound to ETFDH to a considerable extent during purification procedures (Ruzicka and Beinert, 1977), it must also be tightly bound to this apoenzyme.

The binding of FAD to the apoenzyme determines the conformation of many holoflavoenzymes (Weimer and Neims, 1975) and may also stabilise the apoenzyme (Mapson and Isherwood, 1963; Massey, 1963). The presence of FAD in isolation buffers increases recoveries considerably (Dommes and Kunau, 1984); furthermore the activity of short chain acyl-CoA dehydrogenase in mitochondria isolated from riboflavin-deficient rats cannot be regained by the addition of FAD to the assay mixture (Sakurai *et al.*, 1982) and indicates instability of the acyl-CoA dehydrogenase apoenzymes.

THE BIOSYNTHESIS OF FAD

The precursor of FAD is riboflavin (vitamin B_2) and normally supplied in the diet. The amounts required for maintainance of the body's metabolism and for compensating for urinary losses, is dependent on metabolic activity. The minimum requirement for adult man is approximately $1.7 \, mg \, day^{-1}$ (Josko and Levy, 1975). A growing child aged 10–12 years should have a minimum intake of $1.75–2.00 \, mg \, day^{-1}$, depending on the basis for the calculation (weight, calorie or protein intake). Pregnant women require approximately 0.3 mg more riboflavin per day than non-pregnant women (Josko and Levy, 1975). When given in pharmacological

doses perorally the upper limit for absorption is about 25 mg per dose (Josko and Levy, 1975) and the unutilized vitamin is excreted during the following 8–24 h.

Following absorption riboflavin is converted first to flavin mononucleotide (FMN) by the cytosolic enzyme flavokinase (riboflavin kinase, EC 2.7.1.26) and then by the enzyme FAD pyrophosphorylase (flavin mononucleotide adenyltransferase, EC 2.7.7.2) to FAD (McCormick, 1975) which is then transported into the mitochondria by as yet unknown mechanisms.

RIBOFLAVIN-RESPONSIVE MULTIPLE ACYL-CoA DEHYDROGENATION DEFICIENCIES

The first patient with multiple acyl-CoA dehydrogenation deficiency which proved to be clinically and biochemically responsive to pharmacological doses of riboflavin, was a 3-year-old boy who was admitted to the hospital in a semicomatose condition. During the following days he developed a Reye-like syndrome with hypoglycaemia, metabolic acidosis and disturbances of consciousness (Gregersen *et al.*, 1982). The liver was enlarged and liver aminotransferases and lactate dehydrogenase concentrations were elevated in the serum. He recovered rapidly after treatment with glucose and electrolytes. The urinary organic acids were characteristic of multiple acyl-CoA dehydrogenation deficiencies. Quantitatively, the metabolites derived from the acyl-CoA intermediates of fatty acid β-oxidation were the most abundant. After the acute attack the excretion rate of these metabolites fell to a lower, but constant, level. Controlled trials with oral riboflavin [100 mg three times per day, which is considerably above the absorption saturation level (see above)], resulted in dramatic improvement of the metabolic profile, and continuous riboflavin medication proved beneficial for the general development of the child (Gregersen *et al.*, 1982). Rhead showed later that riboflavin-depleted cultured skin fibroblasts from the patient were more sensitive to the consequent FAD deficiency than control cells when fatty acid was oxidised, thus confirming the clinical riboflavin-response (Rhead and Fritchman, 1983).

A metabolic assessment after 3 years of riboflavin treatment showed that the excretion of acyl-CoA ester-derived metabolites has changed (Gregersen *et al.*, unpublished results). Metabolites derived from the longer chain length acyl-CoA esters, i.e. the dicarboxylic acids and 5-hydroxyhexanoic acid, were excreted in lower amounts and excretion of metabolites derived from butyryl-CoA, i.e. ethylmalonic acid, had increased. This might indicate that the deficiency of β-oxidation has moved to a lower chain length, as is the case in the brother of the index case, where ethylmalonic acid is by far the most abundant metabolite (Gregersen *et al.*, 1982). Another change during the 3 year period is that the excretion rate of free and esterified carnitine has decreased markedly, from 60 and 190 μmol (mmol creatinine)$^{-1}$ to 8 and 25 μmol (mmol creatinine)$^{-1}$, respectively. This is as low as control excretion (free carnitine: 3–22 μmol (mmol creatinine)$^{-1}$, esterified carnitine: 10–52 µmol (mmol creatinine)$^{-1}$) and questions the hypothesis that carnitine is trapped in considerable quantities by accumulated acyl-CoA esters and excreted as acyl-carnitine (Gregersen *et al.*, 1985). However, any conclusions based on analyses of urinary excretion of metabolites must be made with great caution. The excretion rates of metabolites vary considerably throughout the day (Gregersen *et al.*, unpublished results). A several hundred per cent increase of excretion between the night, where metabolic rate and muscular activity is low, and that of certain day urines, especially those taken after the first morning meal, can be observed. This preliminary result emphasises the fact that random urine is of no value in the assessment of the metabolic effect of a riboflavin treatment and that at least 24 h urine samples should be used.

Several other patients, who are apparently riboflavin-responsive, have been reported in abstract form. Unfortunately it is difficult to establish whether riboflavin has a beneficial effect in itself from the information given. Two Dutch cases were presented at the SSIEM meeting in Lyon, 1983. One, a 17-year-old girl, who excreted the metabolites characteristic of multiple acyl-CoA dehydrogenation deficiency (glutaric aciduria type II), improved clinically and biochemically on riboflavin medication in combination with diet treatment (Schutgens *et al.*, 1984). It remains to be established whether this patient is truly riboflavin-responsive. The other patient was a 6-week-old boy who excreted urinary organic acids corresponding to the pattern found in glutaric aciduria type II. He showed a decrease in ability to oxidise palmitate in isolated mitochondria (Mooy *et al.*, 1984). Despite the fact that riboflavin treatment produced a decrease in urinary organic acids it is not clear whether this treatment was assessed alone. Therefore riboflavin responsiveness is also not conclusively established in this case. The patient reported by Krieger and Bieber (1984) with a Reye-like syndrome and characteristic organic acid excretion is similar, responding apparently positively to riboflavin therapy but the conditions for this assessment were not reported.

An additional case has been reported by Green *et al.* (1985). A 9-month-old male child presented with a Reye-like syndrome, during which he excreted predominantly ethylmalonic and adipic acids in his urine. At 18 months of age, after six more acute attacks, riboflavin medication was started (100 mg day^{-1}). At 3 years of age he has had one additional attack and has otherwise developed normally.

The only other detailed cases reported are by Harpey *et al.* (1983). The mother of one normal and seven dead infants (one stillborn and the rest dying in the first month of life) had symptoms of fatiguability, mild jaundice and pruritus (during the last trimester of her ninth and tenth pregnancies) and the fetal movements were decreased. The metabolic profile indicated multiple acyl-CoA dehydrogenation deficiency. Low erythrocyte glutathione reductase activity and the beneficial effect of riboflavin (20 mg day^{-1}) suggested some type of "riboflavin deficiency". That the deficiency manifested itself during pregnancy is consistent with the increased riboflavin requirement of pregnant women. The girl from the ninth birth was treated with riboflavin in the first month of life but after 5 months the medication was stopped. The boy from the tenth pregnancy did not require additional riboflavin for the first months of life (Harpey *et al.*, 1983). Later, both children required treatment with 20 mg riboflavin per day (Harpey, personal communication).

These reported cases suggest that a therapeutic trial of riboflavin is indicated in patients with evidence of multiple acyl-CoA dehydrogenation deficiencies. However, since so few patients have been diagnosed at the enzymatic level, the biochemical justification for the treatment is not clear. Rational treatment requires knowledge of the molecular basis of the riboflavin effect and therefore much effort has been devoted to the elucidation of the primary defect(s).

POSSIBLE DEFECTS IN RIBOFLAVIN-RESPONSIVE ACYL-CoA DEHYDROGENATION DEFICIENCIES

The following defects in this type of patient are theoretically possible:–
   (1) Acyl-CoA dehydrogenase apoenzyme "defects".
   (2) ETF/ETF dehydrogenase apoenzyme "defects".
   (3) FAD-related defects:
      (a) riboflavin uptake
      (b) FAD synthesis
      (c) FAD transport
      (d) FAD binding.

Primarily FAD-related defects must be considered in patients with riboflavin-responsive multiple acyl-CoA dehydrogenation deficiencies but deficiencies of the apoenzymes of the acyl-CoA dehydrogenases, ETF and ETF dehydrogenases, cannot be ruled out. However, inborn defects in the acyl-CoA dehydrogenase apoenzymes themselves are extremely unlikely because of the existence of six different and distinct enzymes. However, it is possible that FAD deficiency will result in a large proportion of apoenzymes which are unstable and hence lowering holoenzyme activities. By use of the product formation assay developed by Kølvraa *et al.* (1982) these possibilities were ruled out for the acyl-CoA dehydrogenases by the finding of normal activity of medium chain acyl-CoA dehydrogenase in the presence of 300 µmol l^{-1} FAD in disrupted fibroblasts from the patients described by Gregersen *et al.* (1982) and Harpey *et al.* (1983). For the same reason, deficiencies of ETF and ETF dehydrogenase cannot be excluded.

The activity of the combined electron transport system, including the ETF and ETFDH, in fibroblasts can be measured in an assay based on the CO_2 release assay for glutaryl-CoA dehydrogenase/glutaconyl-CoA decarboxylase (Christensen, 1983). By omitting the electron acceptor methylene chloride the assay will measure the combined activities of glutaryl-CoA dehydrogenase and the electron transport chain. Very low activity was found with this assay in fibroblasts from patients with neonatal glutaric aciduria type II and with glutaryl-CoA dehydrogenase deficiency (Christensen *et al.*, 1984; Christensen, 1984). When fibroblasts of the riboflavin-responsive patient described by Gregersen *et al.* (1982) were tested, normal activity was found. The ETF/ETF dehydrogenase apoenzyme in this patient is therefore unaffected at the FAD concentration of the assay, $100\,\mu mol\,l^{-1}$. With the possibilities of gross apoenzyme defects excluded defects more directly related to the metabolism of riboflavin [(3)a, b] may be considered.

An absorption defect should manifest itself in insufficient total amount of riboflavin and corresponding metabolites (FMN and FAD) in the body. This situation can be assessed by measuring the activity *in vitro* of erythrocyte glutathione reductase, with and without added FAD, in the reaction medium (Glatzle *et al.*, 1968; Beutler, 1969; Bamji, 1969). Glutathione reductase in the erythrocytes from the patient described by Harpey *et al.* (1983) was assayed in this manner and the ratio of enzyme activity with and without FAD was found to be 2.3 (normal approximately 1.4), suggesting riboflavin deficiency. Because of normal urinary output of riboflavin the disease must, however, be different from a simple nutritional deficiency. Further investigations in this patient have not yet been reported. The same analysis in the Danish patient during the riboflavin treatment showed values within the control range (Gregersen *et al.*, unpublished results). This result, together with the fact that the treatment does not fully correct the deficiency, excludes an absorption deficiency for riboflavin with a consequent FAD deficiency. The synthesis of FMN and FAD from riboflavin was studied in fibroblasts from the same patient. Normal incorporation of ^{14}C from [^{14}C]-riboflavin into FMN and FAD was found by the method of Christensen *et al.* (unpublished results).

These investigations leave the last two possibilities [(3)c, d], concerning the transport of FAD through the mitochondrial membrane and the binding of FAD to the apoenzymes to be considered. The only relevant binding studies performed on these types of patients were the measurement of acyl-CoA dehydrogenase activity in fibroblasts from the patient described by Gregersen *et al.* (1982) with the product formation assay (Kølvraa *et al.*, 1982). The assay was performed with added FAD in concentrations from $1-300\,\mu mol\,l^{-1}$ and no difference from the corresponding measurements with control fibroblasts was seen (unpublished results), thus indicating normal tight binding of FAD to the acyl-CoA dehydrogenase. The binding of FAD to ETF and ETF dehydrogenase has not yet been investigated in any patient and neither has the transport of FAD through the mitochondrial membrane. The elucidation of the primary defect in patients with riboflavin-responsive multiple acyl-CoA dehydrogenation deficiency must await the development of appropriate methods.

The author is grateful to Niels Jacob Brandt, Ernst Christensen, Mogens Fjord Christensen, Jean-Paul Harpey, Anne Marie Holm, Inga Knudsen, Steen Kølvraa, Karsten Rasmussen, William Rhead and Vibeke Winter for their contribution to the studies reviewed in this paper. The study has been supported by the Danish Medical Research Council.

References

Bamji, M. S. Glutathione reductase activity in red blood cells and riboflavin nutritional status in humans. *Clin. Chim. Acta* 26 (1969) 263–269

Besrat, A., Polan, C. E. and Henderson, L. M. Mammalian metabolism of glutaric acid. *J. Biol. Chem.* 244 (1969) 1461–1467

Beutler, E. Glutathione reductase: Stimulation in normal subject by riboflavin supplementation. *Science* 165 (1969) 613–615

Christensen, E. Improved assay of glutaryl-CoA dehydrogenase in cultured cells and liver; Application to glutaric aciduria type I. *Clin. Chim. Acta* 129 (1983) 91–97

Christensen, E. Glutaryl-CoA dehydrogenase activity determined with intact electron transport chain: Application to glutaric aciduria type II. *J. Inher. Metab. Dis.* 7, Suppl. 2 (1984) 103–104

Christensen, E. and Brandt, N. J. Studies on glutaryl-CoA dehydrogenase in leucocytes, fibroblasts and amniotic fluid cells. The normal enzyme and the mutant form in patients with glutaric aciduria. *Clin. Chim. Acta* 88 (1978) 267–276

Christensen, E., Kølvraa, S. and Gregersen, N. Glutaric aciduria type II: Evidence for a defect related to the electron transfer flavoprotein or its dehydrogenase. *Pediatr. Res.* 18 (1984) 663–667

Dommes, V. and Kunau, W. H. Purification and properties of acyl coenzyme A dehydrogenases from bovine liver. *J. Biol. Chem.* 259 (1984) 1789–1797

Dusheiko, G., Kew, M. C., Joffe, B. I., Lewin, J. R., Path, F. F., Mantagos, S. and Tanaka, K. Recurrent hypoglycemia associated with glutaric aciduria type II in an adult. *N. Engl. J. Med.* 301 (1979) 1405–1409

Furuta, S., Miyazawa, S. and Hashimoto, T. Purification and properties of rat liver acyl-CoA dehydrogenases and electron transfer flavoprotein. *J. Biochem.* 90 (1981) 1739–1750

Glatzle, D., Weber, F. and Wiss, O. Enzymatic test for the detection of a riboflavin deficiency. NADPH-dependent glutathione reductase of red blood cells and its activation by FAD *in vitro*. *Experimentia* 24 (1968) 1122

Goodman, S. I., McCabe, E. R. B., Fennessey, P. V. and Mace, J. W. Multiple acyl-CoA dehydrogenase deficiency (glutaric aciduria type II) with transient hypersarcosinemia and sarcosinuria: Possible inherited deficiency of an electron transfer flavoprotein. *Pediatr. Res.* 14 (1980) 12–17

Green, A., Marshall, T. G., Bennett, M. J., Gray, R. G. F. and Pollitt, R. J. Riboflavin responsive ethylmalonic–adipic aciduria. *J. Inher. Metab. Dis.* 8 (1985) 67–70

Gregersen, N. Fatty acyl-CoA dehydrogenase deficiency: Enzyme measurement and studies on alternative metabolism. *J. Inher. Metab. Dis.* 7, Suppl. 1 (1984) 28–32

Gregersen, N., Fjord Christensen, M. and Kølvraa, S. Metabolic effects of carnitine medication in a patient with multiple acyl-CoA dehydrogenation deficiency. *J. Inher. Metab. Dis.* (In press) (1985)

Gregersen, N., Kølvraa, S., Rasmussen, K., Christensen, E., Brandt, N. J., Ebbesen, F. and Hansen, F. A. Biochemical studies in a patient with defects in the metabolism of acyl-CoA and sarcosine: Another case of glutaric aciduria type II. *J. Inher. Metab. Dis.* 3 (1980) 67–72

Gregersen, N., Wintzensen, H., Kølvraa, S., Christensen, E., Christensen, M. F., Brandt, N. J. and Rasmussen, K. C_6–C_{10}-dicarboxylic aciduria: Investigations of a patient with riboflavin responsive multiple acyl-CoA dehydrogenation defects. *Pediatr. Res.* 16 (1982) 861–868

Hall, C. L. and Kamin, H. The purification and some properties of electron transfer flavoprotein and general fatty acyl coenzyme A dehydrogenase from pig liver mitochondria. *J. Biol. Chem.* 250 (1975) 3476–3486

Harpey, J. P., Charpentier, C., Goodman, S. I., Darbois, Y., Lefebvre, G. and Sebbah, J. Multiple acyl-CoA dehydrogenase deficiency occurring in pregnancy and caused by a defect in riboflavin metabolism in the mother. *J. Pediatr.* 103 (1983) 394–398

Ikeda, Y., Dabrowski, C. and Tanaka, K. Separation and properties of five distinct acyl-CoA dehydrogenases from rat liver mitochondria: Identification of a new 2-methyl branched chain acyl-CoA dehydrogenase. *J. Biol. Chem.* 158 (1983) 1066–1076

Ikeda, Y. and Tanaka, K. Isolation of 2-Me-branched chain acyl-CoA dehydrogenase from rat liver mitochondria. *Fed. Proc.* 41 (1982) 1192

Ikeda, Y. and Tanaka, K. Purification and characterization of isovaleryl coenzyme A dehydrogenase from rat liver mitochondria. *J. Biol. Chem.* 258 (1983) 1077–1085

Josko, W. J. and Levy, G. Absorption, protein binding, and elimination of riboflavin. In Rivlin, R. S. (ed.) *Riboflavin*, Plenum Press, New York, 1975, pp. 99–152

Kølvraa, S., Gregersen, N., Christensen, E. and Hobolth, N. *In vitro* fibroblast studies in a patient with C_6–C_{10}-dicarboxylic aciduria: Evidence for a defect in general acyl-CoA dehydrogenase. *Clin. Chim. Acta* 126 (1982) 53–67

Krieger, I. and Bieber, L. L. Carnitine metabolism in recurrent Reye syndrome due to defective acetyl-CoA disposal. *Pediatr. Res.* 18 (1984) 294A

McCormick, D. B. Metabolism of riboflavin. In Rivlin, R. S. (ed.) *Riboflavin*, Plenum Press, New York, 1975, pp. 153–198

Mantagos, S., Genel, M. and Tanaka, K. Ethylmalonic–adipic aciduria: *In vivo* and *in vitro* studies indicating deficiency of activities of multiple acyl-CoA dehydrogenases. *J. Clin. Invest.* 64 (1979) 1580–1589

Mapson, L. W. and Isherwood, F. A. Glutathione reductase from germinated peas. *Biochem. J.* 86 (1963) 173–191

Massey, V. Lipoyl dehydrogenase. In Boyer, P. D., Lardy, H.

and Myrback, K. (eds.) *The Enzymes*, Vol. 7, Academic Press, New York, 1963, p. 275

Mooy, P. D., Giesberts, M. A. H., van Gelderen, H. H., Scholte, H. R., Luyt-Houwen, I. E. M., Przyrembel, H. and Blom, W. Glutaric aciduria type II. Multiple defects in isolated muscle mitochondria and deficient β-oxidation in fibroblasts. *J. Inher. Metab. Dis.* 7, Suppl. 2 (1984) 101–102

Noda, C., Rhead, W. J. and Tanaka, K. Isovaleryl-CoA dehydrogenase: Demonstration in rat liver mitochondria by ion exchange chromatography and isoelectric focusing. *Proc. Natl. Acad. Sci. USA* 77 (1980) 2646–2650

Przyrembel, H., Wendel, U., Becker, K., Bremer, H. J., Bruinvis, L., Ketting, D. and Wadman, S. K. Glutaric aciduria type II. Report on a previously undescribed metabolic disorder. *Clin. Chim. Acta* 66 (1976) 227–239

Rhead, W. R. and Fritchman, K. N. Riboflavin-responsive ethylmalonic–adipic aciduria: *In vitro* confirmation of riboflavin responsiveness in intact fibroblasts. *Pediatr. Res.* 17 (1983) 218A

Ruzicka, F. J. and Beinert, H. A new ion-sulfur flavoprotein of the respiratory chain. *J. Biol. Chem.* 252 (1977) 8440–8445

Sakurai, T., Miyazawa, S., Furuta, S. and Hashimoto, T. Riboflavin deficiency and β-oxidation systems in rat liver. *Lipids* 17 (1982) 598–604

Schutgens, R. B. H., Scholte, H. R., Luyt-Houwen, I. E. M., Veder, H. A., De Visser, M. and Bethle, J. Glutaric aciduria type II: Clinical and biochemical observations and riboflavin treatment in four sisters. *J. Inher. Metab. Dis.* 7, Suppl. 2 (1984) 97

Sweetman, L., Nyhan, W. L., Trauner, D. A., Merritt, T. A. and Singh, M. Glutaric aciduria type II. *J. Pediatr.* 96 (1980) 1020–1026

Weimar, W. R. and Neims, A. H. Physical and chemical properties of the flavins; Binding of flavins to protein and conformational effects; Biosynthesis of riboflavin. In Rivlin, R. S. (ed.) *Riboflavin*, Plenum Press, New York, 1975, pp. 1–47

J. Inher. Metab. Dis. 8 Suppl. 1 (1985) 70–75

Thiamine-responsive Inborn Errors of Metabolism

M. DURAN and S. K. WADMAN

University Children's Hospital, 'Het Wilhelmina Kinderziekenhuis', Nieuwe Gracht 137, 3512 LK Utrecht, The Netherlands

Three different inherited disorders are known in which thiamine may exert a beneficial effect: maple syrup urine disease (MSUD), lactic acidaemia and the syndrome of megaloblastic anaemia with sensorineural deafness and diabetes mellitus. The amounts of thiamine which were used for long-term treatment varied from 20 to $2400\,mg\,day^{-1}$. Additional treatment, such as the reduction of dietary branched chain amino acids in MSUD, could not be omitted in some cases. It has been shown that the vitamin improves the stability of the branched chain ketoacid decarboxylase, although some weeks may be needed to observe the *in vivo* effect of treatment. A prolonged trial with high doses of thiamine should always be given.

Thiamine, or vitamin B_1, was isolated for the first time in 1926. The occurrence of beri-beri after a long-term diet of highly milled rice, which has lost most of its thiamine, eventually led to the discovery of this vitamin. It occurs mainly in meat, cereals and dairy products. The human daily need is approximately 1 mg. Thiamine deficiency leads to severe neurologic disease (Wernicke–Korsakoff syndrome). Thiamine is taken up in the gut by a carrier-mediated process, which is limited to $10\,mg\,day^{-1}$. When larger amounts are ingested, a small portion is absorbed by passive diffusion (Davis and Icke, 1983). After intestinal absorption thiamine is readily phosphorylated to thiamine pyrophosphate (TPP). The latter compound acts as a cofactor in several enzyme reactions, such as the oxidative decarboxylation of branched chain 2-ketoacids, pyruvate, 2-ketoglutarate and 2-ketoadipate.

The role of thiamine in the 2-ketoacid dehydrogenase complexes has been studied extensively. TPP loses a proton and consequently is present as a thiazolium ion. This ion forms an adduct with the 2-ketoacid and subsequently allows the decarboxylation reaction to take place. In addition TPP plays a role in the transketolase reaction, a step in the hexose monophosphate shunt and in the metabolism of glyoxylate. TPP can even be further phosphorylated to thiamine triphosphate, a substance which plays a role in nerve conduction. A deficiency of thiamine triphosphate has been associated with subacute necrotizing encephalo-myelopathy (Leigh syndrome) (Cooper *et al.*, 1969).

This review is concerned with thiamine-responsive branched chain ketoaciduria, a well-studied defect. Thiamine-responsive lactic acidaemia and thiamine-responsive megaloblastic anaemia will also be reviewed.

THIAMINE-RESPONSIVE BRANCHED CHAIN KETOACIDURIA

Branched chain ketoaciduria, maple syrup urine disease (MSUD) (McKusick 28460), an inborn error affecting the degradation of the branched chain amino acids leucine, isoleucine and valine has been recognized for almost 30 years. The basic defect lies in the inappropriate functioning of the branched chain ketoacid (BCKA) dehydrogenase complex (EC 1.2.4.4); it results in the accumulation of the branched chain amino acids (leucine, isoleucin and valine), their corresponding keto analogues (2-ketoisocaproic acid, 2-keto-3-methyl-valeric acid and 2-ketoisovaleric acid) and of the corresponding hydroxy acids (Menkes, 1959). The severity of this disease is variable and is related to the amount of residual enzyme activity. The most seriously affected patients (the classical type) have ketoacidosis and seizures in the early neonatal period. Coma and rapid death occur frequently and the surviving patients often have mental and neurological defects. The milder forms of MSUD are characterized by a later onset and higher residual dehydrogenase activity ($> 2\%$ of controls). The thiamine-responsive patients all fall into this category.

After the initial description of thiamine-responsive MSUD by Scriver and colleagues (1971), eight additional patients have been reported (Kodama *et al.*, 1976; Danner *et al.*, 1978; Duran *et al.*, 1978; Pueschel *et al.*, 1979; Elsas *et al.*, 1981; Elsas and Danner, 1982). The clinical presentation of these patients is summarized in Table 1. It can be seen that most of the patients were not diagnosed in the neonatal period and would thus be classified as having the intermittent or intermediate type of MSUD. The enzyme data, either in fibroblasts or in leukocytes (Table 2) further support this.

Prior to the institution of thiamine therapy, several of these patients were treated by dietary restriction of branched chain amino acids, which did not always prevent the occurrence of ketoacidotic attacks. None of the patients who were treated with pharmacological doses of thiamine for prolonged periods had episodes of ketoacidosis. The original patient described by Scriver and colleagues (1971) is still on thiamine and a low protein diet (Scriver, personal communication). She has had one episode of intermittent disadaptation with ataxia and disorientation leading to coma. Aggressive treatment restored homeostasis. The patient described by Kodama and colleagues (1976) had to be readmitted at the age of 15 months because of dermatological problems. Her serum Zn level was low ($15\,\mu g\,dl^{-1}$, controls $82–105\,\mu g\,dl^{-1}$; $2.3\,mmol\,l^{-1}$, controls $2.6–16\,mmol\,l^{-1}$) and she died 2 days later (Kodama, personal communication). The patient had been on thiamine supplements ($100\,mg\,day^{-1}$) and a moderate restriction of dietary branched chain amino acids for 2 months.

Journal of Inherited Metabolic Disease. ISSN 0141-8955. Copyright © SSIEM and MTP Press Limited, Queen Square, Lancaster, UK.

Table 1   Relevant clinical data on patients with thiamine-responsive maple syrup urine disease

Patient	Age of diagnosis	Pretreatment symptoms	Treatment thiamine (mg)	Additional	Outcome
1. Scriver *et al.* (1971)	11 months	neurological impairment	10	low protein	alive
2. Pueschel *et al.* (1979)	13 months	neurological abnormalities; ataxia	10	low protein	unknown
3. Kodama *et al.* (1976)	5 months	odour; mental retardation	100	low BCAA	died (low Zn?)
4. Duran *et al.* (1978)	17 months	vomiting; retardation; ataxia	$10 \rightarrow 100 \rightarrow 1000$	low protein	alive and well
5. Elsas *et al.* (1981) M.C.	7 weeks	seizures; acidosis; failure to thrive	150	low BCAA	retardation; no ketotic attacks
6. Elsas *et al.* (1981) K.C.	birth	none	150	low BCAA	alive and well
7. Elsas and Danner (1982) V.H.	2 years	retardation; ketoacidosis	100	low protein	retardation; no ketotic attacks
8. Elsas and Danner (1982) T.M^c.	2 weeks	infections; ketoacidosis; ataxia	100	low protein + low BCAA	no ketotic attacks
9. Elsas and Danner (1982) J.P.	2 weeks	ketoacidosis; ataxia	100	low protein + low BCAA	no ketotic attacks

The patient described by Pueschel and colleagues (1979) was lost for follow-up investigations. The patient described by Duran and colleagues (1978) appeared to be mentally retarded when he was diagnosed at the age of 17 months (van der Horst and Wadman, 1971). Subsequently he was treated with a diet restricted in branched chain amino acids, after which normal physical and intellectual development was observed. The administration of thiamine was started at the age of 7 years with the simultaneous introduction of a low protein diet consisting of normal foods. The amount of thiamine had to be increased from 10 to 100 and then to 1000 mg day^{-1}, on the basis of recurrent increases of branched chain amino acid and ketoacid concentrations. Clinically the boy remained in excellent condition: he did not have episodes of ketoacidosis or neurological abnormalities. From the age of 11 years a daily oral supplement of 20 mg lipoic acid was given. The addition of this cofactor could theoretically activate the other components of the dehydrogenase complex. However, the introduction of lipoic acid did not lead to any further biochemical improvement in this patient: the mean prelipoate plasma leucine was 656 μmol l^{-1} ($n = 11$); its mean concentration after lipoate was 601 μmol l^{-1} ($n = 19$). The observed difference was statistically not significant. At the age of 18 years the patient was maintained on a low protein diet of 1 g (kg body weight)$^{-1}$, supplemented with 1000 mg thiamine and 20 mg lipoic acid. He was in good mental and physical health (height 181 cm, weight 71 kg). Occasionally during a minor illness the body was noted to have an odour. He then self-restricted his protein intake.

Table 2   Relevant biochemical data in thiamine-responsive maple syrup urine disease

Patient	BCKA dehydrogenase (% of control)	Plasma leucine (μmol l^{-1}) Pre-thiamine	Post-thiamine
1. Scriver *et al.* (1971)	40 (leuk.)	610	<100
2. Pueschel *et al.* (1979)	4.5 (fibr.)	1530	<100
3. Kodama *et al.* (1976)	15 (leuk.)	1040	285
4. Duran *et al.* (1978)	15 (fibr.)	1153	621 ± 187
5. Elsas *et al.* (1981) M.C.	5 (fibr.)	NR	
6. Elsas *et al.* (1981) K.C.	7 (fibr.)	NR	
7. Elsas *et al.* (1982) V.H.	10.9 (lymph.)	435 ± 214	269 ± 59
8. Elsas *et al.* (1982) T.M^c.	3.0 (lymph.)	495 ± 78	117 ± 23
9. Elsas *et al.* (1982) J.P.	4.7 (lymph.)	413 ± 86	196 ± 43

NR, not reported
leuk, leukocytes
fibr, fibroblasts
lymph, lymphocytes

The clinical follow-up of the four thiamine-responsive MSUD patients of the Atlanta group has been reported elsewhere (Elsas *et al.*, 1981; Elsas and Danner, 1982). These patients were treated with a BCAA-restricted diet from the time of diagnosis. This did not prevent the occurrence of episodes of ketoacidosis and ataxia (patients MC, KC, TM^c, JP). After the introduction of supra-physiological amounts of thiamine, episodes of ketoacidosis ceased. Plasma leucine values, which were in the 400–500 μmol l^{-1} range in the prethiamine period, dropped to values between 100 and 300 μmol l^{-1} following the thiamine supplementation (Table 2). Comparable data were obtained for the fasting plasma branched chain 2-ketoacid concentrations. The full effect of thiamine on plasma and urinary levels of branched chain amino acid and ketoacids did not occur until after 3 weeks of treatment. One patient was taken off thiamine for a month without detrimental effects.

In vitro effects of thiamine

Fibroblast or leukocyte branched chain ketoacid dehydrogenase activity in the thiamine-responsive patients ranged from 4 to 40 % of controls (Table 2). The highest value (40 % of controls) was found in the patient described by Scriver and colleagues (1971); measured in the presence of 0.1 mmol l^{-1} leucine, a normal activity was found at a substrate concentration of 5 mmol l^{-1}. Subsequently Chuang and colleagues (1982) demonstrated a reduced affinity of the mutant BCKA dehydrogenase for thiamine pyrophosphate in this patient's fibroblasts using 2-ketoisovalerate as a substrate (K_m 25 μmol l^{-1}; control 1.6 μmol l^{-1}). Surprisingly Danner and colleagues (1978), who analyzed the same cell line, found a normal K_m (1.6 μmol l^{-1}) using isolated fibroblast inner mitochondrial membrane matrix fraction (mitoplasts) and 1-^{14}C-2-ketoisocaproate as substrate. However, the Canadian patient had a much higher capacity to bind thiamine, hence a more rapid response to oral thiamine could occur. Both Kodama's patient and Duran's patient had 15 % residual activity. Neither of these patients' cell lines nor the cells of Pueschel's patient which had 4.5 %

residual activity have been studied in more detail. Much work on the effects of thiamine on the BCKA dehydrogenase complex in normal and mutant cells has been done by the group of Elsas. Their main and most recent conclusion was that TPP exerts a stabilizing effect on the enzyme complex. Using bovine liver mitochondria they have shown (Heffelfinger *et al.*, 1984) that proteolytic digestion of the subunits of the decarboxylase component did not occur when the complex was saturated with TPP. The same group showed that the BCKA dehydrogenase activity in normal human liver increased two-fold after at least 18 days of pharmacological doses of oral thiamine (Elsas and Danner, 1982). They also showed that the virtually complete disappearance of BCKA dehydrogenase activity in fibroblast inner mitochondrial membrane matrix occurring during incubation without TPP, could be prevented by the addition of 0.2 mmol l^{-1} TPP. The same addition to cells from thiamine-responsive patients, however, gave a maximal retention of 34 % of the original activity. Heat inactivation of the decarboxylase at 50 °C proceeded slower in the presence of 0.2 mmol l^{-1} TPP. The protective effect of thiamine on the BCKA dehydrogenase complex suggests that thiamine treatment would benefit all patients with intermediate MSUD. However, there are patients in whom no effect could be observed (Fritsch *et al.*, 1983). In this respect it must be stressed that long-term treatment with high doses of thiamine ($\geq$ 100 mg day^{-1}) may be necessary to observe an effect in some patients. Additional treatment with dietary restriction of protein and/or branched chain amino acids may also be necessary in some cases.

THIAMINE-RESPONSIVE LACTIC ACIDAEMIA

Only a few patients with apparent disorders of pyruvate metabolism reacting favourably to thiamine have been reported (Lonsdale *et al.*, 1969; Brunette *et al.*, 1972; Wick *et al.*, 1977; Krawiecki *et al.*, 1984; Smit *et al.*, 1984). Virtually all patients had neurological abnormalities and were mentally retarded; seizures and ataxia were frequent findings (Table 3). The blood lactate values

Table 3   Thiamine-responsive lactic acidaemia

	Lonsdale et al. *(1969)*	*Brunette* et al. *(1972)*	*Wick* et al. *(1977)*	*Krawiecki* et al. *(1983)*	*Smit* et al. *(1984)*
Age of onset	2 years	1 day	13 months	infancy	8 years
Acidosis	−	+	−	+	
Mental retardation	+	+	+	+	+
Neurological abnormalities	+	+	+	+	+
Seizures	−	+	−	+	+
Ataxia	+	−	+	−	−
Prethiamine blood lactate (mmol l^{-1})	3.2	16.1	3.0	5	5.7
Post-thiamine blood lactate (mmol l^{-1})	NR	2–5	1.4	1.5	2.5
Thiamine dose (mg day^{-1})	300–600	5–20	1800–2400	250	100 kg body weight^{-1}
PDH in fibroblasts	<30%	normal*	40%	normal	†

*Pyruvate carboxylase deficiency
†Determined in liver, decreased

in these patients were only moderately elevated, with the exception of Brunette's patient, who suffered from pyruvate carboxylase deficiency. The pyruvate and alanine concentrations followed roughly the same pattern (data not shown). The 5-year-old boy described by Lonsdale and colleagues (1969) had intermittent episodes of ataxia and mental confusion similar to the symptoms observed in Wernicke's encephalopathy. A spontaneous recovery from these attacks occurred together with a decrease of the level of urinary excretion of alanine and pyruvate (lactate values were not given). High doses of thiamine ($300-600$ mg day^{-1}) led to a further biochemical normalization. Subsequently Blass and colleagues (1970) demonstrated a partial deficiency of pyruvate decarboxylase in the patient's fibroblasts. A comparable clinical presentation was observed in Wick's patient, who was first admitted at the age of 20 months because of mental retardation and hypotonia. Blood pyruvate was 170μmol l^{-1} (controls $40-67 \mu$mol l^{-1}).

Following the administration of large amounts of thiamine (1800 mg day^{-1}) there was a definite clinical improvement. The interruption of the thiamine supplementation at home led to a prompt recurrence of the ataxia. At the age of 12 years the boy was moderately retarded (I.Q. 66); he was on a daily supplement of 2400 mg thiamine. The oxidation of pyruvate in the patient's fibroblasts was decreased to about 30% of the control value.

The patient reported by Krawiecki and colleagues (1983) suffered from chronic lactic acidosis since infancy. At 3 years she showed psychomotor retardation, cortical blindness and spastic tetraparesis. Treatment with 250 mg day^{-1} of thiamine kept the patient free of intermittent episodes of lethargy and tachypnoea. Although the overall activity of the pyruvate dehydrogenase complex in cultured fibroblasts was normal, defects such as a K_m mutant for TPP have not been ruled out. Recently Smith and colleagues (1984) presented the case history of an 8-year-old girl who had convulsions, general hypotonia, areflexia, and abnormalities in the EEG and CT scan. Lactate, pyruvate, and alanine were increased in blood, urine, and CSF. The activity of pyruvate dehydrogenase in a liver biopsy sample was decreased. High doses of thiamine (100 mg kg^{-1}) led to a near-normalization of all biochemical parameters; the abnormalities of the central or peripheral nervous system

disappeared with the exception of the areflexia. Finally the patient of Brunette and colleagues (1972) with a partial deficiency of hepatic pyruvate carboxylase will be discussed briefly. This girl had suffered from severe lactic acidosis from the neonatal period. Seizures and psychomotor retardation had developed at the age 14 months, when she had an acute episode of metabolic acidosis (base excess -25 mmol l^{-1}) leading to prolonged apnoea. An intramuscular injection of 20 mg thiamine cured the acidosis within 12 h. A second milder acidotic episode occurring after a high carbohydrate diet was relieved with 5 mg thiamine i.m. It was thought that the thiamine facilitated the removal of pyruvate towards the tricarboxylic acid cycle in this case where its entry into the gluconeogenic pathway was blocked.

THIAMINE-RESPONSIVE MEGALOBLASTIC ANAEMIA

The combination of megaloblastic anaemia, sensorineural deafness and diabetes mellitus, responding completely only to pharmacologic doses of thiamine, has been described several times (Rogers *et al.*, 1969; Viana and Carvalho, 1978; Haworth *et al.*, 1982; Poggi *et al.*, 1984). The occurrence of two cases in one family favours the heritable character of this condition (Haworth *et al.*, 1982). Parental consanguinity was reported only by Viana and Carvalho (1978). Plasma levels of folate and of vitamin B_{12} were essentially normal in all patients, hence a derangement in the transport of these vitamins could be ruled out. Generally the anaemia was noticed during the first year of life; a temporary effect of iron supplements, indicated by an increase of the haemoglobin level, was noticed once (Haworth *et al.*, 1982). The final diagnosis, however, was only made after a considerable delay (Table 4). Insulin-dependent diabetes was observed in most of the patients, but the girl reported by Viana and Carvalho (1978) only showed glycosuria after a glucose tolerance test preceded by prednisone treatment. Bilateral sensorineural hearing loss was invariably present. In contrast mental retardation was only reported by Rogers *et al.* (1969). The response to thiamine was discovered by accident after giving a multivitamin preparation with success. Following the start of the treatment, a sharp increase of the reticulocyte

Table 4 Thiamine-responsive megaloblastic anaemia

	Rogers et al. (1969)	Viana and Carvalho (1978)	Haworth et al. (1982) 1	Haworth et al. (1982) 2	Poggi et al. (1984)
Age of diagnosis	11 years	6 years	8 years	7 years	5 years
Haemoglobin (mmol l^{-1})*	4.8	4.5	5.2	6.4	4.3
MCV (fl)	102	85	108	96	96
Sensorineural deafness	+	+	+	+	+
Diabetes mellitus	+	(+)	+	+	+
Mental retardation	+	−	−	−	−
Thiamine dose (mg day^{-1})	20	25	25	25	25

* To convert haemoglobin mmol l^{-1} to g/dl divide by 0.6205

count was observed, accompanied by a slow but continuing rise of the haemoglobin level and an improvement of the megaloblastic changes in the bone marrow. One of the patients no longer needed insulin after the start of the thiamine treatment (Poggi *et al.*, 1984).

Various investigations into the nature of the primary metabolic lesion have been performed. Both normal (Rogers *et al.*, 1969) and decreased (Poggi *et al.*, 1984) blood thiamine levels have been reported. The latter authors performed thiamine uptake studies in erythrocytes; it could be shown that the patient's cells had a strongly decreased uptake ($0.81 \, \mathrm{pmol} \, 10^9 \, \mathrm{cells}^{-1} \mathrm{h}^{-1}$; controls $2.03 \pm 0.40 \, \mathrm{pmol} \, 10^9 \, \mathrm{cells}^{-1} \mathrm{h}^{-1}$). No apparent defect in DNA synthesis could be detected in bone marrow cells (Haworth *et al.*, 1982). It is likely that this hitherto unknown primary defect of thiamine metabolism is limited to some cell types only.

CONCLUDING REMARKS

The number of thiamine-responsive MSUD patients is small, especially when taking into account the fact that the protective effect of thiamine on branched chain ketoacid dehydrogenase is a general phenomenon. It is open to question whether all thiamine trials that have been reported in the literature were done with high enough doses and were pursued for a long enough period to observe an effect. Even a slight alleviation of symptoms is worthwhile exploring in a condition which is difficult to treat.

The possibility of thiamine treatment should also be considered in patients with lactic acidaemia, especially in those showing diet-induced changes in lactate and pyruvate concentrations possibly as a result of malfunctioning carboxylation or decarboxylation enzymes. Careful studies will no doubt bring to light future patients with a defective metabolism of 2-ketoglutaric and 2-ketoadipic acid. The possibility of thiamine-responsive hyperoxaluria remains to be investigated.

The majority of thiamine-related problems remain unsolved for the moment, such as the interference of thiamine with bone marrow activity and the exact relation between alcoholism, thiamine deficiency and Wernicke's encephalopathy. No doubt future biochemical investigations will contribute to the solution of these problems.

The following persons are gratefully thanked for their contributions which enabled the updating of previously published case reports: Dr L. J. Elsas II, Atlanta; Dr S. Kodama, Kobe; Dr S. Pueschel, Providence; Dr J. C. M. Stigter, Rotterdam; Dr C. R. Scriver, Montreal; Dr H. Wick, Basel.

References

Blass, J. P., Lonsdale, D., Uhlendorf, B. W. and Avigan, J. Intermittent ataxia with pyruvate decarboxylase deficiency. *Clin. Res.* 18 (1970) 393

Brunette, M. G., Delvin, E., Hazel, B. and Scriver, C. R. Thiamine-responsive lactic acidosis in a patient with deficient low-K_m pyruvate carboxylase activity in liver. *Pediatrics* 50 (1972) 702–711

Chuang, D. T., Ku, L. S. and Cox, R. P. Thiamin-responsive maple syrup urine disease: decreased affinity of the mutant branched-chain α-keto acid dehydrogenase for α-ketoisovalerate and thiamin pyrophosphate. *Proc. Natl. Acad. Sci. USA* 79 (1982) 3300–3304

Cooper, J. R., Itokawa, Y. and Pincus, J. H. Thiamine triphosphate deficiency in subacute necrotizing encephalomyelopathy. *Science* 164 (1969) 74–75

Danner, D. J., Wheeler, F. B., Lemmon, S. K. and Elsas, L. J. *In vivo* and *in vitro* response of human branched chain α-ketoacid dehydrogenase to thiamine and thiamine pyrophosphate. *Pediatr. Res.* 12 (1978) 235–238

Davis, R. E. and Icke, G. C. Clinical chemistry of thiamine. *Adv. Clin. Chem.* 23 (1983) 93–140

Duran, M., Tielens, A. G. M., Wadman, S. K., Stigter, J. C. M. and Kleijer, W. J. Effects of thiamine in a patient with a variant form of branched-chain ketoaciduria. *Acta Paediatr. Scand.* 67 (1978) 367–372

Elsas, L. J. and Danner, D. J. The role of thiamin in maple syrup urine disease. *Ann. N.Y. Acad. Sci.* 378 (1982) 404–427

Elsas, L. J., Danner, D. J., Lubitz, D., Fernhoff, P. M. and Dembure, P. P. Metabolic consequences of inherited defects in branched chain α-ketoacid dehydrogenase: mechanism of thiamine action. In Walser M. and Williamson, J. P. (eds.) *Metabolism and Clinical Implications of Branched Chain Amino and Ketoacids*, Elsevier, Amsterdam, 1981, pp. 369–382

Fritsch, G., Langenbeck, U., Wendel, U., Lehnert, W., Palm, W. and Steger, W. Intermittierende Form der Ahornsirupkrankheit bei einem 12 jährigen Knaben: Klinik, Diagnostik und Therapie. *Klin Pädiat.* 195 (1983) 351–354

Haworth, C., Evans, D. I. K., Mitra, J. and Wickramasinghe, S. N. Thiamine responsive anaemia: study of two further cases. *Br. J. Haematol.* 50 (1982) 549–561

Heffelfiinger, S. C., Sewell, E. T., Elsas, L. J. and Danner, D. J. Direct physical evidence for stabilization of branched chain α-ketoacid dehydrogenase by thiamin pyrophosphate. *Am. J. Hum. Genet.* 36 (1984) 802–808

van der Horst, J. L. and Wadman, S. K. A variant form of branched-chain ketoaciduria. *Acta Paediatr. Scand.* 60 (1971) 594–599

Kodama, S., Seki, A., Hanabusa, M., Morisita, Y., Sakurai, T. and Matsuo, T. Mild variant of maple syrup urine disease. *Eur. J. Pediatr.* 124 (1976) 31–36

Krawiecki, N., Hartlage, P., Roesel, A., Carter, L. and Hommes, F. A. Thiamine responsive lactacidemia. *J. Inher. Metab. Dis.* Suppl. 2 (1984) 98 (title only)

Lonsdale, D., Faulkner, W. R., Price, J. W. and Smeby, R. R. Intermittent cerebellar ataxia associated with hyperpyruvic acidemia, hyperalaninemia, and hyperalaninuria. *Pediatrics* 43 (1969) 1025–1034

Menkes, J. H. Maple syrup urine disease: Isolation and identification of organic acids in the urine. *Pediatrics* 23 (1959) 348–353

Poggi, V., Longo, G., DeVizia, B., Andria, G., Rindi, G., Patrini, C. and Cassandro, E. Thiamin-responsive megaloblastic anaemia: a disorder of thiamin transport? *J. Inher. Metab. Dis.* 7, Suppl. 2 (1984) 153–154

Pueschel, S. M., Bresnan, M. J., Shih, V. E. and Levy, H. L. Thiamine-responsive intermittent branched-chain ketoaciduria. *J. Pediatr.* 94 (1979) 628–631

Rogers, L. E., Stanley-Porter, F. and Sidbury, J. B. Thiamine-responsive megaloblastic anemia. *J. Pediatr.* 74 (1969) 494–504

Scriver, C. R., MacKenzie, S., Clow, C. L. and Delvin, E. Thiamin responsive maple syrup urine disease. *Lancet* i (1971) 310–311

Smit, G. P. A., le Coultre, R., Fernandes, J., Berger, R. and Begeer, J. H. Reversible symptoms of the central and peripheral nervous system in a patient with pyruvate decarboxylase (E_1) deficiency. *Abstr. 22nd Symp. SSIEM, Newcastle* (1984) 71

Viana, M. B. and Carvalho, R. I. Thiamine-responsive megaloblastic anemia, sensorineural deafness, and diabetes mellitus: a new syndrome? *J. Pediatr.* 93 (1978) 235–238

Wick, H., Schweizer, K. and Baumgartner, R. Thiamine dependency in a patient with congenital lacticacidaemia due to pyruvate dehydrogenase deficiency. *Agents Actions* 7 (1977) 405–410

J. Inher. Metab. Dis. 8 Suppl. 1 (1985) 76–83

Recent Advances in the Mechanism of Pyridoxine-responsive Disorders

B. FOWLER

Willink Biochemical Genetics Unit, Royal Manchester Children's Hospital, Pendlebury, Manchester M27 1HA, UK

Pyridoxine metabolism is summarised and speculation on possible defects leading to disease is made. Inherited deficiencies of PLP enzymes, which are known to respond *in vivo* to pharmacologic doses of pyridoxine are listed. The mechanism of pyridoxine responsiveness in homocystinuria due to cystathionine β-synthase deficiency is discussed. There is a correlation in most (but not all) cases between the presence of residual CS activity, which is often stimulated by pyridoxal phosphate much more than control enzyme, in cultured fibroblasts and pyridoxine responsiveness *in vivo*. Exceptional patients have been found and are discussed in the light of more detailed studies on their cell lines. Clearly defined abnormalities of pyridoxal phosphate binding to mutant enzyme have been demonstrated and evidence of reduced intracellular stability of mutant CS and possible modulation by pyridoxal phosphate is presented. Preliminary findings suggest that the tissue level of pyridoxal phosphate achieved following pyridoxine treatment could be one other factor in determining pyridoxine responsiveness.

The metabolism and transport of pyridoxine has been well studied in mammalian systems and is summarised in Figure 1. Some major features are as follows. Intestinal transport (Mehansho *et al.*, 1979; Hamm *et al.*, 1979) and uptake into liver (Mehansho *et al.*, 1980) and erythrocytes (Mehansho and Henderson, 1980) of the non-phosphorylated vitamers is thought to be passive. The liver plays the major role in metabolism of pyridoxine. Pyridoxine, pyridoxal and pyridoxamine are phosphorylated by pyridoxal kinase, (EC 2.7.1.35) which occurs in most tissues although mitochondria contain no kinase and take up pyridoxal 5′-phosphate directly (Lui *et al.*, 1981). Pyridoxine 5′-phosphate is oxidised to the active coenzyme form pyridoxal 5′-phosphate by an enzyme (EC 1.3.4,5), found mainly in liver. Pyridoxal 5′-phosphate interconverts with pyridoxamine 5′-phosphate during enzymic transamination. There is hydrolysis by phosphatases and release to the circulation of all forms (Mehansho *et al.*, 1980) with evidence of binding to plasma proteins (Anderson *et al.*, 1974) and haemoglobin (Mehansho and Henderson,

1980). Indeed plasma levels have been shown to reflect closely liver concentrations in man (Lumeng *et al.*, 1980). Pyridoxal is oxidised to pyridoxic acid, the main excretory form of pyridoxine.

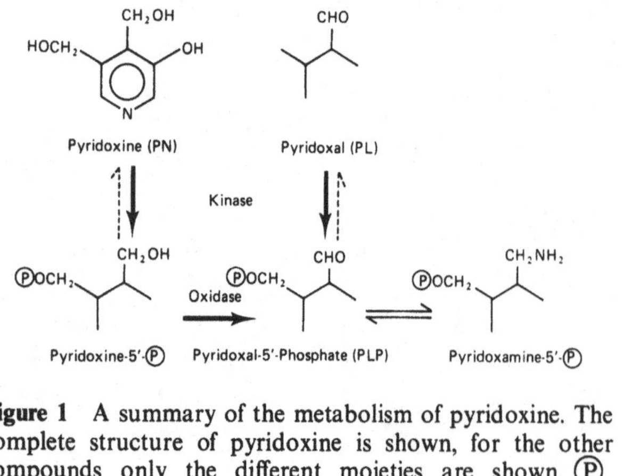

Pyridoxal 5′-phosphate (PLP) is the coenzyme for more than 50 enzymes (Lipson *et al.*, 1980b), with vital roles in intermediary metabolism and therefore at first sight it seems unlikely that a mutation affecting formation or accumulation of PLP would be compatible with life. However, such a possibility cannot yet be excluded since a partial reduction in available PLP may specifically lead to reduced activity of a few enzymes, due to the widely varying degrees of binding of the cofactor to PLP-requiring enzymes (Meister, 1965). Indeed this situation is observed in pyridoxine deficiency (Scriver, 1967). Furthermore, Scriver and Hutchison (1963) described a single patient who excreted cystathionine and following a tryptophan load excessive xanthurenic acid. This patient responded to pyridoxine treatment. Also in a personal communication, Boers has reported two adult patients with vascular disease who show evidence of deranged sulphur-amino acid metabolism after a methionine load, but in whom normal activity of trans-sulphuration enzymes in cultured fibroblasts was found (Boers and Fowler, unpublished observations). These patients are presently being investigated for a possible defect in pyridoxine metabolism and could be examples of heterozygotes as mentioned by Professor Scriver in his paper at this symposium.

Considering the large number of PLP enzymes, relatively few are known to be deficient in humans (Table 1). Homocystinuria (McKusick 23620), cystathioninuria (McKusick 21950), xanthurenic aciduria (McKusick 27860) and ornithinaemia (McKusick 25887) have well-documented forms which are responsive to pyridoxine both *in vivo* and *in vitro*. Primary oxaluria (McKusick 25990) is thought to be caused by deficiency of cytoplasmic α-ketoglutarate: glyoxylate

Figure 1 A summary of the metabolism of pyridoxine. The complete structure of pyridoxine is shown, for the other compounds only the different moieties are shown. Ⓟ = phosphate

Journal of Inherited Metabolic Disease. ISSN 0141–8955. Copyright © SSIEM and MTP Press Limited, Queen Square, Lancaster, UK.

Table 1 Summary of pyridoxine-responsive disorders

Disorder	Enzyme	Reaction		
Homocystinuria	Cystathionine β-synthase (CS)	Homocysteine + serine	→	Cystathionine
Cystathioninuria	γ-Cystathionase (γ-CL)	Cystathionine	→	Cysteine + α-ketobutyrate
Xanthurenic aciduria	Kynureninase (kynase)	(HO-) Kynurenine	→	(HO-) Anthranilic acid + alanine
Ornithinaemia (gyrate atrophy)	Ornithine δ-amino-transferase (OKT)	Ornithine + α-ketoglutarate	→	Glutamic γ-semialdehyde + glutamate
Primary oxaluria	α-Ketoglutarate: glyoxalate carboligase (NOT a PLP enzyme)	? ? Glyoxalate	→	Glycine (requires PLP)

carboligase, which is not a PLP enzyme. In this condition it has been suggested that pyridoxine responsiveness may be due to enhanced activity of the transaminase which converts glyoxylate to glycine (EC 2.6.1.4). Against this, not all patients with hyperoxaluria respond to pyridoxine, so this question remains open (Williams and Smith, 1983).

Although pyridoxine-dependent convulsions in newborns are receiving increasing attention (Bankier *et al.*, 1983; Crowell and Roach, 1983) they are outside the scope of this review since no distinct enzyme deficiency has been demonstrated.

This communication concentrates on homocystinuria due to cystathionine β-synthase (EC 4.2.1.22) deficiency. Since it is the most common of these disorders, it has been studied in most depth and provides the most interesting model of a pyridoxine-responsive disorder.

HOMOCYSTINURIA DUE TO CS DEFICIENCY

Clinical and biochemical aspects

Homocystinuria can be caused by three distinct enzyme deficiencies. The two less common defects cause defective remethylation of homocysteine [5,10-methylenetetrahydrofolate reductase (EC 1.1.99.15) and 5-methyltetrahydrofolate:L-homocysteine methyltransferase (EC 2.1.1.13)]. The more common form is caused by deficiency of cystathionine β-synthase (CS) which catalyses the condensation of serine with homocysteine to form cystathionine. This condition, first described in 1963, is characterised clinically by abnormalities of the ocular, skeletal, nervous and vascular systems with dislocation of lenses occurring in almost all untreated patients. Biochemically, homocystine and methionine concentrations are increased in body fluids with reduced levels of cystine. Approximately half of the patients show amelioration of these biochemical abnormalities when treated with oral pyridoxine in doses ranging from 50 to 1000 mg day^{-1}, the recommended daily intake being less than 1 mg (Mudd and Levy, 1983).

Biochemical response to pyridoxine (folate depletion must be excluded) can be apparently considerable, as shown in Figure 2, with a dramatic fall in plasma homocystine and methionine concentration and a rise in cystine in one patient receiving 750 mg pyridoxine day^{-1}. It must be emphasised, however, that Boers *et al.* (1983) have shown that in patients with a good response to pyridoxine, based on fasting plasma measurements, there is a diurnal increase in plasma homocystine, reflecting protein intake. A much less clear response is observed in some cases, as illustrated by another of our patients detected by newborn screening and treated from birth. Good control of plasma sulphur amino acid concentrations has been maintained on 200 mg day^{-1} of pyridoxine together with a dietary intake of methionine of 400 mg day^{-1}, which is much higher than the 100–200 mg day^{-1} of methionine required for control in our eight non-responsive patients, also treated from birth.

In an attempt to correlate pyridoxine response with clinical severity, 54 patients (21 from our Unit and the rest in whom enzyme studies were performed in this laboratory) were classified clinically, based on presence or absence, or age of development of clinical features. Figure 3 shows the numbers of patients in each group and their response to pyridoxine *in vivo*. In the mild/late

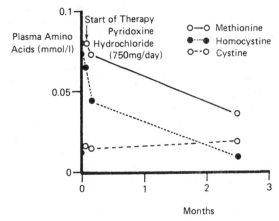

Figure 2 Effect of pyridoxine on plasma levels of sulphur-containing amino acids in a patient with homocystinuria

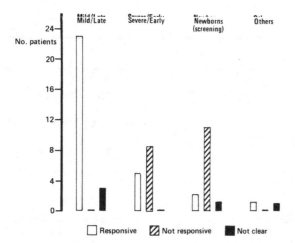

Figure 3 Response to pyridoxine in different clinical groups. Mild/late and severe/early groups defined as in text. Responsive, not responsive and not clear response defined as described in text

presentation group, the great majority of patients were responsive to pyridoxine in contrast to the preponderance of non-responsive patients in the severe/early group. Also most of the patients detected by newborn screening were non-responsive. This reinforces the concept that non-responsive patients tend to have more severe symptoms and are more likely to be detected by newborn screening. Similar conclusions were made by Mudd *et al.* (1985) from a survey of 629 patients.

Residual CS measurements in cultured fibroblasts

There have been a number of approaches to investigation of the nature and mechanism of pyridoxine responsiveness. These include measurement of residual CS activity in cultured fibroblasts; effects of PLP addition on residual CS activity in fibroblasts (Seashore *et al.*, 1972; Kim and Rosenberg, 1974; Fowler *et al.*, 1978) and in liver (Mudd *et al.*, 1970; Gaull *et al.*, 1974); studies of CS activity in cells grown in pyridoxine-depleted medium (Lipson *et al.*, 1980a); heat stability of mutant CS and the effects of PLP on this (Longhi *et al.*, 1977; Fowler *et al.*, 1978; Fleisher *et al.* 1978); and immunologic studies (Skovby *et al.*, 1982). There have been three main studies of residual CS activity in cultured fibroblasts from homocystinuric patients, based on the reasonable assumption that fibroblasts reflect findings in the liver. First by Uhlendorf *et al.* (1973), then by Fowler *et al.* (1978) and more recently, a large series of cell lines have been studied in this laboratory (Fowler, unpublished data) with the results discussed below.

The ability to reliably measure small quantities of CS activity is fundamental to such a study. In this study a radioisotopic assay was used in which the product of the enzyme reaction, [^{14}C]cystathionine, is separated by paper chromatography allowing detection of as little of 0.2% of control CS activity. Assays were performed as previously described (Fowler *et al.*, 1978), with and without addition of the coenzyme, PLP, and modified by using chromatographic development for at least 60 h to

ensure separation of cystathionine from an additional radioactive compound formed in the assay. Figure 4 shows the separation of [^{14}C]cystathionine obtained with assays of four representative mutant cell extracts. In mutants number 22 and 1 appreciable quantities of radioactivity in the region of cystathionine are clearly detected. In mutant number 5, a small but definite peak, corresponding to 0.2% of the mean of control activity, is found compared with the values shown in the dotted lines obtained with a zero-time blank. In the other mutant cell extract no radioactivity above the blank values was obtained, even using a very concentrated cell extract with 670 µg protein compared with approximately 250 µg usually included.

As further validation of the assay there was a clearly demonstrable increase of CS activity with a doubling of the protein used in assays of two mutant cell lines which had 0.3% residual activity assayed both without and with added PLP. Also in four different mutant cell lines, residual CS activity was stimulated by dialysis to a

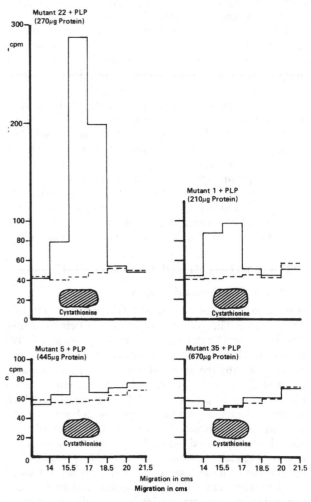

Figure 4 Cystathionine β-synthase activity in representative mutant cell sonicates. Paper chromatographic separation of [^{14}C]cystathionine. Cell culture and assay conditions of Fowler *et al.* (1978) used with the modification described in text. The position of marker cystathionine shown by the hatched area. Mutants 22, 1 and 5 are responsive *in vivo*, mutant 35 is non-responsive *in vivo*

degree similar to that seen in controls (Fowler, unpublished data).

With this assay we have measured residual CS activity in 51 cell lines from patients who are pyridoxine-responsive (complete or partial) or non-responsive, based on careful consideration of plasma sulphur-amino acid levels before and after treatment (Fowler, unpublished data). In five of these patients, the response was inconclusive or information was not sent by the referring centre. Assays were performed in at least two, and usually three or four, different batches of cells taking the average value to minimise effects of variable factors in, for example cell culture conditions. There were clear differences between the groups of cell lines from responsive patients and those from non-responsive patients. Twenty-six out of 30 responsive patients had small but definitely detectable CS in their fibroblasts (ranging from 0.2 to 5% of the mean control value, assayed with added PLP) whereas only three of 16 cell lines from non-responsive patients had any detectable activity (0.2, 0.7 and 0.75% of control). Lower levels of activity but similar differences between the groups were found when assays were performed without added PLP.

In this study, fibroblast CS activity was similar in siblings from six sibships. However, in two sibships both with two *in vivo* responsive patients, residual activity was found in cells from one sibling but not from the other, suggesting that non-genetic factors may affect the expression of CS in fibroblasts in some cases. In one such sibling, whose cells had no activity in the standard assay, residual CS could be demonstrated after dialysis of cell extracts, a finding not seen in representative cell extracts from non-responsive patients so studied. Unfortunately this could not be tried in the cells with no activity from the other sibship. These findings emphasise again the difficulties and need for careful study and consideration of many exogenous factors in studies of very small quantities of residual enzyme activity.

An important question is whether mutant CS can be stimulated by addition of PLP. The percentage increase of activity by added PLP at a concentration of $1000 \mu mol\, l^{-1}$ (Control CS, K_m for PLP approx. $30 \mu mol\, l^{-1}$) was calculated as a measure of the proportion of CS existing as holo- or apoenzyme in each cell line. In controls there was less than 50% stimulation in all except two cell lines with a mean value of 28%. In contrast, in those mutant cell lines with residual activity stimulation by PLP was much higher in most cases,

ranging from 30 to 733% (mean 273%) suggesting reduced binding of PLP to mutant CS.

The findings of residual CS activity measurements in three studies are summarised in Table 2, in which the hypothesis that patients who are responsive *in vivo* have residual CS activity in fibroblasts and conversely that non-responsive patients have no residual CS is considered. In these studies 39 of 46, 10 of 14, and 33 of 35 cell lines fit the hypothesis. However, the exceptions seen in each study, either responsive patients with no activity or non-responsive patients with activity, cannot be ignored. From these studies on residual CS activity measurements in cultured fibroblasts it can be concluded that most pyridoxine-responsive patients do have residual enzyme activity in their fibroblasts and most non-responsive patients do not. Also when mutant CS activity can be detected, it is usually stimulated by PLP addition to a much higher degree than control CS.

Degree of restoration of CS activity by PLP

An important question arising from these studies is whether the degree to which CS activity is increased by PLP is enough to explain the clinical responsiveness and, importantly, is CS activity lost or destroyed during cell processing?

To check whether conditions of cell growth or extract preparation cause losses of mutant CS activity, CS was assayed in cell extracts prepared in various ways from five representative cell lines (Fowler, unpublished data). Assays were done on sonicated cells, the standard procedure; on suspended cells; on cells frozen and thawed; on cells extracted with digitonin at 4°C or at room temperature; and on cells grown for only 24 h after subculture. Although some quantitative differences in CS activity were observed there was no appreciable increase towards the range of control levels of activity in three cell lines with measurable CS activity. Furthermore, in two cell lines with no residual activity when assayed in the standard way, one from a responsive patient, no activity was found with any method of cell extract preparation.

As a different approach, conversion of [^{35}S]homocystine to cysteine was measured in intact fibroblasts in monolayer from patients and controls (Fowler, 1982). As shown in Figure 5, formation of cysteine was considerably reduced in CS mutants compared with controls but was not appreciably higher in fibroblasts from responsive patients compared with

Table 2 Mechanism for pyridoxine responsiveness in CS deficiency

Hypothesis:

Patients responsive *in vivo* have residual CS in fibroblasts
Patients non-responsive *in vivo* have no residual CS in fibroblasts

Study	Number of cell lines	Number which fit hypothesis	Responsive in vivo no CS activity	Non-responsive in vivo with CS activity
Fowler (1982)	46	39	4	3
Fowler *et al.* (1978)	14	10	1	3
Uhlendorf *et al.* (1973)	35	33	1	1

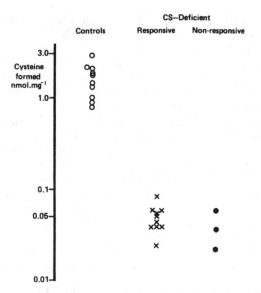

Figure 5 Conversion of [^{35}S]homocystine to cysteine in control and CS-deficient cell lines. NB Logarithmic scale

those from non-responsive patients. This provides further evidence that there is no increased trans-sulphuration in cells from responsive patients which was being lost during cell processing prior to CS assay.

The degree of restoration of enzyme activity by PLP in homocystinuria is compared with that in other disorders in Figure 6. In CS deficiency restoration of activity in responsive cell lines is much smaller than in

the other pyridoxine-responsive conditions, that is an average of 1.2% of the mean control activity and no higher than 5%. This contrasts with much higher restoration of activity in cystathioninuria, in liver (Frimpter, 1965) and lymphoid cells (Pascal *et al.*, 1978); in ornithinaemia, in cultured fibroblasts found more recently by Kennaway *et al.* (1980) and others (Shih *et al.*, 1978; Hayasaka *et al.*, 1981); and in xanthurenic aciduria in liver found by Tada *et al.* (1968). Importantly, however, Mudd and co-workers found restoration of CS in liver by PLP, to 3 and 4%, respectively (Mudd *et al.*, 1970), in two patients with less than 1% of control activity in their fibroblasts (Uhlendorf *et al.*, 1973). This may be a very significant finding but many more liver biopsies would be needed for confirmation. Mudd *et al.* (1970) have argued that since the capacity for trans-sulphuration in normal human liver far exceeds that normally required, a few percent of control CS activity may allow significant handling of methionine in pyridoxine-treated patients.

Interaction of mutant CS with PLP

More detailed studies of mutant CS have concentrated on the effects of PLP addition *in vitro*. Fowler *et al.* (1978) studied the effect of varying PLP concentration on CS activity in three control and five mutant cell lines. Cells were grown in normal medium, which contains 1 μg ml^{-1} of pyridoxal which is at least 100 times that required for normal growth of cells. Holo-CS in control, and all but one mutant cell extract, was converted to the apoenzyme by dialysis against hydroxylamine. In one

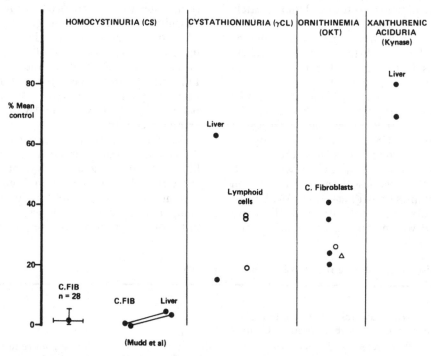

Figure 6 Restoration of enzyme activity by *in vitro* addition of PLP. Values represent maximum activity of the respective enzymes (see Table 1 for key to abbreviations) in mutant samples when assayed with PLP expressed as percentage of mean control activity. Homocystinuria: C.FIB-cultured fibroblasts from 28 responsive patients (Fowler, unpublished observations); other data; C.FIB-cultured fibroblasts (Uhlendorf *et al.*, 1973) liver, (Mudd *et al.*, 1970). For the other conditions values were calculated from reported data. Cystathioninuria: liver (Frimpter, 1965), cultured lymphoid cells (Pascal *et al.*, 1978). Ornithinaemia: ●, Kennaway *et al.* (1980); ○, Shih *et al.* (1978); △, Hayasaka *et al.* (1981). Xanthurenic aciduria: Tada *et al.* (1968)

mutant cell extract CS was unstable to this treatment and dialysis against buffer was used. Holo-CS was reconstituted by incubation with varying amounts of PLP, then assayed as before. Controls showed typical Michaelis–Menten kinetics of reassociation of PLP with apoenzyme. Linear Hill plots were used to calculate a K_m or, more appropriately, a reassociation constant for PLP. Abnormally high reassociation constants for PLP were found for two cell lines from responsive patients (both 4-fold higher than the average of control values) and for two cell lines from non-responsive patients (2- and 10-fold higher). One cell line from a responsive patient had a normal value. In these experiments there was no clear distinction between the cell lines from non-responsive patients and those from the responsive patients, although the highest value observed was from a *non*-responsive patient.

Lipson *et al.* (1980a,b) extended this work by studying PLP kinetics in these and other cell lines in which resolution of PLP from CS was achieved by growth of cells in medium containing very low amounts of pyridoxal. In Figure 7 PLP binding constants obtained in the same cell lines in each study are compared. Two main conclusions can be drawn. First, the cell line from a responsive patient R1, normal before, now shows a clearly abnormal binding constant. Importantly, the values from the non-responsive patients are now considerably higher than those in cells both from

controls and from patients who are responsive *in vivo*. These findings provide the explanation for those exceptional cell lines from non-responsive patients who have residual CS in their fibroblasts. The affinity of the mutant CS for PLP in these patients is reduced to a much higher degree than that in responsive patients and tissue levels of PLP obtained following pyridoxine treatment will be insufficient to modulate CS activity in these mutants.

Preliminary findings from studies in this laboratory (Fowler, unpublished observations) using cultured fibroblasts grown with medium containing zero, normal ($1 \mu g \, ml^{-1}$) and high ($20 \mu g \, ml^{-1}$) concentrations of pyridoxal have revealed an additional effect on CS activity expression. In two control cell lines total CS activity, as well as the proportion of holo-CS, was much lower in low pyridoxal medium than in normal medium, with no further increase in total activity after growth in high pyridoxal medium. Similarly, in four mutant cell lines total residual CS was reduced in low pyridoxal medium and was increased considerably in cells grown in medium with higher quantities of pyridoxal. Cells from a non-responsive patient had no CS activity under any of these conditions. These as yet preliminary results can be compared with studies of thermolability of mutant and control fibroblast CS. First, mutant CS was shown to be far more labile than control enzyme when heated at 54°C. Second, apo-CS from control cells was much more labile than holo-CS (Fowler *et al.*, 1978). Third, during heating at 54°C, control fibroblast CS was protected by the presence of PLP and this effect was specific to this compound and not exhibited by any of eight other derivations of vitamin B_6 (Fowler, unpublished observations). Taken together these findings suggest that PLP may stabilise mutant CS molecules possibly by influencing the proportions of apo- and holo-CS *in vivo*, in a similar manner to that observed for other PLP enzymes. For example, tyrosine aminotransferase (EC 2.6.1.5) in the liver of rats (Snape *et al.*, 1980), serine dehydratase (EC 4.2.1.13) in vitamin B_6-deficient rats (Hunter and Harper, 1976), aspartate aminotransferase (EC 2.6.1.1) in rat tissues (Okada and Hirose, 1979) and, finally, partially purified cystathionase which was protected by PLP against degradation by proteolytic enzymes (Chatagner *et al.*, 1970). Recently, Skovby *et al.* (1984) have reported studies of biogenesis of CS subunits which suggest that there can be a normal rate of synthesis of mutant CS molecules whose stability is much reduced.

Pyridoxal 5′-phosphate levels in homocystinuric patients

As a further aspect of study of pyridoxine-responsive homocystinuria we have started to measure pyridoxal phosphate and other B_6 levels in plasma, using HPLC with fluorescence detection (Coburn and Mahuren, 1983). Plasma PLP levels in seven homocystinuric patients were as follows with the dose of pyridoxine received in mg (kg body weight)$^{-1}$ in brackets: 56 (15), 109 (12), 162 (5.5), 170 (42), 230 (26), 352 (2.8), 485 (42) $nmol \, l^{-1}$; control range ($n = 5$) 20–36 $nmol \, l^{-1}$. The lowest plasma PLP levels of 56 and 109 $nmol \, l^{-1}$ were found in two siblings who had relatively high residual CS

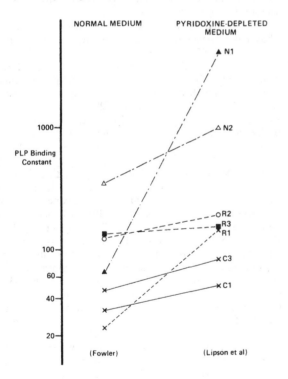

Figure 7 PLP-binding constants of mutant fibroblast CS. Values are replotted from previously reported data; cells grown in normal medium (pyridoxal 1000 ng ml^{-1}) and CS resolved by hydroxylamine treatment (Fowler *et al.*, 1978); cells grown in pyridoxal-depleted medium to resolve PLP from CS (Lipson *et al.*, 1980). C1, C3, controls; R1, R2, R3, responsive *in vivo* mutants; N1, N2, non-responsive *in vivo* mutants. NB Logarithmic scale

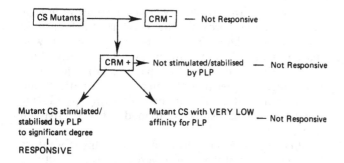

N.B. Ability to accumulate PLP <u>in vivo</u> may influence response to Pyridoxine <u>in vivo</u>

Figure 8 Summary of the mechanism of pyridoxine-responsive homocystinuria (CS deficiency)

activity in fibroblasts of 3 and 2% of control activity, respectively and who showed only a partial response to pyridoxine *in vivo* (Fowler, unpublished observations). Although preliminary, these data suggest that in these two patients, a lack of complete response to pyridoxine *in vivo* may be due to a reduced ability to synthesise or maintain high levels of PLP when receiving high doses of the vitamin.

CONCLUSIONS

Figure 8 shows a summary of our knowledge of pyridoxine responsiveness in homocystinuria due to CS deficiency, based on the findings described, some speculation and immunochemical studies of Skovby *et al.* (1982). These workers studied 20 CS-deficient cell lines by measuring cross-reacting material(CRM) with rabbit antiserum raised against the purified human liver CS. Seventeen cell lines had CRM and all except three of these had detectable residual CS activity. Three cell lines had no CRM and no residual CS activity. Although this study shows no correlation between pyridoxine responsiveness and the presence or absence of CRM it does provide the basis for the scheme shown here.

In final conclusion, there appears to be a correlation between clinical severity, pyridoxine responsiveness and the presence of residual CS activity in patients with homocystinuria due to CS deficiency.

References

Anderson, B. B., Newmark, P. A., Rawlins, M. and Green, R. Plasma binding of vitamin B_6 compounds. *Nature, Lond.* 250 (1974) 502–504

Bankier, A., Turner, M. and Hopkins, I. J. Pyridoxine dependent seizures—a wider clinical spectrum. *Arch. Dis. Child.* 58 (1983) 415–418

Boers, G. H. J., Smals, A. G. H., Drayer, J. I. M., Trijbels, F. J. M., Leermakers, A. I. and Kloppenberg, P. W. Pyridoxine treatment does not prevent homocystinemia after methionine loading in adult homocystinuric patients. *Metabolism* 32 (1983) 390–397

Chatagner, F., Gicquel, Y., Portemer, C. and Tixier, M. Inactivation of cystathionase and of cysteine sulphinic acid decarboxylase by proteolytic enzymes, effect of pyridoxal phosphate. *Experientia* 26 (1970) 602–604

Coburn, S. P. and Mahuren, J. D. A versatile cation-exchange procedure for measuring the seven major forms of vitamin B_6 in biological samples. *Analyt. Biochem.* 129 (1983) 310–317

Crowell, G. F. and Roach, E. S. Pyridoxine-dependent seizures. *Am. Fam. Phys.* 27 (1983) 183–187

Fleisher, L. D., Longhi, R. C., Tallan, H. H. and Gaull, G. E. Cystathionine β-synthase deficiency: Differences in thermostability between normal and abnormal enzyme from cultured human cells. *Pediatr. Res.* 12 (1978) 293–296

Fowler, B. Trans-sulphuration and methylation of homocysteine in control and mutant human fibroblasts. *Biochim. Biophys. Acta* 72 (1982) 201–207

Fowler, B., Kraus, J., Packman, S. and Rosenberg, L. E. Homocystinuria: Evidence for three distinct classes of cystathionine β-synthase mutants in cultured fibroblasts. *J. Clin. Invest.* 61 (1978) 645–653

Frimpter, G. W. Cystathioninuria: Nature of the defect. *Science* 149 (1965) 1095–1096

Gaull, G., Sturman, J. A. and Schaffner, F. Homocystinuria due to cystathionine synthase deficiency: Enzymatic and ultrastructural studies. *J. Pediatr.* 84 (1974) 381–390

Hamm, M. W., Mehansho, H. and Henderson, L. M. Transport and metabolism of pyridoxamine and pyridoxamine phosphate in the small intestine of the rat. *J. Nutr.* 109 (1979) 1552–1559

Hayasaka, S., Saito, T., Nakajima, H., Takaku, Y., Shiono, T., Mizuno, K., Ohmura, K. and Tada, K. Gyrate atrophy with hyperornithinaemia: different types of responsiveness to vitamin B_6. *Ophthalmology* 65 (1981) 478–483

Hunter, J. E. and Harper, A. E. Stability of some pyridoxal phosphate-dependent enzymes in vitamin B_6 deficient rats. *J. Nutr.* 106 (1976) 653–664

Kennaway, N. G., Weleber, R. G. and Buist, N. R. M. Gyrate atrophy of the choroid and retina with hyperornithinemia: Biochemical and histologic studies and response to vitamin B_6. *Am. J. Hum. Genet.* 32 (1980) 529–541

Kim, Y. J. and Rosenberg, L. E. On the mechanism of pyridoxine responsive homocystinuria. II. Properties of normal and mutant cystathionine β-synthase from cultured fibroblasts. *Proc. Natl. Acad. Sci. USA* 71 (1974) 4821–4825

Lipson, M. H., Kraus, J. and Rosenberg, L. E. Affinity of cystathionine β-synthase for pyridoxal 5'-phosphate in cultured cells. A mechanism for pyridoxine-responsive homocystinuria. *J. Clin. Invest.* 66 (1980a) 188–193

Lipson, M. H., Kraus, J., Solomon, L. R. and Rosenberg, L. E. Depletion of cultured human fibroblasts of pyridoxal 5'-phosphate: Effect on activities of aspartate aminotransferase, alanine aminotransferase, and cystathionine β-synthase. *Arch. Biochem. Biophys.* 204 (1980b) 486–493

Longhi, R. C., Fleisher, L. D., Tallan, H. H. and Gaull, G. E. Cystathionine β-synthase deficiency: A qualitative abnormality of the deficient enzyme modified by vitamin B_6 therapy. *Pediatr. Res.* 11 (1977) 100–103

Lui, A., Lumeng, L. and Li, T. Metabolism of vitamin B_6 in rat liver mitochondria. *J. Biol. Chem.* 256 (1981) 6041–6046

Lumeng, L., Lui, A. and Li, T. Plasma content of B_6 vitamers and its relationship to hepatic vitamin B_6 metabolism. *J. Clin. Invest.* 66 (1980) 688–695

Mehansho, H., Buss, D. D., Hamm, M. W. and Henderson, L. M. Transport and metabolism of pyridoxine in rat liver. *Biochim. Biophys. Acta* 631 (1980) 112–123

Mehansho, H., Hamm, M. W. and Henderson, L. M. Transport and metabolism of pyridoxal and pyridoxal phosphate in the small intestine of the rat. *J. Nutr.* 109 (1979) 1542–1551

Mehansho, H. and Henderson, L. M. Transport and accumulation of pyridoxine and pyridoxal by erythrocytes. *J. Biol. Chem.* 255 (1980) 11901–11907

Meister, A. *Biochemistry of the Amino Acids*, Academic Press, New York, 1965, pp. 380, 411

Mudd, S. H., Edwards, W. A., Loeb, P. M., Brown, M. S. and Laster, L. Homocystinuria due to cystathionine synthase deficiency: The effect of pyridoxine. *J. Clin. Invest.* 49 (1970) 1762–1773

Mudd, S. H. and Levy, H. L. Disorders of trans-sulfuration. In Stanbury, J. B., Wyngaarden, J. B., Fredrickson, D. S., Goldstein, J. L. and Brown, M. S. (eds.) *The Metabolic Basis of Inherited Disease*, 5th Edn., McGraw-Hill, New York, 1983, pp. 522–559

Mudd, S. H., Skovby, F., Levy, H., Pettigrew, K. D., Wilcken, B., Pyeritz, R. E., Andria, G., Boers, G. H. J., Bromberg, I. L., Cerone, R., Fowler, B., Grobe, H., Schmidt, H. and Schweitzer, L. The natural history of homocystinuria due to cystathionine β-synthase deficiency. *Am. J. Hum. Genet.* 37 (1985) 1–31

Okada, M. and Hirose, M. Regulation of aspartate aminotransferase activity associated with change of pyridoxal phosphate level. *Arch. Biochem. Biophys.* 193 (1979) 294–300

Pascal, T. A., Gaull, G. E., Beratis, N. G., Gillam, B. M. and Tallan, H. H. Cystathionase deficiency: Evidence for genetic heterogeneity in primary cystathioninuria. *Pediatr. Res.* 12 (1978) 125–133

Scriver, C. R. Vitamin B$_6$ deficiency and dependency in man. *Am. J. Dis. Child.* 113 (1967) 109–114

Scriver, C. R. and Hutchison, J. H. The vitamin B$_6$ deficiency

syndrome in human infancy: Biochemical and clinical observations. *Pediatrics* 31 (1963) 240–250

Seashore, M. R., Durant, J. L. and Rosenberg, L. E. Studies of the mechanism of pyridoxine-responsive homocystinuria. *Pediatr. Res.* 6 (1972) 187–196

Shih, V. E., Berson, E. L., Mandell, R. and Schmidt, S. Y. Ornithine ketoacid transaminase deficiency in gyrate atrophy of the choroid and retina. *Am. J. Hum. Genet.* 30 (1978) 174–179

Skovby, F., Kraus, J., Redlich, C. and Rosenberg, L. E. Immunochemical studies on cultured fibroblasts from patients with homocystinuria due to cystathionine β-synthase deficiency. *Am. J. Hum. Genet.* 34 (1982) 73–83

Skovby, F., Kraus, J. and Rosenberg, L. E. Homocystinuria: Biogenesis of cystathionine β-synthase subunits in cultured fibroblasts and in an *in vitro* translation system programmed with fibroblast messenger RNA. *Am. J. Hum. Genet.* 36 (1984) 452–459

Snape, B. M., Badawy, A. B. and Evans, M. Stabilization of rat liver tyrosine aminotransferase *in vivo* by pyridoxine administration. *Biochem. J.* 186 (1980) 625–627

Tada, K., Yokoyama, Y., Nakagawa, H. and Arakawa, T. Vitamin B$_6$ dependent xanthurenic aciduria. *Tohoku J. Exp. Med.* 95 (1968) 107–114

Uhlendorf, B. W., Conerly, E. B. and Mudd, S. H. Homocystinuria: Studies in tissue culture. *Pediatr. Res.* 7 (1973) 645–658

Williams, H. E. and Smith, Jr., L. H. Primary hyperoxaluria. In Stanbury, J. B., Wyngaarden, J. B., Fredrickson, D. S., Goldstein, J. L. and Brown, M. S. (eds.) *The Metabolic Basis of Inherited Disease*, 5th Edn., McGraw-Hill, New York, 1983, pp. 204–228

J. Inher. Metab. Dis. 8 Suppl. 1 (1985) 84–87

Vitamin E and Muscle Diseases

M. J. JACKSON*, D. A. JONES and R. H. T. EDWARDS*

Department of Medicine, University College London School of Medicine, The Rayne Institute, University Street, London WC1, UK

Studies of the basic biochemical mechanisms underlying muscle damage aimed at finding agents which might reduce the amount of damage occurring in muscular dystrophy and other severe myopathies have been performed. These have suggested three types of agent which might be useful for this purpose, namely calcium antagonists, phospholipase inhibitors, and antioxidants or scavengers of reactive-free radicals. Vitamin E falls into the latter of these three categories and has been shown to reduce the amount of damage which occurs in isolated skeletal muscles following a given stress. It is suggested that, in the absence of calcium antagonists having relatively specific and effective actions on skeletal muscle or suitable inhibitors of muscle phospholipases in man, therapy with vitamin E or other antioxidants may reduce the amount of muscle damage occurring in patients with severe myopathies.

The genetically inherited muscular dystrophies are chronic degenerative diseases of muscle which, in the most severe form (Duchenne), usually result in death in the second or third decade of life. All attempts to modify therapeutically the expression of the defective gene in patients have been limited by a lack of knowledge of the nature of the basic biochemical defect in these disorders. It has been recognised for a number of years that the severe forms of the muscular dystrophies share many characteristics with vitamin E deficiency myopathy in animals (Bicknell, 1940); however, several investigators have been unable to demonstrate any evidence for abnormal vitamin E levels in patients (e.g. see Jackson *et al.*, 1984a) nor has short-term vitamin E treatment been shown to be beneficial to patients (Fitzgerald and McArdle, 1941; Walton and Nattrass, 1954).

One approach to therapy in these diseases would be to reduce the amount of damage to the muscle fibres which results from the basic genetic defect. This requires a knowledge of the biochemical mechanisms underlying muscle damage and to this end we have been studying these mechanisms using an *in vitro* preparation. These studies have revived the possibility that vitamin E therapy might be useful in reducing the extent of muscle damage and hence that a longer term trial of vitamins in patients with degenerative muscle diseases may be worthwhile.

The aim of this paper is to briefly review these studies of the mechanisms of muscle damage and to consider their possible implications for treatment aimed at reducing muscle damage *in vivo*.

MODEL SYSTEMS FOR THE STUDY OF MUSCLE DAMAGE

Despite extensive use of isolated heart preparations to study damage to cardiac muscle there have been relatively few studies using skeletal muscle. Those studies which have been undertaken have primarily relied on only one indicator of the extent of the damage, i.e. either histological and electron microscopic appearance (Duncan, 1978; Publicover *et al.*, 1978) changes in the rate of protein breakdown (e.g. Rodemann *et al.*, 1981) or variations in the rate of efflux of cytoplasmic enzymes (Dawson, 1966; Suarez-Kurtz and Eastwood, 1981). We have developed a system which utilises small mouse soleus or extensor digitorum longus muscles from which the release of intracellular components can be measured as an index of damage (Jones *et al.*, 1983) but muscles for this system can also be taken for examination of their electron microscopic appearance (Jones *et al.*, 1984).

EVIDENCE FOR A ROLE OF VITAMIN E

Addition of vitamin E to perfusion fluids surrounding cardiac muscle preparations has previously been shown to protect them against hypoxic trauma (Guarnieri *et al.*, 1978) but we were unable to demonstrate any similar effect on skeletal muscle. Vitamin E was added to the medium surrounding isolated mouse soleus muscles subjected to damaging excessive contractile activity but no protective effect was seen (Jackson *et al.*, 1983). However, when muscles from mice of differing vitamin E status were used vitamin E-supplemented animals exhibited a dramatic reduction in the damage which occurred following the same amount of contractile activity (Figure 1). In this same piece of work it was also shown that the vitamin E status of a rat influenced its susceptibility to damage resulting from contractile activity *in vivo*, a finding which is supported by the work of Quintanilha and Packer (1983), who have studied the effect of vitamin E status on damage to subcellular organelles during physical exercise. They have also demonstrated a dramatic protective effect of supplemental oral vitamin E in their experiments.

These results suggest that vitamin E supplements may reduce the extent of damage to skeletal muscle but that an increased circulating level within the plasma is unlikely to be effective.

---

*Present address: University Department of Medicine, Royal Liverpool Hospital, P.O. Box 147, Liverpool L69 3BX, UK

Journal of Inherited Metabolic Disease. ISSN 0141–8955. Copyright © SSIEM and MTP Press Limited, Queen Square, Lancaster, UK.

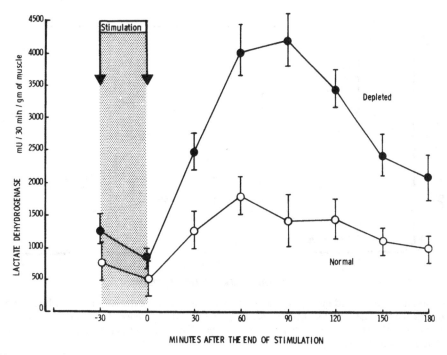

Figure 1 Efflux of intracellular lactate dehydrogenase from soleus muscles of mice fed a low vitamin E diet (●) or the same diet supplemented with vitamin E(○), stimulated for 30 min in oxygenated medium. The efflux from muscles of the vitamin E-depleted mice was significantly ($p < 0.001$) greater than that from the control group, at all times after the end of stimulation. Reprinted with permission from Jackson *et al.* (1983)

STUDIES OF THE GENERAL MECHANISMS UNDERLYING MUSCLE DAMAGE

Most of the work on mechanisms of muscle damage has concentrated on the role which calcium plays in this process. A raised intracellular calcium content has been described in Duchenne muscular dystrophy (Bodenstein and Engel, 1978; Maunder-Sewry *et al.*, 1980; Bertorini *et al.*, 1982) and experiments with the calcium ionophore A23187 and caffeine have demonstrated that increased intracellular levels of calcium can lead to disruption of the internal structure of the muscle fibre (Duncan, 1978). Furthermore, it has also been shown that increasing the extracellular calcium concentration augments the leakage of enzymes from mouse muscle (Soybell *et al.*, 1978). We have shown that the enzyme efflux and ultrastructural damage seen after excessive contractile activity were markedly reduced when the extracellular calcium was withdrawn (Figure 2). Low extracellular calcium also protected against the large enzyme efflux seen after treatment with low concentrations of detergent (Jones *et al.*, 1984).

These data imply that an influx of external calcium occurs during the damaging process and that this induces further biochemical changes leading to damage. There has been considerable speculation concerning the mechanism by which this excess intracellular calcium induces damage. We have recently obtained evidence that one of the sequelae of calcium accumulation involves activation of membrane-bound phospholipases (Jackson *et al.*, 1984b), probably phospholipase A_2. An increase in the products of phospholipase activity would mean liberation of free fatty acids from the membrane

phospholipids and the appearance of lysophospholipids within the membrane bilayer. Both of these would be deleterious to the membrane. This is likely to be the area where vitamin E plays a protective role since its function is thought to be as a stabilising component of membranes (Diplock, 1982) and as a non-specific antioxidant preventing free radical mediated peroxidation of lipids (Tappel, 1962). The free fatty acids liberated into the cytoplasm away from the protective effect of membrane-bound vitamin E may therefore be more susceptible to free radical-mediated lipid peroxidation (Gutteridge, 1977; Jain and Shohet, 1981).

PROPOSED SCHEME FOR THE BIOCHEMICAL MECHANISMS UNDERLYING MUSCLE DAMAGE

These studies using *in vitro* muscle preparations have led us to propose a scheme for the biochemical mechanisms underlying muscle damage, which is shown in Figure 3 and on which is also shown the various points at which vitamin E may exert a controlling action.

IMPLICATIONS OF THESE STUDIES FOR THERAPY IN PATIENTS WITH DEGENERATIVE MUSCLE DISEASE

The *in vitro* studies suggest that agents having one or more of the following actions may reduce muscle damage in patients:

(1) Inhibition of calcium movements into muscle cells.
(2) Inhibition of muscle phospholipase activity.

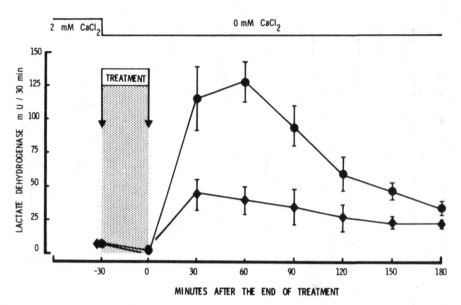

Figure 2 Enzyme release from stimulated muscles in the presence and absence of external calcium. Muscles were stimulated under hypoxic conditions during the treatment period. Muscles were incubated in the presence of $CaCl_2$ throughout the experiment (●) or in calcium-free medium from the start of the treatment period (◆). Reprinted by permission from Jones *et al.* (1984), p. 318. Copyright © 1984 The Biochemical Society, London

(3) Scavenging of free radicals and inhibition of lipid peroxidation.

Vitamin E falls primarily into the third of these categories although it may also influence the plasma membrane permeability to calcium. It therefore seems reasonable to attempt a long-term therapeutic trial of this agent in patients with muscle diseases. A long-term trial may be necessary because most trials of vitamin E therapy in myopathic disorders have been of a relatively short duration (Fitzgerald and McArdle, 1941; Walton

and Nattrass, 1954; Edwards *et al.*, 1984) whereas in the only human disorder where vitamin E has been shown to be an effective treatment (i.e. abetalipoproteinaemia) therapy was continued for several years before benefit was seen (Muller *et al.*, 1983).

The authors should like to thank Dr E. J. Harris and Dr D. P. Brenton for helpful discussions, Miss C. Forte for the excellent technical assistance and the Muscular Dystrophy Group of Great Britain for financial support.

PROPOSED MECHANISMS OF MUSCLE DAMAGE

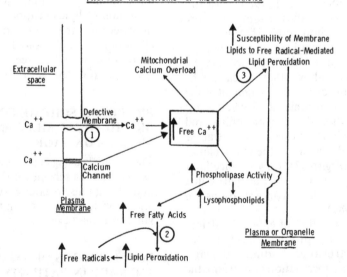

Figure 3 It is proposed that an influx of external calcium raises the free intracellular calcium level. This leads to a breakdown of membrane organisation either by altering the conformation of membranes making them more susceptible to free radical-mediated lipid peroxidation or by activation of membrane bound phospholipases. This latter process may also lead to increased free radical mediated peroxidation of the liberated fatty acids. Vitamin E may exert a controlling role over this process at the three numbered sites: (1) Stabilisation of membranes reducing calcium influx. (2) Inhibition of free radical-mediated peroxidation of lipids liberated by phospholipase activity. (3) Prevention of calcium-induced increase in susceptibility of membrane lipids to free radical-mediated peroxidation

References

Bertorini, T. E., Bhattacharya, S. K., Palmieri, G. M. A., Chesney, C. M., Pifer, D. and Baker, B. Muscle calcium and magnesium content in Duchenne muscular dystrophy. *Neurology* 32 (1982) 1088–1092

Bicknell, F. Vitamin E in the treatment of muscular dystrophies and nervous diseases. *Lancet* i (1940) 10–13

Bodenstein, J. B. and Engel, A. G. Intracellular calcium accumulation in Duchenne dystrophy and other myopathies: a study of 567000 muscle fibres in 114 biopsies. *Neurology* 28 (1978) 439–446

Dawson, D. M. Efflux of enzymes from chicken muscle. *Biochim. Biophys. Acta* 113 (1966) 144–157

Diplock, A. T. The modulating influence of vitamin E in biological membrane unsaturated phospholipid metabolism. *Acta Vit. Enzymol.* 4 (1982) 303–309

Duncan, C. J. Role of intracellular calcium in promoting muscle damage: a strategy for controlling the dystrophic condition. *Experientia* 34 (1978) 1531–1535

Edwards, R. H. T., Jones, D. A. and Jackson, M. J. An approach to treatment trials in muscular dystrophy with particular reference to agents influencing free radial damage. *Med. Biol.* 62 (1984) 143–147

Fitzgerald, G. and McArdle, B. Vitamin E and B$_6$ in the treatment of muscular dystrophy and motor neurone disease. *Brain* 64 (1941) 19–42

Guarnieri, C., Ferrari, R., Visioli, O., Caldarera, C. M. and Nayler, W. G. Effect of α-tocopherol on hypoxic-perfused and reoxygenated rabbit heart muscle. *J. Molec. Cell. Cardiol.* 10 (1978) 893–906

Gutteridge, J. M. C. The effect of calcium on phospholipid peroxidation. *Biochem. Biophys. Commun.* 74 (1977) 529–537

Jackson, M. J., Jones, D. A. and Edwards, R. H. T. Vitamin E and skeletal muscle. In *Ciba Foundation Symposium Series No. 101. Biology of Vitamin E*, Pitman Press, London, 1983, pp. 224–239

Jackson, M. J., Jones, D. A. and Edwards, R. H. T. Techniques for studying free radical damage in muscular dystrophy. *Med. Biol.* 62 (1984a) 135–138

Jackson, M. J., Jones, D. A. and Edwards, R. H. T. Experimental skeletal muscle damage: the nature of the calcium-activated degenerative processes. *Eur. J. Clin. Invest.* 14 (1984b) 366–374

Jain, S. K. and Shohet, S. B. Calcium potentiates the peroxidation of erythrocyte membrane lipids. *Biochim. Biophys. Acta* 642 (1981) 46–54

Jones, D. A., Jackson, M. J. and Edwards, R. H. T. Release of intracellular enzymes from an isolated mammalian skeletal muscle preparation. *Clin. Sci.* 65 (1983) 193–201

Jones, D. A., Jackson, M. J., McPhail, G. and Edwards, R. H. T. Experimental mouse muscle damage: the importance of external calcium. *Clin. Sci.* 66 (1984) 317–322

Maunder-Sewry, C. A., Gorodetsky, R., Yaron, R. and Dubowitz, V. Elemental analysis of skeletal muscle in Duchenne muscular dystrophy using X-ray fluorescence spectrometry. *Muscle and Nerve* 3 (1980) 502–508

Muller, D. P. R., Lloyd, J. K. and Wolf, O. H. Vitamin E and neurological function: abetalipoproteinaemia and other disorders of fat absorption. In *Ciba Foundation Symposium Series No. 101. Biology of Vitamin E*, Pitman Press, London, 1983, pp. 106–121

Publicover, S. J., Duncan, C. J. and Smith, J. L. The use of A23187 to demonstrate the role of intracellular calcium in causing ultrastructural damage in mammalian muscle. *J. Neuropath. Exp. Neurol.* 37 (1978) 544–557

Quintanilha, A. T. and Packer, L. Vitamin E, physical exercise and tissue oxidative damage. In *Ciba Foundation Symposium Series No. 101. Biology of Vitamin E*, Pitman Press, London, 1983, pp. 56–69

Rodemann, H. P., Waxman, L. and Goldberg, A. L. The stimulation of protein degradation in muscle by Ca^{2+} is mediated by prostaglandin E_2 and does not require the calcium activated protease. *J. Biol. Chem.* 257 (1981) 8716–8723

Soybell, D., Morgan, J. and Cohen, L. Calcium augmentation of enzyme leakage from mouse skeletal muscle and its possible site of action. *Res. Commun. Chem. Pathol. Pharmacol.* 20 (1978) 317–329

Suarez-Kurtz, G. and Eastwood, A. B. Release of sarcoplasmic enzymes from frog skeletal muscle. *Am. J. Physiol.* 241 (1981) C98–C105

Tappel, L. Vitamin E as the biological lipid antioxidant. *Vitamins and Hormones* 20 (1962) 493–510

Walton, J. N. and Nattrass, F. J. On the classification, natural history and treatment of the myopathies. *Brain* 77 (1954) 169–231

J. Inher. Metab. Dis. 8 Suppl. 1 (1985) 88–92

The Role of Vitamin E in the Treatment of the Neurological Features of Abetalipoproteinaemia and Other Disorders of Fat Absorption

D. P. R. MULLER[1], J. K. LLOYD[2] and O. H. WOLFF[1]
[1]*Institute of Child Health, 30 Guilford Street, London WC1N 1EH, UK*
[2]*St. Georges Hospital Medical School, Cranmer Terrace, London SW17 0RE, UK*

Studies in patients with abetalipoproteinaemia and other chronic and severe fat malabsorptive states, and neuropathological studies in the vitamin E-deficient human, monkey and rat indicate that vitamin E is important for normal neurological function. Appropriate vitamin E supplementation is, therefore, advisable for all patients with chronic fat malabsorption who have low serum vitamin E concentrations.

Vitamin E was discovered in 1922 by Evans and Bishop when they found that a fat-soluble factor was necessary for normal reproduction in the rat. Since that time a number of vitamin E-deficient syndromes have been produced experimentally in several animal species (Wasserman and Taylor, 1972) but with the possible exception of haemolytic anaemia in some premature infants (Oski and Barness, 1967; Ritchie *et al.*, 1968; Bell and Filer, 1981), the role of vitamin E in human nutrition has remained disputed. A major reason for the discrepancy between human and animal studies has been the difficulty in achieving total deficiency in humans.

Vitamin E is a highly hydrophobic fat-soluble compound and serum concentrations tend to be reduced in disorders of fat absorption (Muller *et al.*, 1974). The most severe deficiency reported in man occurs in abetalipoproteinaemia, where the vitamin is undetectable in serum (Kayden *et al.*, 1965; Muller *et al.*, 1974). A deficiency of vitamin E that is almost as severe occurs in certain other chronic disorders of fat absorption, especially those associated with a reduced intraluminal concentration of bile salts which are necessary for the efficient solubilization and absorption of vitamin E (Harries and Muller, 1971). Such conditions therefore provide useful models for investigating the role of vitamin E in human nutrition.

Three lines of evidence will be presented which indicate that vitamin E has an important role in the maintenance of normal neurological structure and function: studies in patients with abetalipoproteinaemia; studies in patients with other severe and chronic disorders of fat absorption; and comparative neuropathological studies in man and animals.

ABETALIPOPROTEINAEMIA (McKUSICK 20010)

Abetalipoproteinaemia is a rare inborn error of lipoprotein metabolism (Herbert *et al.*, 1978) which is inherited in an autosomal recessive mode. From birth, patients have steatorrhoea and spiky red cells (acanthocytes) and they typically develop a severe and progressive ataxic neuropathy and pigmentary retinopathy toward the end of the first decade of life. The primary abnormality is an absence of apoprotein B (Gotto *et al.*, 1971) which is an essential component of chylomicrons, low density lipoprotein and very low density lipoprotein. All these lipoproteins are absent from the serum of affected patients, resulting in greatly reduced concentrations of serum lipids. Chylomicrons are necessary for the absorption of vitamin E and low density lipoprotein is an important carrier of the vitamin; the absence of these lipoproteins results therefore in the severe deficiency of vitamin E.

The neurologic and retinal features of abetalipoproteinaemia were comprehensively reviewed by Herbert *et al.* (1978) who concluded that they were "devastating", that at least a third of affected children had developed a symptomatic, neurologic disorder before the age of 10 years and that virtually all had ataxia by the age of 20. There have been no reports of spontaneous improvement of neurological function in untreated patients. A hypothesis to explain the pathogenesis of the neurological features is that they result from a prolonged deficiency of a fat-soluble compound normally transported by an apoprotein B-containing lipoprotein. Vitamin E could be such a substance, especially as neurological lesions have been described in the vitamin E-deficient rat and monkey (Wasserman and Taylor, 1972; Nelson *et al.*, 1981) and the vitamin E-deficient chick develops a cerebellar disorder with ataxia (Pappenheimer and Goettsch, 1931). We therefore decided to treat children with abetalipoproteinaemia with very large oral doses of vitamin E (approximately $100\,mg\,kg^{-1}\,day^{-1}$ of tocopheryl acetate [Ephynal], supplied by Hoffmann-La Roche and Co.) and have now followed eight patients who have been receiving such therapy for periods of 12–18 years. Vitamin E status has been assessed by estimating serum concentrations and by *in vitro* tests of red cell haemolysis (autohaemolysis or peroxide haemolysis), as described previously (Muller *et al.*, 1974).

After supplementation with large oral doses of vitamin E, absorption could be demonstrated in all eight

Journal of Inherited Metabolic Disease. ISSN 0141-8955. Copyright © SSIEM and MTP Press Limited, Queen Square, Lancaster, UK.

patients. A summary of the pre- and post-treatment serum vitamin E concentrations and *in vitro* haemolysis values is given in Table 1. In all patients the serum concentrations, which were initially undetectable, became measurable after supplementation, though they never reached the normal range because of the absence of low density lipoprotein. *In vitro* haemolysis was abnormally high in all patients in whom it was measured before treatment, and was within normal limits in all eight patients after supplementation.

The long-term clinical results of vitamin E therapy in the eight patients have been reported in detail elsewhere (Muller *et al.*, 1977; Muller and Lloyd, 1982). The five patients who first received vitamin E supplements before the age of 16 months all attend normal schools and show no clinical abnormalities; motor nerve conduction studies and electrodiagnostic tests of retinal function remain normal. The three other patients (Table 2) already showed some neurological dysfunction before supplementation with vitamin E in later childhood.

Patient 6* had absent tendon reflexes when diagnosed at 18 months of age. He received vitamin E from the age of 3 years. At 11 years he had slight diminution in vibration sense in all limbs and by 18 he had minimal reduction in proprioception in the limbs and a slight reduction of the action potential in the sural and radial nerve but no other neurological or retinal abnormalities have developed. He now works in a car body repair workshop and attends a college of further education.

Patient 7 was initially reported by Salt *et al.* (1960), when it was first demonstrated that β-lipoprotein (low density lipoprotein) was absent in this clinical syndrome. Her parents had reduced serum lipid and low density lipoprotein concentrations and she, therefore, probably has homozygous hypobetalipoproteinaemia which is inherited as an autosomal dominant (Herbert *et al.*, 1978; Muller and Lloyd, 1982) rather than classical abetalipoproteinaemia. The two conditions appear to be clinically and biochemically indistinguishable. At

---

*Case numbers are the same as in previous reports (Muller *et al.*, 1977, 1983; Muller and Lloyd, 1982)

diagnosis at the age of 18 months she had absent tendon reflexes; at 5 years she developed a mild pigmentary retinopathy, even though normal serum concentrations of vitamin E had been maintained. Since the start of vitamin E supplementation at 8 years, the retinal appearance has remained unchanged. She is now 26 years of age and has no neurological or visual symptoms; retinal function is normal and the only neurological findings are absent tendon reflexes and a slight reduction in the sural nerve action potential. She is a secondary school teacher with a university degree and has recently married.

The eldest patient is now 28 years old (patient 8). He was diagnosed at 7 years and first received vitamin E at the age of 10, by which time he already had marked ataxia, absent tendon reflexes, delayed motor nerve conduction velocities, a pigmentary retinopathy and abnormal retinal function. Within 2 years of starting vitamin E supplementation his gait, motor nerve conduction velocities and the electro-oculogram had improved, although his fundal appearances remained unchanged and his tendon reflexes absent. Since then there has been further improvement in his gait, and his motor nerve conduction velocities and retinal function tests have returned to normal. He is currently employed making furniture in a sheltered workshop and is able to drive a car.

Other investigators have subsequently reported the beneficial effects of large doses of vitamin E in abetalipoproteinaemia (Herbert *et al.*, 1978; Azizi *et al.*, 1978; Miller *et al.*, 1980; Malloy *et al.*, 1981).

OTHER CHRONIC DISORDERS OF FAT ABSORPTION

Any chronic disorder of fat absorption, and in particular those conditions with a reduction in intraluminal bile salt concentrations, may be expected to have an associated severe deficiency of vitamin E with the development of similar neurological findings to those described in abetalipoproteinaemia. A number of such reports have now appeared (e.g. Rosenblum *et al.*, 1981;

Table 1 Long-term response to oral vitamin E in abetalipoproteinaemia

Patient*	Oral vitamin E (mg kg^{-1} day^{-1})	Serum vitamin E (µmol l^{-1})		In vitro RBC haemolysis (%)	
		Before	After†	Before	After‡
1	65–122	0	4.8	93 ‖	0 ‖
2	64–172	0	6.9	15 §	0 ‖
3	90–100	0	4.6	ND	5 ‖
4	47–100	0	3.0	33 §	0 ‖
5	70–105	0	6.9	85 ‖	0 ‖
6	53–105	0	4.6	15 §	0 ‖
7	25–86	0	5.5	17 §	0 ‖
8	33–144	0	4.1	33 ‖	10 ‖
Normal		11.5–35.0		< 5 §	< 10 ‖

ND, not done
*Case numbers are the same as in the previous reports (Muller *et al.*, 1977, 1983; Muller and Lloyd, 1982)
†Maximum concentration
‡Minimum percentage
§Autohaemolysis
‖Peroxide haemolysis

Table 2 Long-term progress in abetalipoproteinaemia: patients starting vitamin E in later childhood

| Patient* | Age at diagnosis (yr) | Age at start of vitamin E (yr) | Age at examination (yr) | Clinical features | Neurological status | | Visual function |
					Nerve conduction	Ophthalmoscopy	
6	1½	13½	1½	Absent tendon reflexes	Normal	Normal	Normal
			11	Reduced vibration sense	Reduced sensory action potential	Normal	Normal
			18	Reduced proprioception	Unchanged	Normal	Normal
7	1½	8¾	1½	Absent tendon reflexes	Normal	Normal	Normal
			5	Unchanged	Normal	Slight retinal pigmentation	Normal
			23	Unchanged	Reduced sural action potential	Unchanged	Normal
8	7¼	10¼	7¼	Absent tendon reflexes ataxic	Not done	Pigmentary retinopathy	Not done
			10	Reflexes unchanged, ataxia worse	Reduced motor nerve conduction velocities	Unchanged	Abnormal electro-diagnostic tests
			12	Reflexes unchanged, ataxia improved	Normal	Unchanged	Improved
			17	Reflexes unchanged, ataxia improved	Normal	Unchanged	Normal
			25	Reflexes unchanged, ataxia improved	Normal	Unchanged	Normal

*Case numbers are the same as in the previous reports (Muller *et al.*, 1977, 1983; Muller and Lloyd, 1982)

Elias *et al.*, 1981; Guggenheim *et al.*, 1982, 1983; Alvarez *et al.*, 1983). In some patients, supplements of vitamin E which typically have had to be given by intramuscular injection, have resulted in marked clinical improvement.

The majority of reported patients have been children with cholestatic liver disease with intra- or extrahepatic biliary atresia. Howard *et al.* (1982), however, described a 64-year-old man who had multiple resections for Crohn's disease and chronic steatorrhoea, who developed ataxia and a visual field defect with pigmentary degeneration of the retina. Only trace amounts of vitamin E were detectable in his serum and vitamin E therapy over a 2 year period corrected both the visual field defect and the ataxia.

We have studied 10 patients with a spinocerebellar disorder, undetectable or trace concentrations of serum vitamin E and an interrupted enterohepatic circulation of bile salts. Six of these patients, all adults, have been described in detail elsewhere (Elias *et al.*, 1981; Harding *et al.*, 1982). Two had chronic cholestatic liver disease, two had cystic fibrosis and two had multiple ileal resections. Long-term vitamin E therapy has led to marked clinical improvement in two of these patients (case 1 of Elias *et al.*, 1981, and case 2 of Harding *et al.*, 1982). Of the other four patients, two had cystic fibrosis together with complications (multiple intestinal resections and chronic active hepatitis, respectively) which would further impair fat malabsorption. The other two patients were a 70-year-old male who, 10 years

previously, had 23 ft of bowel removed for Crohn's disease, and a 14-year-old boy with a congenital rubella syndrome, congenital glaucoma and intrahepatic biliary atresia.

NEUROPATHOLOGICAL STUDIES

Neuropathological studies have been reported in the vitamin E-deficient human, rat and monkey. In all three species degeneration of the axons of the posterior columns and a selective loss of large calibre myelinated sensory axons in the spinal cord and peripheral nerves, which is particularly severe in the posterior columns, has been reported (Nelson *et al.*, 1981). As a result of these observations, Nelson *et al.* (1981) suggested that chronic and severe vitamin E deficiency in the rat, monkey and human leads to degeneration and loss of sensory axons in the posterior columns, sensory roots, and peripheral nerves. He also postulated that this degeneration results from axonal membrane injury and then develops as a distal and dying-back type of axonopathy.

Additional evidence to support a causal relationship between vitamin E deficiency and neurological lesions comes from the observations of Sung (1964) and Sung *et al.* (1980). They found that the incidence at necropsy of axonal dystrophy in the gracile nucleus of patients with cystic fibrosis who died between 1970 and 1980 was lower than that for similar patients dying between 1952 and 1969. This fall coincided with the introduction of vitamin E supplementation into the management of patients with cystic fibrosis in the mid-1960s.

TREATMENT WITH VITAMIN E

We believe that the evidence linking vitamin E deficiency with neurological abnormalities is now sufficiently strong to recommend vitamin E supplementation for all patients with chronic fat malabsorption who have reduced serum concentrations of the vitamin. It is, however, essential that the vitamin is administered appropriately. In patients with abetalipoproteinaemia it is necessary to give very large oral doses of about $100 \, \text{mg} \, \text{kg}^{-1} \, \text{day}^{-1}$ if an adequate vitamin E status is to be achieved. In patients with greatly reduced luminal bile salt concentrations, it is likely that oral preparations will not be absorbed and that the vitamin will have to be given intramuscularly. Before, however, embarking on long-term, regular, intramuscular treatment it is our practice to assess intestinal absorption by giving a large oral load of tocopheryl acetate (1–2 g) and monitoring serum concentrations of the vitamin at regular intervals over the following 24 h. If there is evidence of absorption, as judged by a significant increase in serum concentrations, large oral doses are given and serum levels carefully monitored to ensure that normal concentrations are reached. If no absorption of the oral load can be shown, intramuscular therapy needs to be given.

CONCLUSIONS

The evidence from the long-term study of patients with abetalipoproteinaemia and other conditions with chronic fat malabsorption, together with neuropathological data from the vitamin E-deficient rat, monkey and human, strongly suggests that vitamin E is essential for normal neurological structure and function. If patients with fat malabsorption have low serum vitamin E concentrations it is important to initiate appropriate vitamin E therapy, with the aim of restoring and maintaining normal serum concentrations and preventing long-term neurological disability. This problem is likely to become more frequent with the increasing survival of patients with chronic fat malabsorptive states. In addition, it may be advisable to measure serum vitamin E concentrations in all patients with spinocerebellar disorders, whatever the aetiology.

D.P.R.M. is grateful to Hoffmann-La Roche and Co. for continued financial support and interest.

References

Alvarez, F., Landrieu, P., Laget, P., Lemonnier, F., Odievre, M. and Alagille, D. Nervous and ocular disorders in children with cholestasis and vitamin A and E deficiencies. *Hepatology* 3 (1983) 410–414

Azizi, E., Zaidman, J. L., Eschar, J. and Szeinberg, A. Abetalipoproteinaemia treated with parenteral and oral vitamin A and E and with medium chain triglycerides. *Acta Pediatr. Scand.* 67 (1978) 797–801

Bell, E. F. and Filer, L. J. The role of vitamin E in the nutrition of premature infants. *Am. J. Clin. Nutr.* 34 (1981) 414–422

Elias, E., Muller, D. P. R. and Scott, J. Association of spinocerebellar disorders with cystic fibrosis or chronic childhood cholestasis and very low serum vitamin E. *Lancet* 2 (1981) 1319–1321

Evans, H. M. and Bishop, K. S. On the existence of a hitherto unrecognized dietary factor essential for reproduction. *Science (Wash DC)* 56 (1922) 650–651

Gotto, A. M., Levy, R. I., John, K. and Fredrickson, D. S. On the nature of the protein defect in abetalipoproteinaemia. *N. Engl. J. Med.* 284 (1971) 813–818

Guggenheim, M. A., Jackson, V., Lilly, J. and Silverman, A. Vitamin E deficiency and neurologic disease in children with cholestasis: a prospective study. *J. Pediatr.* 102 (1983) 577–579

Guggenheim, M. A., Ringel, S. P., Silverman, A. and Grabert, B. E. Progressive neuromuscular disease in children with chronic cholestasis and vitamin E deficiency: diagnosis and treatment with alpha tocopherol. *J. Pediatr.* 100 (1982) 51–58

Harding, A. E., Muller, D. P. R., Thomas, P. K. and Willison, H. J. Spinocerebellar degeneration secondary to chronic intestinal malabsorption. A vitamin E deficiency syndrome. *Ann. Neurol.* 12 (1982) 419–424

Harries, J. T. and Muller, D. P. R. Absorption of vitamin E in children with biliary obstruction. *Gut* 12 (1971) 579–584

Herbert, P. N., Gotto, A. M. and Fredrickson, D. S. Familial lipoprotein deficiency. In Stanbury, J. B., Wyngaarden, J. B. and Fredrickson, D. S. (eds.) *The Metabolic Basis of Inherited Diseases*, 4th Edn., McGraw-Hill, New York, 1978, pp. 544–588

Howard, L., Ovesen, L., Satya-Murti, S. and Chu, R. Reversible neurological symptoms caused by vitamin E deficiency in a patient with short bowel syndrome. *Am. J. Clin. Nutr.* 36 (1982) 1243–1249

Kayden, H. J., Silber, R. and Kossmann, C. E. The role of vitamin E deficiency in the abnormal autohemolysis of acanthocytosis. *Trans. Assoc. Am. Phys.* 78 (1965) 334–342

Malloy, M. J., Kane, J. P., Hardman, D. A., Hamilton, R. L. and Dalal, K. B. Normotriglyceridemic abetalipoproteinaemia. Absence of the B-100 apolipoprotein. *J. Clin. Invest.* 67 (1981) 1441–1450

Miller, R. G., Davis, C. J. F., Illingworth, D. R. and Bradley, W. The neuropathy of abetalipoproteinaemia. *Neurology* 30 (1980) 1286–1291

Muller, D. P. R., Harries, J. T. and Lloyd, J. K. The relative importance of the factors involved in the absorption of vitamin E in children. *Gut* 15 (1974) 966–971

Muller, D. P. R. and Lloyd, J. K. Effect of large oral doses of vitamin E on the neurological sequelae of patients with abetalipoproteinaemia. *Ann. N.Y. Acad. Sci.* 393 (1982) 133–144

Muller, D. P. R., Lloyd, J. K. and Bird, A. C. The long-term management of abetalipoproteinaemia. Possible role for vitamin E. *Arch. Dis. Child.* 52 (1977) 209–214

Muller, D. P. R., Lloyd, J. K. and Wolff, O. H. Vitamin E and neurological function. *Lancet* 1 (1983) 225–228

Nelson, J. S., Fitch, C. D., Fischer, V. W., Brown, G. O., Jr and Chou, A. C. Progressive neuropathologic lesions in vitamin E-deficient rhesus monkeys. *J. Neuropathol. Exp. Neurol.* 40 (1981) 166–186

Oski, F. A. and Barness, L. A. Vitamin E deficiency, a previously unrecognized cause of hemolytic anemia in the premature infant. *J. Pediatr.* 70 (1967) 211–220

Pappenheimer, A. M. and Goettsch, M. A cerebellar disorder

in chicks, apparently of nutritional origin. *J. Exp. Med.* 53 (1931) 11–26

Ritchie, J. H., Fish, M. B., McMasters, V. and Grossman, M. Edema and hemolytic anemia in premature infants: a vitamin E deficiency syndrome. *N. Engl. J. Med.* 279 (1968) 1185–1190

Rosenblum, J. L., Keating, J. P., Prensky, A. L. and Nelson, J. S. A progressive neurologic syndrome in children with chronic liver disease. *N. Engl. J. Med.* 304 (1981) 503–508

Salt, H. B., Wolff, O. H., Lloyd, J. K., Fosbrooke, A. S., Cameron, A. H. and Hubble, D. V. On having no beta-lipoprotein. A syndrome comprising a-beta-lipoprotein-

aemia, acanthocytosis and steatorrhoea. *Lancet* 2 (1960) 325–329

Sung, J. H. Neuroaxonal dystrophy in mucoviscidosis. *J. Neuropathol. Exp. Neurol.* 23 (1964) 567–583

Sung, J. H., Park, S. H., Mastri, A. R. and Warwick, W. J. Axonal dystrophy in the gracile nucleus in congenital biliary atresia and cystic fibrosis (mucoviscidosis): beneficial effect of vitamin E therapy. *J. Neuropathol. Exp. Neurol.* 39 (1980) 584–597

Wasserman, R. H. and Taylor, A. N. Metabolic roles of fat-soluble vitamin D, E and K. *Ann. Rev. Biochem.* 41 (1972) 179–202

Preface to Short Communications

This issue is devoted to short communications based on oral and poster presentations at the free sessions of the Annual Meeting of the Society for the Study of Inborn Errors of Metabolism held in Newcastle upon Tyne, 5–8 September 1984. Most of the communications selected for oral presentation were related to the main topics of the symposium but recent advances in many other aspects of the study of inherited metabolic disease were presented in the large display of posters which, following the trend of recent years, was an important feature of the meeting. Those presentations not reported elsewhere in this issue are listed below. Many of the short communications were submitted for the Noel Raine Award which commemorates the founding editor of the *Journal of Inherited Metabolic Disease*. This year the prize was awarded to S. K. Wadman, R. Berger, M. Duran, P. K. de Bree, S. A. Stoker de Vries, F. A. Beemer, J. J. Weits-Binnerts, T. J. Penders and J. K. van der Woude for their paper 'Dihydropyrimidine dehydrogenase deficiency leading to thymine-uraciluria. An inborn error of pyrimidine metabolism'.

With pressure on space in all scientific journals we hope that contributors and users will accept our suggestion that these papers be generated and used as short communications rather than as preliminary abstracts, at least in part. Since all must be subjected to critical scrutiny by an informed committee and by an international audience at the meeting some element of appraisal is inherent in their production. It is clear to the editors that some are preliminary communications which allow priority to be established. However, others are worthwhile additional records which are adequate in themselves as contributions to our accumulated experience and may not require additional recording.

We shall try to produce these short communications rapidly and we hope that they can continue to be an open channel of communication for members of the SSIEM and their colleagues.

R. A. Harkness
R. J. Pollitt
G. M. Addison

Free communications

Biopterin deficiency: tetrahydrobiopterin monotherapy or combined treatment with neurotransmitter precursors? *W. Endres, A. Niederwieser and H.-Ch. Curtius*

Screening for biopterin defects: experience with 387 patients with hyperphenylalaninaemia. *R. Matalon and K. Michals*

Clinical and biochemical aspects of tetrahydrobiopterin deficiencies. Current status of an international survey. *J. L. Dhondt*

Reduced concentrations of CSF biopterins and neurotransmitter amine metabolites in methylene tetrahydrofolate reductase deficiency. *P. T. Clayton, J. V. Leonard, I. Smith, R. Leeming, K. Hyland and J. Perry*

Transport characteristics of biotin by the small intestine in man. Preliminary evidence for defective *in vitro* absorption of biotin in biotinidase deficiency. *A. Munnich, E. Grasset, M. Gaudry, A. M. Crain, J. F. Desjeux and J. M. Saudubray*

Lipid metabolism in multiple carboxylase deficiency. *Maria del Carmen Gonzalez-Rios and S. Packman*

A case of riboflavin-responsive ethylmalonic–adipic aciduria. *A. Green, R. G. F. Gray and R. J. Pollitt*

Ehlers–Danlos syndrome type VI: response to ascorbate. *P. Dembure, A. Janko, J. Priest and L. Elsas*

Therapeutic attempts in a new case of infantile methylene tetrahydrofolate reductase deficiency. *H. Ogier, J. Zittoun, F. Herve, C. Charpentier, P. Parvy, J. Bardet and J. M. Saudubray*

Effect of arginine supplementation in neonatal citrullinaemia. *M. Matsuo, K. Sano, H. Nakamura, T. Matsuo and H. Takemine*

Biopterins and neurotransmitter amine metabolites in children on methotrexate. *G. R. Pinkerton, I. Smith, R. Leeming, G. Sarner and K. Hyland*

Clinical and biochemical study of mild dihydropteridine reductase deficiency. *H. Nakabayashi, M. Owada, Y. Yoshida, T. Sakiyama and T. Kitagawa*

Clinical and biochemical observation in a case with congenital defect of folate absorption. *T. Sakiyama, M. Tsuda, H. Nakabayashi, H. Shimizu, M. Owada and T. Kitagawa*

Therapeutical trial of 6R-tetrahydrobiopterin in a patient with defect biopterin biosynthesis. *B. Beck, E. Christensen, N. J. Brandt and A. Niederwieser*

The measurement of pterins of all oxidation states in a single run using high performance liquid chromatography. *K. Hyland*

Seven-year follow-up in a child with early-treated dihydropteridine reductase (DHPR) deficiency. *J. P. Harpey, F. Rey and R. J. Leeming*

Neonatal hyperphenylalaninaemia due to GTP cyclohydrolase I deficiency. *J. L. Dhondt, J. P. Farriaux, C. Largilliere and J. Ringel*

Homovanillic acid (HVA) and 5-hydroxyindoleacetic acid (5HIAA) in CSF in 'classical' phenylketonuria. *I. Smith, K. Hyland and D. Brenton*

Four offspring of treated maternal PKU pregnancies. *K. Fishler, R. Koch, C. Crowley and K. Jew*

Maternal phenylketonuria. *R. Koch, E. Wenz, K. Jew, C. Crowley, K. N. F. Shaw, F. Gilles, K. Fishler, L. Platt and G. DeVore*

West syndrome in a 10-month PKU child—complete reversal of symptoms shortly after the initiation of dietary treatment. *G. Krajewska, F. Carnevale and G. Di Bitonto*

Molecular heterogeneity in phenylalanine hydroxylase in rat, monkey and human. *D. M. Danks, J. F. B. Mercer, S. Smith, W. McAdam, A. Grimes, I. Walker and R. G. H. Cotton*

Trace elements in PKU children in the course of dietary treatment. *B. Cabalska, J. Skorkowska-Zieleniewqwska, D. Banas, B. Zachara, W. Wasowicz, J. Gromadzinska*

Increased adiposity in phenylketonuria. *L. S. Taitz, W. T. Houlsby and R. A. Primhak*

Unusual skin disorder during treatment of a baby with propionic acidaemia. *J. R. Rajnherc, A. H. Van Gennip, J. J. E. M. De Nef and C. A. J. M. Jakobs*

A functional test for evaluation of biotin requirement in multi-carboxylase deficient (MCD) patients. *A. Munnich, C. Marsac, H. Ogier, C. Charpentier, C. Augereau, E. Saliba and J. M. Saudubray*

Biotin responsive stridor etcetera. *M. King*

A continuous flow procedure for determining biotinidase activity in serum. *G. S. Heard, K. A. Weissbecker and B. Wolf*

C_6–C_{10} Dicarboxylic aciduria responsive to riboflavin. *J. P. Harpey, C. Charpentier and I. Ceballos*

The diagnosis and management of a case of glutaric aciduria type I presenting in early infancy. *R. A. Chalmers, T. Edwards, H. Losty and A. Westwood*

A case of glutaric aciduria type I – previously diagnosed as Leigh's encephalopathy and cerebral palsy. *P. Stutchfield, M. A. Edwards, R. G. F. Gray, P. Cawley and A. Green*

Congenital malformations in glutaric aciduria. *N. J. Brandt, H. Pedersen and E. Christensen*

Nocturnal UCS (uncooked cornstarch) therapy in medium chain acyl-CoA deficiency. *G. P. A. Smit, H. Schierbeek, J. Fernandes and R. Berger*

Pyridoxal 5'-phosphate concentration in human cerebrospinal fluid. Implication to vitamin B_6 dependent seizures in newborn infants. *Y. S. Shin, R. Rasshofer and W. Endres*

Effects of intensive 1-hydroxyvitamin D_3-phosphate treatment during postsurgical immobilization in children with familial hypophosphataemic rickets. *E. Pronicka, E. Wieczorek, H. Kulczycka, A. Jelonek, D. Tylman, I. Pomierna and S. Fijalkowski*

Deficiency of 3-methylglutaconyl-CoA hydratase in cultured skin fibroblasts from two siblings with 3-methylglutaconic aciduria. *K. Narisawa, K. M. Gibson, L. Sweetman and W. L. Nyhan*

A defect of cobalamin metabolism – biochemical studies of various therapeutic regimens. *B. Wilcken, J. Hammond, D. Wilckenn and N. Dudman*

Haemolytic–uraemic syndrome revealing a congenital derangement in B_{12} metabolism. *H. Ogier, C. Charpentier, P. Parvy, F. Beaufils, J. Laugier and J. M. Saudubray*

Vitamin-responsiveness disorders: epidemiological data. *R. Cerone, F. M. Pistone, G. F. Gargani and C. Romano*

Thiamin unresponsive maple syrup urine disease resulting from the absence of branched chain acyl transferase. *D. J. Danner, S. Litwer and L. J. Elsas*

L-Carnitine treatment in methylmalonicacidaemia: *in vivo* estimation of enhanced long-chain fatty acid oxidation. *J. Kneer, M. Brockstedt, H. Paust, C. Jakobs, D. Penn, E. Monch and H. Helge*

Heterogeneity of familial carnitine deficiency. *V. Barash, N. Brand, Y. Shapira, A. Boneh and A. Gutman*

Effect of L-carnitine and L-glutamic acid on serum isovaleric acid levels during oral loading with L-leucine in a patient with isovaleric acidaemia. Urinary metabolic profile under L-carnitine and L-glutamic acid therapy. *W. Lehnert, E. Niemeyer and D. Penn*

Serum carnosinase deficiency: a benign phenotype? *P. L. Hartlage, N. Krawiechi, M. Cohen, R. A. Roesel, A. L. Carter and F. A. Hommes*

Prenatal diagnosis and DNA analysis in citrullinaemia. *P. Berman, J. Davidson and E. H. Harley*

Brittle hair, intellectual impairment, decreased fertility and short stature (BIDS) syndrome in three sibs. *S. Przedborski, A. Ferster, M. Song, R. Wolter and E. Vamos*

Biochemical studies and follow up of five children with maple syrup urine disease. *F. Roman, C. Perez-Cerda, B. Merinero, M. J. Garcia, M. Ugarte, M. Martinez-Pardo, C. Ludena, R. Lama and A. Verdu*

Prenatal diagnosis of maple syrup urine disease in uncultured amniotic fluid cells. *A. Zenker and U. Wendel*

High speed amino acid analysis by HPLCC in the investigation of inborn errors of metabolism. *S. J. Price, T. Palmer, M. Griffin and V. G. Oberholzer*

A case of hereditary fructose intolerance due to fructose-1-phosphate aldolase deficiency, accidentally discovered by breath hydrogen test on saccharose loading. *H. D. Bakker, A. H. Van Gennip and N. G. Abeling*

Neonatal isovaleric acidaemia treated by glycine and MSUD diet supplemented with valine and isoleucine. *L. Hagenfeldt, J.-I. Henter and U. von Dobeln*

Adenine phosphoribosyl transferase deficiency: a case diagnosed by GC-MS identification of 2,8-dihydroxyadenine in urinary crystals. *E. Christensen, N. J. Brandt and T. Laxdal*

Familial psuedohyperkalaemia: a case report. *D. Stansbie, D. James and S. Leadbeatter*

Urinary galactitol as a diagnostic acid in galactosaemia. *L. Dorland, J. B. C. de Klerk, M. Duran, F. J. van Sprang and S. K. Wadman*

Elevated plasma or serum α-N-acetyl glucosaminidase as a potential indicator of San Filippo A disease. *J. Toone and D. Applegarth*

Piperacillin – the source of another artifact in the diagnosis of organic acid disorders. *J. Hammond and L. Hick*

Biochemical findings in patients with Morquio disease of different severity. *D. M. Broadhead, J. Nelson and J. Mossman*

Detection of type III glycogenosis in erythrocytes with a simplified method of amylo-1,6-glucosidase assay. Elevated debrancher activity in phosphorylase B kinase deficiency. *Y. S. Shin, T. Witt, R. Ungar, M. Rieth and W. Endres*

Complementation of steroid sulphatase in somatic cell hybrids of X-linked ichthyosis and multiple sulphatase deficiency fibroblasts. *A. Ballabio, G. Parenti, E. Napolitano, P. Di Natale and G. Andria*

Type II and type III glycogenosis screening by thin layer chromatography of oligosaccharides in urines. *S. Boyer, I. Maire, C. Vianey-Liaud and P. Divry*

Reversible symptoms of the central and peripheral nervous system in a patient with pyruvate decarboxylase (E1) deficiency. *G. P. A. Smit, R. le Coultre, J. Fernandes, R. Berger and J. H. Begeer*

Dietary therapy in two patients with propionic acidaemia: differences derived from leucine restriction. *C. Perez-Cerda, M. J. Garcia, F. Roman, B. Merinero, M. Ugarte, R. Lama and M. S. Martin Romero*

A disturbance in the mitochondrial respiratory chain at the level of ubiquinone in a patient with convulsions. *J. C. Fischer, F. J. M. Gabreels, W. Ruitenbeek, J. M. F. Trijbels, R. C. A. Sengers, A. J. M. Janssen, A. M. Stadhouders and H. J. ter Laak*

An X-linked (cardio)myopathy and granulocytopenia, with a low succinate cytochrome-C-reductase and cytochrome-C-oxidase activity in skeletal muscle. *C. J. de Groot, G. C. M. Beaufort-Krol, H. R. Scholte, I. E. M. Luyt-Houwen, W. F. Arts and W. Blom*

Prenatal diagnosis of MPS I: conflicting results by chorion biopsy and amniocentesis. *A. Cooper, B. Fowler, I. B. Sardharwalla, P. Donnai and J. Tracy*

Maple syrup urine disease: branched chain aminoacid levels during the first two days life. *C. Romano, R. Cerone and U. Caruso*

Non-ketotic hyperglycinaemia: treatment with protein restriction, benzoate and folic acid. *C. Ramano, F. M. Pistone, M. Cotellessa, U. Caruso and R. Cerone*

Quantitative assay of amino acids: electronic elaboration of results and graphic translation. *U. Caruso, E. Della Foglia, S. Gatti and C. Romano*

A method for the estimation of galactose-1-phosphate. *J. A. Dobbie and J. B. Holton*

Anomalous eosinophils in blood and bone marrow: a diagnostic marker for infantile GM_1 gangliosidosis? *R. Gitzelmann, M. A. Spycher, B. Steinmann and K. Baerlocher*

Unexpected biochemical findings in a child with persistent mild methylmalonic aciduria. *A. H. Van Gennip, H. D. Bakker and S. K. Wadman*

Malonyl-CoA decarboxylase deficiency – a further case with an unusual pattern of organic acids in the urine. *D. M. Danks, G. K. Brown, E. A. Haan, S. Hunt and R. Scholem*

Leprechaunism: an inborn error of insulin receptor function. *L. Elsas and F. Endo*

Galactosaemia due to UDPGal-4-epimerase deficiency. *R. Longhi, R. Valsasina, G. Panigada, E. Riva and M. Giovannini*

Complementation studies with pyruvate carboxylase deficiencies in cultured fibroblasts. *C. Augereau, C. Marsac, D. Dinh Pham, A. Moncion, J. M. Saudubray and J. P. Lepoux*

Beneficial effect of pyridoxine and folate on dietary management of apparently non-B_6-responsive homocytinuria due to cystathionine synthetase deficiency. *A. G. F. Davidson, C. L. Ireton, L. T. K. Kirby*

Bicarbonate–chloride exchange in pancreatic secretions from cystic fibrosis patients. *D. A. Applegarth, A. G. F. Davidson, P. Sorensen and L. T. K. Wong*

J. Inher. Metab. Dis. 8 Suppl. 2 (1985) 95–96

Short Communication

Biopterin, Neopterin and Tyrosine Responses to Combined Oral Phenylalanine and Tetrahydrobiopterin Loading Tests in Two Normal Children and in a Girl with Partial Biopterin Deficiency

C. Lykkelund, H. C. Lou, V. Rasmussen and F. Güttler
The John F. Kennedy Institute, Gl. Landevej 7, DK-2600 Glostrup, Denmark

A. Niederwieser
Department of Pediatrics, University of Zürich, Steinwiesstrasse 75, CH-8032 Zürich, Switzerland

Phenylketonuria (McKusick 26160, 26163, 26164) is caused by a genetic defect in the enzyme system that catalyzes the conversion of phenylalanine to tyrosine. The enzyme system involves two enzymes, phenylalanine hydroxylase (EC 1.14.16.1) and dihydropteridine reductase (EC 1.6.99.7), and a reduced cofactor 6R-L-*erythro*-5,6,7,8-tetrahydrobiopterin (Curtius *et al.*, 1979; Kaufman, 1983).

Biopterin deficiency is due to a defect in the biosynthesis of tetrahydrobiopterin. This genetic defect may occur in the enzyme guanosine triphosphate cyclohydrolase (EC 3.5.4.16), which catalyzes the conversion of guanosine triphosphate to dihydroneopterin triphosphate, or it may be located to one of the enzymatic steps that convert dihydroneopterin triphosphate to tetrahydrobiopterin (Curtius *et al.*, 1982; Neiderwieser *et al.*, 1984). Recently *partial* defects in the biosynthesis of tetrahydrobiopterin have been described. Children with this partial defect are characterized by a slightly elevated fasting serum phenylalanine, a delayed elimination of a phenylalanine load, and a decreased urinary excretion of biopterin. They may be mentally retarded or have a normal intelligence (Rey *et al.*, 1983; Güttler *et al.*, 1984). The present paper describes a method for the detection of partial biopterin deficiency using combined phenylalanine and tetrahydrobiopterin loading tests, and it is shown that tetrahydrobiopterin is a rate limiting factor in the hydroxylation of phenylalanine *in vivo*.

SUBJECTS AND METHODS

The patient (H.V.J.) was a 10-year-old girl with normal appearance, normal intelligence, and an abnormal electroencephalogram with focal spikes. Her case story has been described earlier (Güttler *et al.*, 1984). Two normal girls (I.L. and A.L.) aged 6 and 10 years, respectively served as controls. They were sisters and unrelated to the patient.

Two oral phenylalanine loading tests (75 mg kg^{-1}) were carried out on two consecutive days. The second day the phenylalanine load was preceded for 1 h by oral (6R,S)-L-*erythro*-tetrahydrobiopterin dihydrochloride (BH$_4$). The dose was 6.5 mg kg^{-1}. Urinary neopterin and biopterin were determined by high performance liquid chromatography with fluorimetric detection. For a given parameter the response was defined as the difference between the actual value and the basal level.

RESULTS AND DISCUSSION

The patient had slightly elevated fasting serum phenylalanine (145 μmol l^{-1}), and during an oral phenylalanine load she showed a low elimination rate of serum phenylalanine and almost no change in serum tyrosine (Figure 1), pointing to a decreased conversion of phenylalanine to tyrosine. Her basal urinary excretion of biopterin was decreased to 27% of the mean excretion of the controls. The biopterin response to oral phenylalanine was two-phased in the unaffected girls, whereas the patient lacked the first phase. During the second phase the patient's response increased to 26% of the mean response of the controls. Her maximum urinary neopterin excretion during the phenylalanine load was greatly increased (11 times) when compared to the mean maximum excretion of the controls. These results are compatible with a partial defect in the patient's biopterin biosynthesis occurring in the enzymatic steps between dihydroneopterin triphosphate and tetrahydrobiopterin.

The possibility that the patient is merely heterozygous for complete biopterin deficiency must be considered. This is not likely, however, since the 11 times elevated maximum excretion of neopterin during the phenylalanine load and the simultaneous 42 times increase in the molar ratio of excreted neopterin and biopterin, when compared to the controls, point to a much more pronounced block in the conversion of dihydroneopterin triphosphate to tetrahydrobiopterin than the expected 50%.

When the phenylalanine load was preceded by oral BH$_4$ a large increase in the tyrosine response was observed in the patient and in the two normal girls. The patient's tyrosine response integrated over the first 4 h after oral phenylalanine increased from −6 to 248 μmol h l^{-1} and the integrated responses of the controls (I.L. and A.L.) increased from 113 to 448 μmol h l^{-1} and from 273 to 445 μmol h l^{-1}, respectively, which implies that the mean increase of the controls (254 μmol h l^{-1}) is equal to the increase in the

Journal of Inherited Metabolic Disease. ISSN 0141-8955. Copyright © SSIEM and MTP Press Limited, Queen Square, Lancaster, UK.

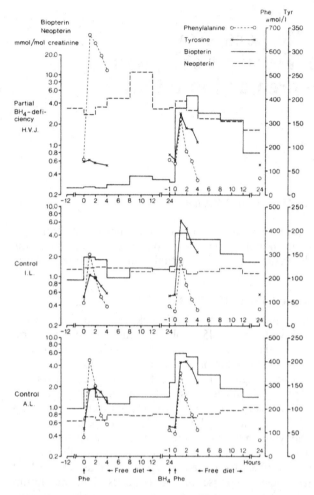

Figure 1 Biopterin, neopterin and tyrosine responses to an oral phenylalanine load and to a combined tetrahydrobiopterin (BH₄)-phenylalanine loading test in a girl with partial biopterin deficiency and in two controls

partially blocked. The patient's urinary excretion of neopterin and biopterin reached a maximum in the fraction collected 8–12 h after the phenylalanine load. These observations indicate that induction of *de novo* biosynthesis of dihydroneopterin triphosphate and tetrahydrobiopterin is a slow process requiring 8–12 h before the biosynthesis reaches a maximum, at least, in the patient. In the same period urinary excretion of biopterin showed a second peak in the two normal girls. This observation is consistent with the hypothesis mentioned above, stating that the second peak is due to *de novo* biosynthesis. It cannot be ruled out, however, that the second peak may at least partly be caused by mobilization of biopterin depots induced by the free diet consumed 4 h after the oral phenylalanine load.

The authors are grateful to Mrs Maj-Britt Lund for typing the manuscript and to the staff at the John F. Kennedy Institute for technical assistance and for the collection of urine samples. The present work was supported by grants from the Danish Health Insurance Foundation, the Danish Parkinson Society, the Foundation of 1870, the Foundation of 15th January 1972, the Krista and Viggo Petersen's Fund, the P. Carl Petersen's Fund, and Privatbanken's Fund.

patient's integrated tyrosine response. These observations indicate that tetrahydrobiopterin is a rate-limiting factor in the conversion of phenylalanine to tyrosine during a phenylalanine load in normal individuals, as well as in partial biopterin deficiency. Thus the observation by Milstien and Kaufman (1975) in the normal rat has been confirmed in man.

The biopterin response in the unaffected girls was two-phased, whereas the patient lacked the first phase. It is tentatively proposed that the first peak was caused by mobilization of biopterin depots, and that the second was due to *de novo* biosynthesis. Dhondt and Farriaux (1982) have reported that serum biopterin increased and liver biopterin decreased in the rat 30 min after an intraperitoneal phenylalanine load. Similar results were obtained by perfused canine liver. These observations lend support to the present hypothesis as far as the first peak is concerned.

In the patient, urinary excretion of neopterin may be used as a rough measure of *de novo* biosynthesis of dihydroneopterin triphosphate, since the conversion of the latter compound to tetrahydrobiopterin is at least

References

Curtius, H. Ch., Häusermann, M., Niederwieser, A. and Ghisla, S. Tetrahydrobiopterin biosynthesis. In Wachter, H., Curtius, H. Ch. and Pfleiderer, W. (eds.) *Biochemical and Clinical Aspects of Pteridines*, Vol. I, Walter de Gruyter, Berlin, 1982, pp. 27–50

Curtius, H. Ch., Niederwieser, A., Viscontini, M., Otten, A., Schaub, J., Scheibenreiter, S. and Schmidt, H. Atypical phenylketonuria due to tetrahydrobiopterin deficiency. Diagnosis and treatment with tetrahydrobiopterin, dihydrobiopterin and sepiapterin. *Clin. Chim. Acta* 93 (1979) 251–262

Dhondt, J. L. and Farriaux, J. P. Relationships between phenylalanine and biopterin metabolisms. In Wachter, H., Curtius, H. Ch. and Pfleiderer, W. (eds.) *Biochemical and Clinical Aspects of Pteridines*, Vol. I, Walter de Gruyter, Berlin, 1982, pp. 319–328

Güttler, F., Lou, H., Lykkelund, C. and Niederwieser, A. Combined tetrahydrobiopterin–phenylalanine loading test in the detection of partially defective biopterin synthesis. *Eur. J. Pediatr.* 142 (1984) 126–129

Kaufman, S. Phenylketonuria and its variants. In Harris, H. and Hirschhorn, K. (eds.) *Advances in Human Genetics*, Vol. 13, Plenum Press, New York, 1983, pp. 217–297

Milstien, S. and Kaufman, S. Studies on the phenylalanine hydroxylase system in liver slices. *J. Biol. Chem.* 250 (1975) 4777–4781

Niederwieser, A., Blau, N., Wang, H., Joller, P., Antarés, M. and Cardesa-Garcia, J. GTP cyclohydrolase I deficiency, a new enzyme defect causing hyperphenylalaninemia with neopterin, biopterin, dopamine, and serotonin deficiencies and muscular hypotonia. *Eur. J. Pediatr.* 141 (1984) 208–214

Rey, F., Saudubray, J. M., Leeming, R. J., Niederwieser, A., Curtius, H. Ch. and Rey, J. Les déficits partiels en tétrahydrobioptérine. *Arch. Fr. Pédiatr.* 40 (1983) 237–241

J. Inher. Metab. Dis. 8 Suppl. 2 (1985) 97–98

Short Communication

Phenylketonuria due to Dihydropteridine Reductase Deficiency: Presentation of Two Cases

R. Longhi, E. Riva, R. Valsasina, S. Paccanelli and M. Giovannini
V Pediatric Department, University of Milan, S. Paolo Hospital, 8 di Rudiní, 20142 Milan, Italy

1–3% of all hyperphenylalaninaemias are due to an impairment of the metabolism of tetrahydrobiopterin (BH_4), the cofactor of the hydroxylases of phenylalanine (Phe), tyrosine and tryptophan (BH_4 deficiency). As a consequence, plasma Phe increases and dopamine, noradrenalin and serotonin are produced at a reduced rate. Known causes of BH_4 deficiency are: dihydropteridine reductase (DHPR, EC 1.6.99.7) deficiency (McKusick 26163), dihydrobiopterin synthetase (DHBS) deficiency and guanosine triphosphate cyclohydrolase (EC 3.5.4.16) deficiency. We present the cases of two girls with DHPR deficiency.

MATERIALS AND METHODS

BH_4 tablets were purchased from Dr Schirks (Wettswill, Switzerland). Amino acids were analyzed by column chromatography, using a Liquimat (Kontron LMT, Zurich, Switzerland). Urinary pterins were quantified by high pressure liquid chromatography (Niederwieser *et al.*, 1980). DHPR activity was assayed on dried spotted blood in Dr Arai's laboratory (Arai *et al.*, 1982).

CASE REPORTS

Case 1

D.G., female, was born at term of unrelated parents, body wt 3320 g. The neonatal Guthrie screening test showed plasma Phe 20 mg dl^{-1}, without ketonuria. At

three weeks plasma Phe was 13.9 mg dl^{-1}. A low Phe diet (50 mg kg^{-1} day^{-1}) was started and, since then, carefully followed by the parents (Guthrie test between 2 and 8 mg dl^{-1}). Evident developmental delay with decreased spontaneous motility and increased muscle tone became manifest. At 16 months EEG and cranial CAT scan were normal. A month later, on the basis of her urinary pterin excretion (Figure 1) and unresponsiveness to an oral BH_4 loading test, DHPR deficiency was diagnosed. The diagnosis was confirmed by the absent activity of red cell DHPR.

Substitutive therapy with L-dopa, 5-hydroxytryptophan and carbidopa was started. Over the following two months progressive improvement of the symptoms was evident. She could sit up well and stand with support, she smiled more frequently and held objects, but at 21 months major seizure activity, controlled by phenobarbital, was noticed. The EEG showed generalized hypsarhythmic activity and the cranial CAT scan showed diffuse atrophy and ventricular dilation. Psychomotor retardation and the neurological picture have progressively worsened with the appearance of transient choreoathetosis, complete loss of head control and absence of voluntary movements.

Case 2

G.C., a Sicilian female, was born at term of unrelated parents, body wt 3300 g. No neonatal screening tests were obtained. At 3 months seizure activity and at 4 months psychomotor retardation were already evident.

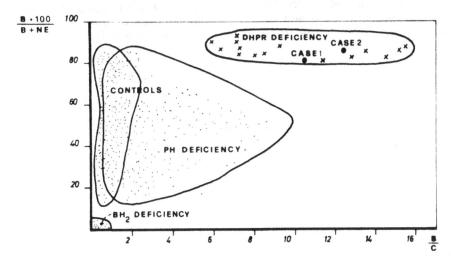

Figure 1 Percentage urinary excretion of biopterin in relation to the urinary biopterin/creatinine ratio. The diagram shows a complete separation of DHPR and DHBS deficient patients from PH deficient patients and the control population. (Determinations by Niederwieser)

Journal of Inherited Metabolic Disease. ISSN 0141-8955. Copyright © SSIEM and MTP Press Limited, Queen Square, Lancaster, UK.

The EEG showed diffuse sharp wave activity with right temporal prevalence and cranial CAT scan generalized atrophy. Phenobarbital and clonazepam therapy partially controlled the crises. At 10 months hyperphenylalaninaemia was found ($19.8\,mg\,dl^{-1}$). She was sent to our department for dietary treatment. On admission horizontal nystagmus, strabismus, slow pupillary reflex and generalized hyperactivity were noticed. A low Phe diet ($30\,mg\,kg^{-1}\,day^{-1}$) was started and good metabolic control was achieved without an improvement of the clinical symptoms. A cranial CAT scan showed calcifications of the basal ganglia. DHPR deficiency was diagnosed following determination of the pattern of excretion of urinary pterins (Figure 1) and oral BH_4 loading test (Phe from 235 to $80\,\mu mol\,l^{-1}$ after 8 h). No red cell DHPR activity was found. 5-Hydroxytryptophan, L-dopa and carbidopa were given, at increasing doses, without satisfactory results. Now, after 1 year of full dosage neurotransmitter therapy, the child has frequent crises of absence, severe tetraparesis and mental retardation.

DISCUSSION

We wish to present these cases to stress the paramount importance of screening all newborns with even slightly raised Phe values for defects of biopterin metabolism. The history of our patients confirms previous reports (Dhondt, 1984) of extremely poor clinical results obtained with the precursors of the lacking neurotransmitters if the therapy is begun after the first few months of life. In both our cases substitution therapy was started after the first year of age. In case 1, there was a significant clinical improvement that lasted only for 2 months. Case 2 did not respond at all. Both cases, after respectively 12 and 16 months of treatment ($8-15\,mg\,kg^{-1}\,day^{-1}$ L-dopa, $5-10\,mg\,kg^{-1}\,day^{-1}$ 5-hydroxytryptophan, $1\,mg\,kg^{-1}\,day^{-1}$ carbidopa), showed a progressive worsening of the neurological condition and of the mental status. Like many other DHPR deficient patients, their Phe tolerance increased with time, so that, in the second year of life, they tolerated more than $120\,mg\,kg^{-1}\,day^{-1}$. Biochemical diagnosis of DHPR and DHBS deficiency is easy to perform, even in the neonatal period, by high pressure liquid chromatographic analysis of urinary pterins. In 1983 Narisawa set up a method that allows for the analysis of urine absorbed on paper, simplifying storage and shipping procedures (Narisawa *et al.*, 1983). Enzymatic diagnosis is possible only for DHPR deficiency. Dried blood can be utilized with excellent results (Arai *et al.*, 1982). The same material has been utilized by Leeming (Leeming *et al.*, 1984) for biopterin determination. This test can screen for DHBS deficiency, since these patients present low values of plasma biopterins even with high values of plasma Phe, unlike classic PKU and DHPR deficient patients. If the method proves to be effective in a larger number of subjects, the diagnosis of DHPR deficiency can be positively made and of DHBS deficiency strongly suspected, utilizing the same Guthrie card obtained at birth.

References

Arai, N., Narisawa, K., Hayakawa, H. and Tada, K. Hyperphenylalaninemia due to dihydropteridine reductase deficiency: diagnosis by enzyme assay on dried blood spots. *Pediatrics* 70 (1982) 426–430

Dhondt, J. L. Tetrahydrobiopterin deficiencies: preliminary analysis from an international survey. *J. Pediatr.* 104 (1984) 501–508

Leeming, R. J., Barford, P. A., Blair, J. A. and Smith, I. Blood spots on Guthrie card can be used for inherited tetrahydrobiopterin deficiency screening in hyperphenylalaninemic infants. *Arch. Dis. Child.* 59 (1984) 58–61

Narisawa, K., Hayakawa, H., Arai, N., Matsuo, N., Tanaka, T., Naritomi, K. and Tada, K. Diagnosis of variant forms of hyperphenylalaninemia using filter paper spots of urine. *Pediatrics* 103 (1983) 577–579

Niederwieser, A., Curtius, H., Gitzelman, R., Otten, A., Baerlocher, K., Bleove, B., Berlow, S., Grobe, H., Rey, F., Schaub, J., Scheibernreiter, S., Schmidt, H. and Viscontini, M. Excretion of pterins in phenylketonuria and phenylketonuria variants. *Helv. Paediatr. Acta* 35 (1980) 335–342

J. Inher. Metab. Dis. 8 Suppl. 2 (1985) 99–100

Short Communication

Neonatal Screening for Dihydropteridine Reductase Deficiency

A. Sahota, J. A. Blair and P. A. Barford
Department of Chemistry, University of Aston, Birmingham B4 7ET, U K

R. J. Leeming
Department of Haematology, General Hospital, Birmingham B4 6NH, U K

A. Green
Department of Clinical Chemistry, Children's Hospital, Birmingham B16 8ET, U K

R. J. Pollitt
Neonatal Screening Laboratory, Middlewood Hospital, Sheffield S6 1TP, U K

Dihydropteridine reductase (DHPR, EC 1.6.99.7) deficiency (McKusick 26163) is a rare cause of hyperphenylalaninaemia and neurological disease. It is important to distinguish it from the more prevalent cause of these, phenylalanine hydroxylase deficiency (McKusick 26160), as the treatment in the two cases is different (for review see Danks *et al.*, 1978; Dhondt, 1984). DHPR activity can be readily measured in dried blood spots on Guthrie cards (Arai *et al.*, 1982; Leeming *et al.*, 1984). We have used this technique to screen for DHPR deficiency in control and hyperphenylalaninaemic neonates.

METHODS

Guthrie cards from newborn children (aged up to 1 month) with raised blood phenylalanine (0.20–$2.0 \, mol \, l^{-1}$) were sent us from metabolic screening centres in the United Kingdom and abroad. Cards from children with normal blood phenylalanine (age 4–7 days) were obtained from the Neonatal Screening Laboratory, Sheffield. The cards were sealed in plastic bags and stored at $-20°C$ until assay. The enzyme was stable under these conditions for at least 2 months. Two 8 mm discs were punched out and eluted with 1 ml water and the enzyme assayed by a slight modification of the method of Arai *et al.* (1982) at 37°C. Fifty samples a day could be analysed using a spectrophotometer (Pye Unicam 8800) equipped with a cell programmer. The assay mixture in a total of 1 ml contained $50 \, mmol \, l^{-1}$ Tris–HCl (pH 7.5), $50 \, \mu mol \, l^{-1}$ ferricytochrome *c* (Sigma, type III), $100 \, \mu mol \, l^{-1}$ NADH, $10 \, \mu mol \, l^{-1}$ 6-methyl-5,6,7,8-tetrahydropterin and $100 \, \mu l$ haemolysate. Batches of cytochrome other than type III were found to give unsatisfactory reproducibility. Enzyme activity was expressed in nmol NADH oxidised min^{-1} ml^{-1} whole blood. One disc typically contained $16.7 \, \mu l$ whole blood.

RESULTS AND DISCUSSION

DHPR activity in 500 apparently normal neonates was 232 ± 60 (SD) (range 64–440) nmol min^{-1} ml^{-1} (Table 1). The distribution of activity showed no kurtosis but had significant negative skewness ($\chi^2 = 98.24$, 17 df; $p < 1\%$). The removal of values below 100 nmol min^{-1} ml^{-1} gave a normal distribution ($\chi^2 = 23.8$, 15 df: NS) without kurtosis. The observed frequencies in the range 60–99 nmol min^{-1} ml^{-1} were significantly higher than expected from this normal distribution (60–79 nmol min^{-1} ml^{-1}, observed 2, calculated 0.07; $\chi^2 = 53.2$, $p < 0.1\%$: 80–99 nmol min^{-1} ml^{-1}, observed 13, calculated 3.83; $\chi^2 = 21.95$, $p < 1.0\%$). These low levels of activity are similar to those in known DHPR heterozygotes (Leeming *et al.*, 1984). If this 2.5–3% of a normal population proves to be heterozygotes for DHPR deficiency, this would be a greater frequency than that calculated (about 1 in 700) from the frequency of occurrence of the live homozygotes. The significance of this partial DHPR deficiency, and its possible relationships to other disorders, is under study. The only report of a pathological state with a significant reduction in DHPR activity is senile dementia of the Alzheimer type where DHPR activity in the lymphocytes is significantly reduced (Young *et al.*, 1982). Enzyme activity was within the range 78–370 nmol min^{-1} ml^{-1} in 48 infants with hyperphenylalaninaemia (presumed to be due to phenylalanine hydroxylase deficiency). There

Table 1 Dihydropteridine reductase (DHPR) activity in newborn children (nmol NADH min^{-1} (ml whole blood)$^{-1}$)

Group	Number	DHPR Mean	SD	Range
Controls	500	232	60	64–440
Hyperphenylalaninaemia	48	206	72	78–370
DHPR deficiency	4	0	—	—

Journal of Inherited Metabolic Disease. ISSN 0141-8955. Copyright © SSIEM and MTP Press Limited, Queen Square, Lancaster, U.K.

was no correlation between blood phenylalanine level and DHPR activity. Activity was undetectable in three known cases of DHPR deficiency and a new case was recently identified using this assay. No false positive or false negative results were observed.

DHPR deficiency has been previously diagnosed by enzyme assay in whole blood, separated blood cells, and cultured fibroblasts and by the protozoological or high performance liquid chromatographic analysis of biopterin derivatives in body fluids (see Dhondt, 1984). The present study shows that DHPR deficiency can be positively identified by enzyme assay in dried spots containing only few µl of blood. The technique is rapid, simple and can be automated. It can be used for the differential diagnosis of DHPR deficiency in hyperphenylalaninaemic neonates identified in the initial screening programmes. The stability of DHPR ensures that samples may be sent by ordinary mail to the screening laboratory.

We are grateful to Dr R. A. Armstrong for helping with the statistical evaluation of data. This work was supported by a grant from the Medical Research Council. R. J. Pollitt is a member of the external scientific staff of the MRC.

References

Arai, N., Narisawa, K., Hayakawa, H. and Tada, K. Hyperphenylalaninaemia due to dihydropteridine reductase deficiency: Diagnosis by enzyme assays on dried blood spots. *Pediatrics* 70 (1982) 426–430

Danks, D. M., Bartholome, K., Clayton, B. E., Curtius, H., Grobe, H., Kaufman, S., Leeming, R. J., Pfleiderer, W., Rembold, H. and Rey, F. Malignant hyperphenylalaninaemia: Current status (June 1977). *J. Inher. Metab. Dis.* 1 (1978) 49–53

Dhondt, J. L. Tetrahydrobiopterin deficiencies. Preliminary analysis from an international survey. *J. Pediatr.* 104 (1984) 501–508

Leeming, R. J., Barford, P. A., Blair, J. A. and Smith, I. Blood spots on Guthrie cards can be used for inherited tetrahydrobiopterin deficiency screening in hyperphenylalaninaemic infants. *Arch. Dis. Child.* 59 (1984) 58–61

Young, J. H., Kelly, B. and Clayton. B. E. Reduced levels of biopterin and dihydropteridine reductase in Alzheimer type dementia. *J. Clin. Exp. Gerontol.* 4 (1982) 389–402

J. Inher. Metab. Dis. 8 Suppl. 2 (1985) 101–102

Short Communication

A Bioassay for Determining Biotinidase Activity and for Discriminating Biocytin from Biotin using Holocarboxylase Synthetase-deficient Cultured Fibroblasts

D. L. WEINER, R. E. GRIER and B. WOLF
Department of Human Genetics and Department of Pediatrics, Children's Medical Center, Medical College of Virginia, Richmond, VA 23298, USA

Biotinidase [EC 3.5.1.12] catalyzes the removal of biotin from biocytin (ϵ-N-biotinyl-lysine) or from the ϵ-amino group of the lysyl residue in partially degraded carboxylases (Thoma and Petersen, 1954). We have recently shown that most individuals with late-onset multiple carboxylase deficiency (MCD) have deficient activity of serum biotinidase by measuring colorimetrically the liberation of p-aminobenzoate from the artificial substrate, N-biotinyl-p-aminobenzoate (Wolf et al., 1983a). We now report the development of a sensitive bioassay for the determination of biotinidase activity using a fibroblast line derived from a patient with a primary deficiency in the activity of holocarboxylase synthetase (Burri et al., 1981). This enzyme links biotin covalently to the various apoenzymes forming their respective holocarboxylases. Fibroblasts from this patient are secondarily deficient in the activities of the various biotin-dependent enzymes, including propionyl-CoA carboxylase (PCC), when cultured in medium containing 10 % fetal calf serum and no supplemental biotin (Feldman et al., 1981). PCC activity increases to normal when these cells are incubated in high concentrations of biotin. In the absence of serum, there is no increase in PCC activity when biocytin is substituted for biotin in the medium. However, there is an increase in PCC activity when cells are incubated in medium with biocytin in the presence of small volumes of normal serum, which contains biotinidase that liberates the biotin from biocytin. The increase in PCC activity is proportional to the concentration of serum added and is therefore a sensitive bioassay for biotinidase activity. Using this method, which incorporates the enzyme's natural substrate, we have confirmed that serum from patients with late-onset MCD have deficient biotinidase activity and that heterozygotes exhibit activities which are intermediate between the normal and deficient values.

METHODS

Fresh human serum was obtained from nine normal donors, from six unrelated patients shown previously to have deficient serum biotinidase activity using the colorimetric assay (Wolf et al., 1983a, b) and from eight parents of affected patients.

Holocarboxylase synthetase-deficient (HSD) fibroblasts (Camden Cell Repository, NJ; GM 3522) were incubated at confluence (1.2×10^6 cells/60 mm plate) in minimal essential medium (MEM) and 10 % fetal calf serum for 24 h at 37°C. The cultures were then washed three times with Hank's salt solution and reincubated in MEM and the various supplements described below for 8 h at 37°C. Cultures were subsequently harvested with trypsin, washed once with Hank's salt solution and once with normal saline. The cell pellet was suspended in 50 mmol l^{-1} Tris–HCl buffer, pH 8.0, 10 mmol l^{-1} reduced glutathione, 0.01 mmol l^{-1} sodium EDTA and 0.5 % Triton X-100 (Sigma, St. Louis, MO), and then disrupted in an Ultramet 3 sonicating water bath for 15 min in ice water. The extract was centrifuged for 2 min at 2000 g to remove cellular debris. PCC activity was determined in the supernatant as previously described (Wolf et al., 1977) and is expressed as pmol of $^{14}CO_2$ incorporated into methylmalonyl-CoA min^{-1} (mg protein)$^{-1}$ of fibroblast extract.

RESULTS

PCC activity in HSD fibroblasts incubated in MEM containing 1 % human serum was 65 pmol min^{-1} (mg protein)$^{-1}$ or 8 % of mean control values. PCC activity increases linearly for at least 16 h in extracts of cultures in which biotin (0.41 μmol l^{-1}) is added with or without serum. The increase in PCC activity in extracts of HSD cells incubated in medium containing biocytin (0.41 μmol l^{-1}) instead of biotin was linear with up to 1.4 % serum (volume of serum:volume of medium). An increase in PCC activity was detectable in medium containing as little as 0.2 % serum. However, little or no increase in PCC activity occurred in cells incubated in medium with biocytin, but without serum. In addition, there was essentially no difference between the PCC activity in cells incubated in MEM with only biocytin and those incubated with only MEM and serum.

HSD cells were incubated in MEM containing 0.41 μmol l^{-1} biocytin and 1 % serum from the children with biotinidase deficiency or from their parents. Identical cultures with cells in MEM and the various sera, but without biocytin, were also prepared. After incubation for 8 h at 37°C the cells were harvested and PCC activity measured in the cell extracts. The net increase in PCC activity was determined by subtracting the PCC activity in extracts of HSD cells incubated in medium with only biocytin from that containing

Journal of Inherited Metabolic Disease. ISSN 0141-8955. Copyright © SSIEM and MTP Press Limited, Queen Square, Lancaster, UK.

biocytin and serum (Table 1). The mean net PCC activity in the cultures containing normal serum was 42.3 pmol min^{-1} (mg protein)$^{-1}$, representing 100% activity. A direct proportionality can then be used to calculate the biotinidase in the various samples. The bioassay is approximately 100 times more sensitive than the colorimetric assay. The mean net PCC activity in the cultures containing serum from the biotinidase-deficient children was 8% of mean normal activity, whereas the mean net activity in those cultures containing serum from the parents were intermediate between deficient and normal activity, 58% of mean normal activity.

DISCUSSION

Activation of PCC by biotin in HSD cells occurs whether or not the cells are incubated in medium containing serum. This would suggest that the cellular uptake of biotin, when the biotin is added to the medium in high concentrations, does not require a specific serum factor. Biocytin, when added to HSD cell cultures results in activation of PCC apoenzyme, but only in the presence of serum. Normal human serum has considerable biotinidase activity (Pispa, 1965), but there was only barely detectable biotinidase activity in very concentrated fibroblast extracts using the colorimetric assay (Wolf *et al.*, 1983a). These findings suggest that the activation of PCC is principally due to the liberation of biotin from biocytin by serum biotinidase and the subsequent uptake of biotin by the cells.

Using the bioassay we have confirmed biotinidase deficiency in the children diagnosed previously by the colorimetric method. Most significantly, the bioassay uses the natural substrate, biocytin, rather than an artificial substrate. Furthermore, sera from obligate

heterozygotes were shown to have activities intermediate between those of normal and enzyme-deficient subjects. These results confirm the nature of the basic defect in late-onset MCD and establish the sensitivity of the bioassay. This method may also be used to distinguish between biotin and biocytin or biotinyl-peptides in concentrated samples of urine or tissue of biotinidase-deficient patients. For example, using urines obtained from individuals prior to biotin therapy as the source of substrate for biotinidase, the increase in PCC activity in cultures incubated without biotinidase (serum) reflects free biotin in urine, whereas the increase in PCC activity of cultures incubated with purified biotinidase or normal serum is attributable to both free and bound vitamin. The net increase in enzyme activity represents bound biotin. The relative concentrations of free to bound biotin can, therefore, be compared in urine of normal and affected individuals. Moreover, this culture system promises to be useful in elucidating other aspects of biotinidase and biotin metabolism.

The authors thank the various physicians who sent us blood specimens from their patients and their patient's parents. This work was supported by grants from NIH (AM 25675 and AM 33022) and from the National Foundation-March of Dimes (6-342).

References

Burri, B. J., Sweetman, L. and Nyhan, W. L. Mutant holocarboxylase synthetase. Evidence for the enzyme defect in early infantile biotin-responsive multiple carboxylase deficiency. *J. Clin. Invest.* 68 (1981)1491–1495

Feldman, G. L., Hsia, Y. E. and Wolf, B. Biochemical characterization of biotin-responsive multiple carboxylase deficiency: Heterogeneity within the *bio* genetic complementation group. *Am. J. Hum. Genet.* 33 (1981) 692–701

Pispa, J. Animal biotinidase. *Ann. Med. Exp. Biol. Fenn.* 43 (1965) 5–39

Thoma, R. M. and Petersen, W. H. The enzymatic degradation of soluble protein bound biotin. *J. Biol. Chem.* 210 (1954) 569–579

Wolf, B., Grier, R. E., Allen, R. J., Goodman, S. I. and Kien, C. L. Biotinidase deficiency: The enzymatic defect in late-onset multiple carboxylase deficiency. *Clin. Chim. Acta* 131 (1983a) 273–281

Wolf, B., Grier, R. E., Allen, R. J., Goodman, S. I., Kien, C. L., Parker, W. D., Howell, D. M. and Hurst, D. L. Phenotype variation in biotinidase deficiency. *J. Pediatr.* 103 (1983b) 233–241

Wolf, B., Hsia, Y. E. and Rosenberg, L. E. Biochemical differences between mutant propionyl CoA carboxylases from two complementation groups. *Am. J. Hum. Genet.* 30 (1977) 455–464

Table 1 Net increase in PCC activity in holocarboxylase synthetase deficient fibroblasts incubated with biocytin and serum from the various subjects

Subjects	Number studied	Net increase in PCC activity		
		Mean	Range	% of mean normal activity
Normal individuals	9	42.3	31.9–78.0	100
Affected children	6	3.3	−6.2–12.4	8
Parents	8	24.7	16.1–33.8	58

J. Inher. Metab. Dis. 8 Suppl. 2 (1985) 103–104

Short Communication

Biotin-responsive 3-Methylcrotonylglycinuria with Biotinidase Deficiency

J. Greter, E. Holme and S. Lindstedt
Department of Clinical Chemistry, Gothenburg University, Sahlgren's Hospital,
S-413 45 Gothenburg, Sweden

M. Koivikko
Department of Pediatrics, University of Tampere, Central Hospital,
SF-33520 Tampere 52, Finland

Functional deficiency of biotin-dependent carboxylases may have two biochemical causes, i.e. either deficiency of the apoenzymes, or deficient synthesis of the holo-enzymes, due to defects in holocarboxylase synthase (EC 6.3.4.10) or due to biotin deficiency induced by biotinidase (EC 3.5.1.12) deficiency or malnutrition.

The symptomatology of multiple carboxylase deficiency (MCD) is very variable but the cases have traditionally been divided into "early-onset" and "late-onset" MCD. The existence of biotinidase deficiency as a cause of MCD was not realized until 1983 (Wolf *et al.*, 1983a). Consequently, cases described before this date have not been adequately classified and it has been difficult to relate clinical picture to biochemical defect. From published descriptions it is now apparent that symptoms may vary considerably from case to case even in patients with the same verified biochemical defect.

Wolf *et al.* (1983b) have reported on a number of cases with biotinidase deficiency—usually classified as "late-onset" MCD. Neurological symptoms, such as seizures, ataxia, and hypotonia were common as were also alopecia and skin rash. Only one of six patients was considered to have a developmental delay. Cases have been described which have presented with lactic acidosis and significant excretion of organic acids such as 3-hydroxyisovaleric acid and 3-methylcrotonylglycine while in others there has been no significant organic aciduria (Swick *et al.*, 1983).

The multifaceted clinical picture and the varying biochemistry may lead to delayed diagnosis and therapy resulting in irreversible brain damage. We describe a case which illustrates this point.

CASE HISTORY

The boy is the second child born to healthy unrelated parents. The first child, now 4 years old, is healthy. Pregnancy and delivery were normal, birth weight 3.4 kg. The child was referred to the outpatient clinic at 4 weeks of age, when it had been noted that the head circumference had increased from 37 to 41 cm. He was slightly hypotonic and dull but no other significant abnormalities were found. He was readmitted 2 weeks later. The body temperature was 34.2°C. He was somnolent, had very little spontaneous activity and an abnormal cry. No eye contact could be established. He was also hypotonic and had occasional tremor in the extremities. A CT-scan showed cerebral oedema and an EEG showed reduced brain activity. He had an increased concentration of lactate in serum, $6.5\,\mathrm{mmol\,l^{-1}}$, with a base deficit of $2.5\,\mathrm{mmol\,l^{-1}}$. One month later he was readmitted. The body temperature now varied between 34 and 38°C, he had tonic seizures and repeated episodes of apnoea. The EEG was highly abnormal, with periods of paroxysmal activity in an otherwise low activity pattern. EMG showed prominent denervation. No diagnosis could be made.

The condition deteriorated at home and at the age of $4\frac{1}{2}$ months he was admitted to the hospital without spontaneous respiration and placed in a respirator. The results of a GC–MS study of organic acids in urine became available the following day. Biotin therapy was started and the condition improved with spontaneous breathing and less frequent seizures.

At the age of $1\frac{1}{2}$ years the child is severely spastic and mentally retarded and does not react on visual or auditory stimuli. He has seizures and the EEG is highly abnormal.

MATERIALS AND METHODS

Organic acids were analyzed by capillary GC–MS as their methoxylimine–trimethylsilyl derivatives. Quantitation was done by mass chromatography. The ion intensities were corrected for their differences in total ion current proportion.

The activities of pyruvate carboxylase (PC) (EC 6.4.1.1), propionyl-CoA carboxylase (PCC) (EC 6.4.1.3) and 3-methylcrotonyl-CoA carboxylase (MCC) (EC 6.4.1.4) in fibroblasts were determined by measuring substrate-dependent $^{14}CO_2$-fixation. Skin fibroblasts were cultured in minimum essential medium with Earl's salts and 18% fetal bovine serum (FBS). Biotin-depleted medium was obtained by treating the FBS with avidin–Sepharose. Biotin supplementation was done by adding sterile filtered biotin solution to the medium, $0.82\,\mu\mathrm{mol\,l^{-1}}$. Serum biotinidase activity was determined according to Knappe *et al.* (1963).

103

RESULTS

Excretion of organic acids

A urine specimen collected when the child was 3.5 months old was analyzed by GC–MS. The following acids were quantified (results expressed as mmol mol creatinine^{-1}): 3-hydroxyisovaleric acid, 2100; 3-methylcrotonylglycine, 620; methylcitrate, 100. Ten urine samples were collected in the period from 2 to 8 weeks after start of treatment. The excretions were (mmol mol creatinine^{-1}): 3-hydroxyisovaleric acid, 3–25; 3-methylcrotonylglycine, 4–16; methylcitrate, 0.4–8. A urine sample collected at $1\frac{1}{2}$ months of age was later shown to contain about 200 mmol mol creatinine^{-1} of 3-methylcrotonylglycine.

Carboxylase activities

PC, PCC and MCC activities were normal in fibroblasts cultured in media without biotin supplementation. Fibroblasts were also cultured in a biotin-free medium to deplete the carboxylase activities before reactivation with biotin. No difference in the biotin concentration-dependent MCC activation could be found between patient and control.

Serum biotinidase activity

The enzyme activity in the patient's serum was <1 nkat l^{-1} (control subjects 60–115 nkat l^{-1}; $n = 20$), in the father's serum 40 nkat l^{-1}, and in the mother's serum 29 nkat l^{-1}.

DISCUSSION

A skin rash and alopecia are often mentioned as the most characteristic signs of biotin deficiency (Bonjour, 1977; Heard et al., 1984), but these important diagnostic clues were absent in our patient. The clinical picture was instead dominated by symptoms from the central nervous system, including a poor temperature regulation and repeated attacks of apnoea—symptoms which have not previously been described in these patients. The symptoms started in the first few weeks of life and one has to consider the possibility that biotin deficiency was already present at birth. Initiation of biotin therapy—probably life-saving—was too late to prevent irreversible brain damage although the organic aciduria disappeared. Cutaneous symptoms are known to disappear after biotin therapy but rapidly developing severe brain damage is more likely to be irreversible. The experience from this case with its uncharacteristic symptomatology suggests that one should include an assay of biotinidase in neonatal screening programs. An easy and cheap assay suitable for this purpose has been described (Heard et al., 1984). An alternative to screening for biotinidase would be to use very wide indications for analysis of urine by GC–MS. Biotinidase deficiency without organic aciduria has, however, been described (Wolf et al., 1983b). In any case, results from this type of analysis is not always available within the short time that may be necessary to prevent irreversible damage.

This work was supported by a grant from the Swedish Medical Research Council (03X-585).

References

Bonjour, J. P. Biotin in man's nutrition and therapy—a review. *Int. J. Vitam. Nutr. Res.* 47 (1977) 107–118

Heard, G. S., Secor McVoy, J. R. and Wolf, B. A screening method for biotinidase deficiency in newborns. *Clin. Chem.* 30 (1984) 125–127

Knappe, J., Brümmer, W. and Biederbick, K. Reinigung und Eigenschaften der Biotinidase aus Schweinenieren und Lactobacillus Casei. *Biochem. Zeitschr.* 338 (1963) 599–613

Swick, H. M. and Kien, C. L. Biotin deficiency with neurologic and cutaneous manifestations but without organic aciduria. *J. Pediatr.* 103 (1983) 265–267

Wolf, B., Grier, R. E., Allen, R. J., Goodman, S. I. and Kien, C. L. Biotinidase deficiency: the enzymatic defect in late-onset multiple carboxylase deficiency. *Clin. Chim. Acta* 131 (1983a) 273–281

Wolf, B., Grier, R. E., Allen, R. J., Goodman, S. I., Kien, C. L., Parker, W. D., Howell, D. M. and Hurst, D. L. Phenotypic variation in biotinidase deficiency. *J. Pediatr.* 103 (1983b) 233–237

J. Inher. Metab. Dis. 8 Suppl. 2 (1985) 105–106

Short Communication

Organic Aciduria in Late-onset Biotin-responsive Multiple Carboxylase Deficiency

C. ERASMUS
Department of Paediatrics, University of Pretoria, Pretoria, 0001, South Africa

L. J. MIENIE and C. J. REINECKE[1]
Department of Biochemistry, Potchefstroom University for Christian Higher Education, Potchefstroom 2520, South Africa

S. K. WADMAN
Universiteitskinderkliniek, Wilhelmina Kinderziekenhuis, University of Utrecht, Utrecht, The Netherlands

Late-onset, biotin-responsive, multiple carboxylase deficiency (McKusick 21021) is an inherited autosomal recessive disorder. The major symptoms of the disease are alopecia skin rash, seizures, ataxia, hypotonia and developmental delay, which typically appear at about 6 months of age, with a range from 3 weeks to 24 months (Wolf *et al.*, 1983b). The primary biochemical defect in this disease was identified as deficient activity of the enzyme biotinidase (biotin-amide amidohydrolase, EC 3.5.1.12; Wolf *et al.*, 1983c). This enzyme catalyzes the removal of biotin from the ε-amino group of a lysine side chain of proteolytic degradation products of the carboxylase holoenzyme, thereby regenerating biotin for reutilization. In biotinidase-deficient patients this biotin-salvage pathway is not operative, and high concentrations of dietary biotin are thus required to prevent the symptoms of the biotin-deficient state (Wolf *et al.*, 1983a).

Organic aciduria is a very general, but surprisingly not a consistent, feature of late-onset multiple carboxylase deficiency. Analysis of the urine of most of these patients have shown the presence of various organic acids associated with the catabolic pathways of the branched chain amino acids (Cowan *et al.*, 1979), whereas pathological amounts of some organic acids only appeared in urine of other patients after a high protein diet (Munnich *et al.*, 1981). In some patients no organic aciduria could be detected (Swick and Kien, 1983; Wolf *et al.*, 1983b).

In this communication we present results of a new case of late-onset multiple carboxylase deficiency. The clinical features were more pronounced than those usually found for individual cases of the disease.

CASE HISTORY

Z.C. is the first child of healthy non-consanguineous parents. Her mother suffered from a resistant diarrhoea during the pregnancy. The delivery and perinatal period were uncomplicated, and she developed normally for the first 10 weeks of life. The onset of resistant myoclonic seizures heralded a relentless downhill course. She lost all social responses and ceased to react to visual or auditory stimuli. She became severely hypotonic and had few voluntary movements. Repeated respiratory infections were troublesome. She developed alopecia, a maculopapular rash and keratoconjunctivitis. Her urine had a pungent feline-like odour. The patient was seen by us at the age of 7 months. At that time she was unresponsive, apart from a startle to loud noise and withdrawal response to pain. The fundi were normal. She had hepatosplenomegaly. Computed tomography showed cerebral atrophy and low attenuation of the white matter. The background activity of the EEG was normal, but epileptiform activity was present over both hemispheres. ERG was normal. VER showed no response and brainstem auditory evoked potential was absent up to 90 dB stimulation. Blood samples for extensive analysis were collected in the fasting state and hourly for 3 h after a load of 1 g protein (kg body weight)$^{-1}$. The plasma pyruvate concentration increased from $135\,\mu\text{mol}\,l^{-1}$ in the fasting state to a maximum of $241\,\mu\text{mol}\,l^{-1}$ at 2 h after the protein load. Likewise the serum lactate increased from $7.5\,\text{mmol}\,l^{-1}$ to $8\,\text{mmol}\,l^{-1}$ at 1 h after the protein load. The values for the blood ammonia were 73.8, 79.6 and $51.8\,\mu\text{mol}\,l^{-1}$, respectively in the fasting state and 1 and 2 h after the protein load. There was an increased anion gap and a compensated metabolic acidosis. Analysis of the urinary organic acids helped to establish the diagnosis of multiple carboxylase deficiency.

Treatment with biotin ($10\,\text{mg}\,\text{day}^{-1}$) was initiated, and increased within 2 weeks to $20\,\text{mg}\,\text{day}^{-1}$. Six weeks after commencing therapy the patient was re-examined. There was a dramatic clinical improvement. She responded socially. Head control, flexor and tensor tone had improved markedly and she was able to sit unsupported. She was fit-free and off antiepileptic medication. The rash, conjunctivitis and respiratory infections had cleared. The EEG and VER had normalized.

---

[1]Author to whom correspondence should be addressed

Journal of Inherited Metabolic Disease. ISSN 0141-8955. Copyright © SSIEM and MTP Press Limited, Queen Square, Lancaster, UK.

METHODS AND RESULTS

The organic acids were extracted with ethyl acetate and diethyl ether from 1.0 ml acidified urine according to standard procedures. TMS derivatives of the extracted organic acids were analyzed by capillary column (25 m × 0.25 mm, SE 30) gas chromatography. Organic acids were identified by comparing the MU values with authentic standards and by mass spectrometry (GLC–MS) using a Ribermag R10-10 (Rueil Malmaison, France) quadrupole mass spectrometer, combined with a Digital (DEC, Maynard, MA, USA) PDP-11/23 minicomputer. A quantitative determination of urinary organic acids prior to biotin treatment is shown in Table 1. The increased lactic acid content is associated with a deficiency in pyruvate carboxylase (EC 4.6.1.1), while the presence of succinic acid, fumaric acid and 2-ketoglutaric acids is regarded as a secondary response to the deficiency in this enzyme (Van Biervliet *et al.*, 1977). Only 3-hydroxyisovaleric acid and trace amounts to 3-methylcrotonylglycine could be related to a deficiency in the activity of 3-methylcrotonyl-CoA carboxylase (EC 4.6.1.4). No 3-methylcrotonic acid could be detected. The presence of 3-hydroxypropionic acid and low concentrations of methylcitric acid indicated a deficiency in propionyl-CoA carboxylase (EC 4.6.1.3). After treatment with 10 mg biotin day^{-1}, lactic acid and 3-hydroxyisovaleric acid at respective concentrations of 2.3 and 0.33 mmol (g creatinine)$^{-1}$ were still present. After treatment with 20 mg biotin day^{-1} the organic acids associated with the disease were absent, and a gas chromatogram of the normal state was obtained.

DISCUSSION

The clinical presentation and biochemical characteristics of the patient studied were suggestive of late-onset multiple carboxylase deficiency due to biotinidase deficiency. The phenotypical presentation of this disease is variable (Wolf *et al.*, 1983b). The variety and extent of clinical symptoms of our patient exceed those normally found for a single affected individual, and include the less frequently found symptoms like conjunctivitis and hearing loss. Moreover, the pattern of organic acids resembled those of other cases, like increased lactic and 3-hydroxyisovaleric aciduria. On the other hand, very low concentrations of 3-methylcrotonylglycine, methylcitrate and 3-hydroxypropionate were present, and no 3-methylcrotonic acid was detectable. This implies that multiple carboxylase deficiency might remain undetected in a given patient. Oral loading with extra protein will provoke the excretion of the typical metabolites and might be useful in patients that are clinically suggestive of multiple carboxylase deficiency, lacking the chemical characteristics. Our observations

Table 1 Concentration of the organic acids, diagnostic for multiple carboxylase deficiency, in a urine sample of the patient prior to biotin treatment

Organic acid	Concentration (mmol (g creatinine)$^{-1}$)
Lactic acid	8.4
Succinic acid	1.6
Fumaric acid	2.1
2-Ketoglutaric acid	7.3
3-Hydroxyisovaleric acid	17.2
3-Methylcrotonic acid	Not detectable
3-Methylcrotonylglycine	Trace
3-Hydroxypropionic acid	0.7
Methylcitric acid	Trace

finally indicate that clinical and genetic heterogeneity will probably also be a characteristic of multiple carboxylase deficiency, and demonstrate once more the variability in the presentation of inborn errors of metabolism.

This research was supported by a grant from the South African Medical Research Council.

References

Cowan, M. J., Wara, D. W., Packman, S., Ammann, A. J., Yoshino, M., Sweetnam, L. and Nyhan, W. Multiple biotin-dependent carboxylase deficiencies associated with defects in T-cell and B-cell immunity. *Lancet* 2 (1979) 115–118

Munnich, A., Saudubray, J. M., Cotisson, A., Coude, F. X., Ogier, H., Charpentier, C., Marsac, C., Carre, G., Bourgeay-Causse, M. and Frezal, J. Biotin dependent multiple carboxylase deficiency presenting as a congenital lactic acidosis. *Eur. J. Pediatr.* 137 (1981) 203–206

Swick, H. M. and Kien, C. L. Biotin deficiency with neurologic and cutaneous manifestations but without organic aciduria. *J. Pediatr.* 103 (1983) 265–267

Van Biervliet, J. P. G. M., Bruinvis, L., Van der Heiden, C., Ketting, D., Wadman, S. K., Willemse, J. L. and Monnens, L. A. H. Report of a patient with severe chronic lactic acidaemia and pyruvate carboxylase deficiency. *Devl. Med. Child Neurol.* 19 (1977) 392–401

Wolf, B., Grier, R. E., Allen, R. J., Goodman, S. I. and Kien, C. L. Biotinidase deficiency: the enzymatic defect in late-onset multiple carboxylase deficiency. *Clin. Chim. Acta* 131 (1983a) 273–278

Wolf, B., Grier, R. E., Allen, R. J., Goodman, S. I., Kien, C. L., Parker, W. D., Howell, D. M. and Hurst, D. L. Phenotypic variation in biotinidase deficiency. *J. Pediatr.* 103 (1983b) 233–237

Wolf, B., Grier, R. E., Parker, W. D., Goodman, S. I. and Allen, R. J. Deficient biotinidase activity in late-onset multiple carboxylase deficiency. *N. Engl. J. Med.* 308 (1983c) 161

J. Inter. Metab. Dis. 8 Suppl. 2 (1985) 107–108

Short Communication

Successful Nicotinamide Treatment in an Autosomal Dominant Behavioral and Psychiatric Disorder

W. BLOM, G. B. VAN DEN BERG and J. G. M. HUIJMANS
Department of Pediatrics, Metabolic Laboratory, Sophia Children's Hospital, Erasmus University Rotterdam, The Netherlands

J. A. R. SANDERS-WOUDSTRA
Department of Child-Psychiatry, Sophia Children's Hospital, Erasmus University Rotterdam, The Netherlands

During the last decade many attempts have been made to correlate behavioral or psychiatric disorders with abnormalities in neurotransmission. Interest and extensive laboratory investigation have centred upon noradrenaline, 5-hydroxytryptamine and dopamine. An obstacle to investigation of such correlation is the impossibility of directly studying central neurotransmission in living patients. Advances have been achieved but results tend to be conflicting (*The Lancet*, editorial review, 1981).

The study of tryptophan metabolism to understand 5-hydroxytryptamine biosynthesis and breakdown is clouded by nutrition, intestinal resorption plus bacterial metabolism, liver metabolism, and the transport mechanisms of tryptophan. Abnormalities of tryptophan transport and metabolism, detectable in plasma, urine or platelets, are not necessarily a reflection of dysfunction of 5-hydroxytryptamine neutrotransmission. However, we have discovered five families with an autosomal dominant behavioral and psychiatric disorder, in which a number of affected family members showed intestinal tryptophan malabsorption, or an abnormal tryptophan metabolism on a tryptophan loading test. These abnormalities prompted us to try nicotinamide therapy. As a result we observed in treated patients a remarkable improvement or normalisation of their behavioral and psychiatric abnormalities.

METHODS

Indoles in urine were examined by TLC, HPLC and GC–MS. TLC of indoles was performed by concentrating the urine 10 times, spotting on a Merck Silicagel plate 10×10 cm, layer thickness 0.25 mm, the amount of urine spotted depending on creatinine concentration and age, and two-dimensional chromatography with the solvents: (1) abs. ethanol/NH_3/H_2O (87.5:1.5:12.0), and (2) butanol/acetic acid/H_2O (60:15:25). The indoles were stained with Ehrlich reagent. HPLC of indoles in urine were done essentially according to the method of Krustulovic and Matzura (1979). Organic acids, including tryptophan metabolites, were analysed in urine by GC–MS. In the salt-saturated urine at pH 1–2 ketone functions were ethoximed with ethoxylamine. The organic acids were extracted with ethyl acetate. The extract was dried and evaporated to dryness. The residue

was dissolved in methanol-ether and the organic acids were methylated with diazomethane. The derivatised organic acids were analysed by GC (packed column SP2250, 70–300°C, 8°C min^{-1}) and identified with MS (Varian MAT CH7A + Varian MAT SS188).

Tryptophan loading tests were performed with an oral load of 110 mg kg^{-1} of L-tryptophan followed by the collection of two 12 h urine samples. During collection and until analysis the urines were deeply frozen.

FAMILY HISTORY

The pedigree of our first discovered family is shown in Figure 1. Examples of the behavioral and psychiatric abnormalities are given in the following family members:

III 3: Hot-tempered, alcohol abuse.

III 4: As a child difficult, uncommunicative, contact disability, hot-tempered, atopic eczema.

IV 4: As a child fits of crying and temper tantrums; was treated by a child psychologist. Now restless, overactive and overtalkative. Sometimes dizziness. Slight ataxia.

IV 6: As a child fits of crying and temper tantrums. Later labile, stress-sensitive. Was admitted to a psychiatric institute for one year.

IV 7: As a child difficult. Now intermittently depressive with temper tantrums.

V 1, 2 and 3 in general: Unmanagable behavior, contact and play disability, hyperactive, restless, chaotic, stress sensitive, fits of crying and temper

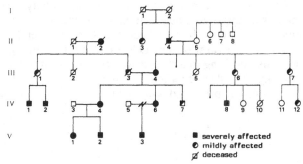

Figure 1 Pedigree of our first family with an autosomal dominant inherited behavioral and psychiatric disorder

Journal of Inherited Metabolic Disease. ISSN 0141-8955. Copyright © SSIEM and MTP Press Limited, Queen Square, Lancaster, UK.

tantrums. Defecation problems. In addition:

V 1: Hypothermia during the first months of life. Extreme sleep difficulties. Atopic eczema. with self-destructive scratching. At the age of 5 years she wanted to be dead.

V 2: Ataxia and intention tremor.

V 3: Extreme sleep difficulties. Wanted to be a girl.

RESULTS

The children V 1, 2 and 3 showed, in a basal urine, metabolites typical of tryptophan malabsorption with increased indican excretion. On a tryptophan loading test they showed, in the first 12 h urine, a high excretion of kynurenine, *N*-acetylkynurenine, 3-hydroxy-kynurenine, kynurenic acid and xanthurenic acid, suggesting a partial enzyme block in the kynurenine pathway at the level of kynureninase. On a tryptophan loading test the mothers IV 4 and 6 excreted the same high amounts of kynurenine and metabolites as the children V 1, 2 and 3.

On nicotinamide treatment ($20 \, mg \, kg^{-1}$ in six doses) the children V 1, 2 and 3 improved dramatically. After 1 month of therapy they were nearly normalised in most of their clinical abnormalities. Patient V 1 is still suffering from atopic eczema, but without self-destructive scratching. She was more definitely improved since her mother IV 4 was also on nicotinamide treatment. Mother IV 4 is quieter now and less dominating. For the first time in her life she feels she has internal peace. Defecation problems and tryptophan malabsorption, as observed in the children V 1, 2 and 3, disappeared with nicotinamide therapy.

DISCUSSION

The pedigree, the fact that in different affected family members metabolic abnormalities could be detected, and the positive results of nicotinamide therapy suggest an autosomal dominant inheritance. The behavioral and psychiatric abnormalities in our families at first view resemble Hartnup disease, but we could not observe the typical amino aciduria and pellagra described in Hartnup disease.

From a genetic point of view it seems unlikely that there is an enzymatic defect in an autosomal dominant inherited disorder. In our affected families we therefore assume a structural protein defect in the serotoninergic neurons. resulting in a disturbed serotonin neurotrans-mission. The affected patients must be heterozygous for the structural protein defect. If there is no enzymatic defect it is reasonable that we or other investigators cannot find striking metabolic abnormalities. The metabolic abnormalities in tryptophan transport or metabolism that we observed in a number of our affected patients must be secondary. We have to realize that about 85% of the total-body 5-hydroxytryptamine is located in the intestinal serotoninergic system. A structural protein defect in the serotoninergic neurons might certainly also affect the intestinal serotoninergic system. Most probably this explains why, in our young affected patients, we observed defecation problems: (patients V 1 and 2 had thin defecation from birth, as patient V 3 had obstipation with intermittent diarrhoea). These defecation problems may be the explanation of the observed tryptophan malabsorption with increased urinary indican excretion. We have to do further investigations to see if an abnormal kynurenine and kynurenine metabolite production after a tryptophan loading test is a significant metabolic parameter in this behavioral and psychiatric illness or not.

From a theoretical point of view there are three possibilities for the treatment of these patients:

(1) tryptophan or 5-tryptophan supplement to the diet;
(2) treatment with vitamin B6 or nicotinamide;
(3) carbohydrate rich, poor fat and protein diet + tryptophan supplement.

We chose nicotinamide therapy, because it can be prescribed in high doses and is supposed to have a broad mode of action:

(1) stimulation of intestinal tryptophan absorption;
(2) inactivation of tryptophan pyrrolase (first enzymatic step in kynurenine pathway);
(3) stimulation of energy metabolism ($NAD^+ / NADP^+$);
(4) possible antiepileptic properties.

In conclusion we want to emphasize that autosomal dominant inherited behavioral and psychiatric illness, such as we have discovered, is unknown in the literature. Thus, a careful family history in every child with abnormal behavior is of great importance. Nicotinamide therapy can be of excellent benefit for the patient.

References

Editorial review. 5-Hydroxytryptamine and psychiatric illness. *Lancet* 2 (1981) 788–789

Krustulovic, A. M. and Matzura, C. Rapid analyses of tryptophan metabolites using reversed-phase high performance liquid chromatography with fluorometric detection. *J. Chromatogr.* 163 (1979) 72–76

J. Inher. Metab. Dis. 8 Suppl. 2 (1985) 109–110

Short Communication

Folic Acid Responsive Rages, Seizures and Homocystinuria

J. V. MURPHY and L. M THOME
Milwaukee Pediatric Neurology, 2040 W Wisconsin Ave., Milwaukee, WI 53233, USA

K. MICHALS and R. MATALON
Department of Pediatrics, University of Illinois School of Medicine, 840 South Wood Street, Chicago, IL 60612, USA

Homocystinuria can be secondary to defects in the conversion of homocysteine either to cystathionine or to methionine. Osteoporosis and ectopia lentis are common features in the former entity (Mudd and Levy, 1983). There has been one patient described with a defect in the conversion of homocysteine to methionine who had a diagnosis of schizophrenia and who improved with folic acid therapy (Freeman *et al.*, 1975). In the past year we have evaluated two unrelated children with periodic rages, seizures, and homocystinuria. Both patients improved dramatically when treated with folic acid.

CASE REPORTS

Case 1, B.V.

At the age of 4 years, this otherwise normal boy demonstrated periodic and unprovoked rages lasting several hours and followed by sleep. Recall was denied. Examples included throwing a chest of drawers down a flight of stairs, attacking his father with a knife, and prolonged temper tantrums with throwing objects, yelling and screaming. His EEG demonstrated polyspikes, and irregular generalized spike and slow wave bursts. Anticonvulsant therapy improved the EEG, but not the patient's symptoms. Prior to psychiatric hospitalization a urinary amino acid analysis was performed. The only abnormality was the presence of 3.5 mg homocystine (g creatinine)$^{-1}$. Urinary methionine concentration was within normal limits.

Treatment with folic acid, 0.8 mg daily, produced a remarkable improvement within a week. After 3 months on this therapy his behavior insidiously deteriorated. Homocystine, which was absent from his urine following the start of folic acid therapy, was once more present, 9.9 mg homocystine (g creatinine)$^{-1}$ (Figure 1). Biochemical and symptomatic improvement occurred after starting a low protein diet, and doubling the dose of folic acid. The only relative with homocystinuria is the patient's 7 year old brother, who is moderately hyperactive.

Case 2, J.W.

Generalized tonic–clonic seizures at the age of 3 years prompted medical attention for this adopted child of Korean ancestry. Her EEG demonstrated generalized bursts of polyspikes during sleep without accompanying

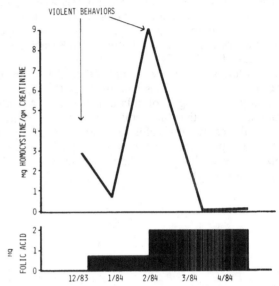

Figure 1 Correlation of urinary homocystine, violent behavior and folic acid therapy in patient 1. Folic acid alone provided only transient clinical and biochemical benefit

clinical seizures. Concurrent with the unsuccessful use of anticonvulsant therapy the patient developed unprovoked, unusual and periodic behavior followed by sleep and amnesia for the event. Examples of such behavior included pinching herself or someone next to her repetitively for an hour, running from home in the predawn hours, repetitively playing two notes on the piano for 45 min, and temper tantrums. At other times she was a model child. Her family reported that she had a distinctive odour which others did not recognize. When all medicinal approaches to her behavioral problems failed metabolic studies were undertaken. Her urinary concentrations of homocystine were 33.8 and 25.8 mg (g creatinine)$^{-1}$. Methionine concentrations were normal. Folic acid (3 mg day^{-1}) produced resolution of seizures and inappropriate behavior, loss of her distinctive odour, and a reduction of urinary homocystine to 7.2 mg. This improvement lasted 2 months. Following the addition of betaine and a low protein diet these improvements have been maintained for over 6 months. Recently no homocystine has been detected in her urine. Rare dietary indiscretions are associated with behavioral deterioration.

No siblings are available for testing.

Journal of Inherited Metabolic Disease. ISSN 0141-8955. Copyright © SSIEM and MTP Press Limited, Queen Square, Lancaster, UK.

DISCUSSION

The above cases appear to be a variant of the previously described patient with folate-responsive homocystinuria and "schizophrenia" (Freeman *et al.*, 1975). Their patient demonstrated a thought disorder at the age of 15 years, which resolved with folic acid therapy. It is interesting to note that their patient deteriorated, as did ours, despite the maintenance of folate therapy (personal communication).

The biochemical defect in our patients appears to be one of conversion of homocysteine to methionine. The absence of ocular defects and osteoporosis, as well as the presence of normal concentrations of methionine in the urine, indicate that our two patients do not have a deficiency of cystathionine synthase (McKusick 23620; Mudd and Levy, 1983).

An alternate etiology would be a defect in the metabolism of folate. This is unlikely as these patients lack any other signs of folate deficiency. A better explanation for this biochemical defect is a deficient 5,10-methylenetetrahydrofolate reductase activity which is partially responsive to folate therapy. Appropriate studies on cultured fibroblasts are underway to validate this theory.

This disorder is a unique example of a correlation between the accumulation of a specific amino acid, homocystine, and a behavior disorder. In the first patient we were able to relate behavioral deterioration with the reappearance of large amounts of homocystine in his urine. Increasing the dose of folic acid and restricting protein intake resulted in improvement.

The therapeutic benefit of folic acid in these patients warrants the consideration of this form of homocystinuria in young children with seizures and periodic behavioral deteriorations. Considering that an older sibling of patient 1 is asymptomatic it is quite possible that the symptoms described above are only variably expressed in patients with this disorder.

References

Freeman, J. M., Finkelstein, J. D. and Mudd, S. H. Folate-responsive homocystinuria and "schizophrenia." *N. Engl. J. Med.* 292 (1975) 491–496

Mudd, S. H. and Levy, H. L. Disorders of transsulfuration. In Stanbury, J., Wyngaarden, J. and Fredrickson, D. (eds.) *The Metabolic Basis of Inherited Disease*, 5th edn., McGraw-Hill, New York, 1983, pp. 522–559

J. Inher. Metab. Dis. 8 Suppl. 2 (1985) 111–112

Short Communication

The Effect of Phytol upon Skeletal Muscle Damage in Vitamin E-Deficient Animals

S. KRYWAWYCH, M. J. JACKSON, C. FORTE, P. J. GARROD, D. K. WALKER and D. P. BRENTON
Department of Medicine, University College London School of Medicine, The Rayne Institute, London WC1E 6JJ, UK

The long-term treatment of Refsum's disease (McKusick 26650) overwhelmingly relies on dietary management with a low phytanate and phytol intake. Although this diet successfully depletes the accumulated phytanate in patients with Refsum's disease, the clinical improvement is incomplete (Steinberg *et al.*, 1970; Sahgal and Olsen, 1975; Gibberd *et al.*, 1979). This raises the question as to whether the persisting clinical problems may be caused by some other undefined and untreated pathology rather than by the direct accumulation of phytanate and its incorporation into myelin (Steinberg *et al.*, 1967).

Cerebral ataxia, retinitis pigmentosa, muscle weakness and peripheral neuropathy are specific clinical features common to both Refsum's disease and abetalipoproteinaemia. In the latter condition these clinical problems can be prevented and reversed with vitamin E therapy (Muller *et al.*, 1983). Furthermore, as there is also a very close structural resemblance between the molecules of phytanate and vitamin E with the unusual branched phytol chain being common to both, it is conceivable that a competitive elimination of vitamin E from nerve and muscle membrane by phytanate could be important in the pathogenesis of Refsum's disease. This report describes the results of the *in vivo* investigations of the effect of phytol upon skeletal muscle damage in vitamin E-deficient animals.

METHODS

Animals and diets

Weanling Wistar female rats were fed *ad libitum* (a) a yeast-based vitamin E-deficient diet, or (b) the same diet but supplemented with vitamin E (250 mg α-tocopheryl-acetate kg diet^{-1}). The composition of the diet was 25% vitamin E-deficient yeast (Distillers Co. Ltd., London) 10% corn oil, 36% starch, 25% sucrose and 4% salt, mineral and vitamin mix. The animals were fed these diets for 90–95 days, then for a further month half the animals on a vitamin E-deficient diet and half the animals on a vitamin E-supplemented diet had 1% phytol added to the diets.

In vivo contractile activity

The animals were fully anaesthetised with intraperitoneal injections of pentobarbitone. Hindlimbs were then stimulated via surface electrodes located below the knee and round the thigh adjoining the gluteal region. Stimulation was with 0.2 ms pulses at 50 Hz and 70 V for 0.5 s, repeated every 2 s for 15 min. Blood was sampled from the tail vein, immediately before stimulation, and then 0 min, 120 min and 24 h after stimulation.

Enzyme and metabolite estimations

Plasma creatine kinase (CK) was assayed at 25°C by using a linked enzyme assay and following the production of NADPH. Plasma vitamin E was estimated as total α-tocopherol fluorometrically by the method of Hansen and Warwick (1966). The malonaldehyde content of muscle homogenates, an indicator of lipid peroxidation, was measured by the method of McMurray and Dormandy (1974).

Phytanate was measured as its trimethylsilyl ester by gas liquid chromatography using 25 m long BP10 capillary columns with an internal diameter of 0.22 mm and temperature programming from 80 to 250°C at 5°C min^{-1}. Animals were killed 14 days after the stimulation investigations had been completed and muscle was removed for histology and biochemistry.

RESULTS

Plasma vitamin E

The plasma vitamin E concentration in vitamin E-supplemented rats was $25.1 \pm 6.8 \, \text{mg} \, \text{l}^{-1}$ (mean ± SD, $n = 9$) and $8.8 \pm 3.1 \, \text{mg} \, \text{l}^{-1}$ (mean ± SD, $n = 9$) in vitamin E-deficient animals. These results were not significantly changed by the addition of phytol to the diet.

Plasma and muscle phytanate

Phytanate was undetected in plasma and muscle in animals whose diet excluded phytol. In phytol-fed rats plasma phytanate concentrations in vitamin E-deficient animals were 20–138 µmol l^{-1} (mean 92, $n = 6$) and 12–158 µmol l^{-1} (mean 78, $n = 4$) in vitamin E-supplemented animals.

Muscle phytanate concentrations in vitamin E-deficient animals fed phytol were 100–240 µmol kg wet wt^{-1} (mean 160, $n = 3$) and 100–160 µmol kg wet wt^{-1} (mean 140, $n = 3$) in vitamin E-supplemented animals fed phytol.

The plasma and muscle phytanate values given above expressed differently as a percentage of total fatty acid similarly did not reveal any differences between vitamin E-deficient or supplemented animals fed phytol.

Muscle malonaldehyde

Malonaldehyde was elevated [21.5 ± 12.1 (SD) nmol g wet wt^{-1} ($n = 4$)] only in the muscle from some animals fed a vitamin E-deficient diet with phytol; animals maintained on alternative diets demonstrated normal malonaldehyde concentrations [vitamin E-deficient

Journal of Inherited Metabolic Disease. ISSN 0141-8955. Copyright © SSIEM and MTP Press Limited, Queen Square, Lancaster, UK.

without phytol, 14.2 ± 3.6 nmol g wet wt^{-1} $(n = 3)$; with vitamin E, 10.4 ± 2.6 nmol g wet wt^{-1} $(n = 3)$; with vitamin E and phytol, 7.9 ± 0.3 nmol g wet wt^{-1} $(n = 4)$].

Resting plasma CK concentrations

The resting plasma CK values were similar in all four groups. Vitamin E-deficient, 91 ± 26.1 IU l^{-1} (mean $\pm$ SD, $n = 7$); vitamin E-supplemented, 101 ± 59 IU l^{-1} (mean $\pm$ SD, $n = 5$); vitamin E-deficient plus phytol, 78 ± 26.1 IU l^{-1} (mean $\pm$ SD, $n = 5$); vitamin E-supplemented plus phytol, 96 ± 31 IU l^{-1} (mean $\pm$ SD, $n = 4$).

Poststimulation plasma CK values

Vitamin E-supplemented animals showed only a small rise in CK. Vitamin E-deficient animals showed a greater rise of CK which had returned to normal by 120 min. Phytol supplementation in vitamin E-deficient animals resulted in a more prolonged rise in CK and a delay in returning to resting values (Figure 1).

Histopathology

No histopathological changes were seen in the mixed muscles from animals fed vitamin E-deficient diets with and without phytol.

DISCUSSION

The increased susceptibility of skeletal muscle to contraction-induced damage in vitamin E-deficient rats is indicated by the significantly elevated rise in their plasma CK immediately after stimulation (Figure 1). This confirms the observation of other workers who employed longer stimulation periods and sampled for a shorter duration on completion of stimulation (Jackson *et al.*, 1983). The rise of plasma CK is similarly abnormal in the phytol-fed vitamin E-deficient animals, in this case, unlike those not fed phytol, the CK continued to increase for at least 2 h into the recovery period.

The function of vitamin E in biological systems is somewhat uncertain, but it is currently thought to have both an important protective and structural role in maintaining the integrity of membranes (Burton *et al.*, 1983). By inactivating potentially hazardous free radicals the cyclic head of vitamin E protects the membrane polyunsaturated fatty acids from oxidation. Free radicals are generated during muscular contraction and, in the absence of vitamin E, would ultimately result in muscle membrane damage with the leakage of CK into the plasma. The augmented muscle damage, induced by phytanate in the vitamin E-deficient animals reported here, may represent a more extreme deficiency of this vitamin in the muscle membrane because of its displacement by competing phytanate. Support for the enhanced free radical damage in this group of animals is attained from their elevated muscle malonaldehyde content.

Such a competitive process between vitamin E and phytanate may operate and be important in the pathogenesis of Refsum's disease; and this disease could therefore lend itself to treatment with vitamin E administration.

References

Burton, G. W., Cheeseman, K. H., Doba, T., Ingold, K. U. and Slater, T. F. Vitamin E as an antioxidant *in vitro* and *in vivo*. In Porter, R. and Whelan, J. (eds.) *Biology of Vitamin E*, Ciba Foundation Symposium 101, Pitman, London, 1983, pp. 4–18

Gibberd, F. B., Page, N. G. R., Billimoria, J. D. and Retsas, S. Heredopathia atactica polyneuritiformis (Refsum's disease) treated by diet and plasma exchange. *Lancet* 1 (1979) 575–578

Hansen, L. G. and Warwick, W. J. A fluorimetric micromethod for serum tocopherol. *Am. J. Clin. Pathol.* 46 (1966) 133–138

Jackson, M. J., Jones, D. A. and Edwards, R. H. T. Vitamin E and skeletal muscle. In Porter, R. and Whelan, J. (eds.) *Biology of Vitamin E*, Ciba Foundation Symposium 101, Pitman, London, 1983, pp. 224–239

McMurray, W. and Dormandy, T. Lipid antioxidation in human skeletal muscle. *Clin. Chim. Acta* 52 (1974) 105–114

Muller, D. P. R., Lloyd, J. K. and Wolff, O. H. Vitamin E and neurological function. *Lancet* 1 (1983) 225–228

Sahgal, V. and Olsen, W. O. Heredopathia Atactica Polyneuritiformis (phytanic acid storage disease). A new case with special reference to treatment. *Arch. Int. Med.* 135 (1975) 585–587

Steinberg, D., Mize, C. E., Herndon Jr, J. H., Fales, H. M., Engel, W. K. and Vroom, F. Q. Phytanic acid in patients with Refsum's syndrome and response to dietary treatment. *Arch. Int. Med.* 125 (1970) 75–87

Steinberg, D., Vroom, F. Q., Engel, W. K., Cammermeyer, J., Mize, C. E. and Avigan, J. Refsum's disease—a recently characterised lipodosis involving the nervous system. *Ann. Int. Med.* 66 (1967) 365–395

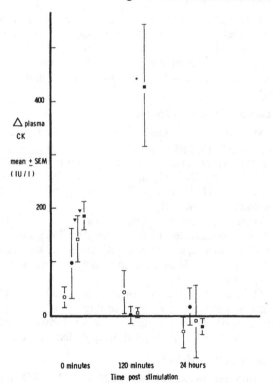

Figure 1 Effect of stimulation upon the changes in plasma CK in rats maintained on differing vitamin E and phytol intakes. ○ + vitamin E $(n = 5)$; ● + vitamin E + phytol $(n = 4)$; □ − vitamin E $(n = 7)$; ■ − vitamin E + phytol $(n = 5)$; ▼ significantly different from + vitamin E animals $(p = 0.005)$; *significantly different from + vitamin E, + vitamin E + phytol and − vitamin E animals $(p = 0.001)$

J. Inher. Metab. Dis. 8 Suppl. 2 (1985) 113–114

Short Communication–Noel Raine Award

Dihydropyrimidine Dehydrogenase Deficiency Leading to Thymine-uraciluria. An Inborn Error of Pyrimidine Metabolism

S. K. Wadman[1], R. Berger[2], M. Duran[1], P. K. de Bree[1], S. A. Stoker-de Vries[2], F. A. Beemer[1], J. J. Weits-Binnerts[3], T. J. Penders[4] and J. K. van der Woude[5]

[1]*University Children's Hospital, "Het Wilhelmina Kinderziekenhuis", Nieuwe Gracht 137, 3512 LK Utrecht, The Netherlands*
[2]*Department of Pediatrics, University of Groningen, The Netherlands*
[3]*Centre for Mental Retardation, Assen, The Netherlands*
[4]*Stichting Streekziekenhuis Koningin Beatrix, Winterswijk, The Netherlands*
[5]*Hospital "De Stadsmaten", Enschede, The Netherlands*

The number of known inherited defects of pyrimidine metabolism is small. At least for a part this may be due to the fact that there is no typical end product, such as uric acid in purine metabolism. Furthermore, urinary pyrimidines are not easily accessible for simple chromatographic screening. However, metabolites such as uracil, thymine and orotic acid can be detected with the routine gas–liquid chromatography procedure for organic acids using ethyl acetate extraction and trimethylsilylation (Wadman *et al.*, 1984) if their concentrations are strongly elevated. By this method we established a persistently excessive excretion of thymine and uracil in a 4-year-old boy, whose urine was screened for inborn errors of metabolism. Later another patient was discovered in the same way. In a third patient the same abnormality was found using 2-dimensional thin layer chromatography according to van Gennip *et al.* (1978). This metabolite profile suggested a deficiency of dihydropyrimidine dehydrogenase (EC 1.3.1.2) (DHPDH) as the underlying defect. The main site of DHPDH is the liver, but the enzyme has also been demonstrated in leukocytes (Goedde *et al.*, 1968). In the present paper the establishment of DHPDH-deficiency in the leukocytes of the three patients is described. Excretory levels of thymine, uracil and of a third metabolite, 5-hydroxymethyluracil, are given.

PATIENTS

Index patient, R.E.*, a boy, diagnosed at the age of 4 years had transient seizures, speech retardation and behavioural problems. When he grew older he developed favourably. The first child of the family is healthy, the second one died of perinatal asphyxia. The second patient, M.S., a girl and only child of parents who are first cousins, was diagnosed at the age of 14 years. Clinical features are mental retardation, solitary behaviour and epileptic absences. The third patient, a Turkish boy, B.B., was presented for screening at the age

of 15 months because of severe growth retardation, diarrhoea and feeding difficulties. Mentally the child seems to be retarded. A second child of the family is normal.

METHODS

Urinary pyrimidines were determined by automated cation exchange column chromatography, using a Technicon TSM1 autoanalyser combined with a Schoeffel model SF 770 UV spectroflow monitor (10 mm cell, wavelength setting 260 nm), an Infotronics CRS 309 integrator and a printer. The column (39.5 cm, dia. 5 mm) was packed with Technicon spherical resin Chromobeads C3 (12 μ). Urine volume applied 10 μl; pump rate 0.45 ml min^{-1}. Elution was performed with sodium citrate (0.066 M)–HCl buffers according to the following scheme. Buffer 1: pH 3.40, 50°C, 24 min. Buffer 2: pH 4.00, 50°C, 32 min. Buffer 3: pH 6.60, 50°C, 68 min. NaOH 0.2 M, 12 min. Buffer 1: 22 min. The retention times of 5-hydroxymethyluracil was 24 min; uracil, 28.5 min; thymine, 37 min.

DHPDH activity in leukocytes was determined by the method of Piper *et al.* (1980), a radiochemical procedure measuring the production of [*methyl*-³H]dihydro-thymine from [*methyl*-³H]thymine after separation by paper chromatography.

RESULTS

All three patients excreted persistently excessive amounts of uracil (2.0–10.5 mmol (g creatinine)$^{-1}$), thymine (2.3–7.5 mmol (g creatinine)$^{-1}$) as well as substantial quantities of 5-hydroxymethyluracil (0.2–0.9 mmol (g creatinine)$^{-1}$), a metabolite of thymine. In normal urine uracil is below 0.30 mmol (g creatinine)$^{-1}$, whilst thymine and 5-hydroxymethyluracil are not detected. Parents and sibs and a normal profile of their urinary pyrimidines.

After loading index patient R.E. with uracil, 1 mmol (kg b.wt)$^{-1}$, 74% of the administered dose was excreted during 24 h. When dihydrouracil was given

---

* Presented at the poster session of the international meeting 1980 at Interlaken

Journal of Inherited Metabolic Disease. ISSN 0141-8955. Copyright © SSIEM and MTP Press Limited, Queen Square, Lancaster, UK.

only 7% of the load was excreted unaltered during 24 h and no free β-alanine was detected.

On oral loading of R.E. with thymine, 1 mmol (kg b.wt)$^{-1}$, 73% of the dose was excreted (as thymine + 5-hydroxymethyluracil). After loading with R,S-dihydrothymine 40% was recovered in the 24 h urine. Also β-aminoisobutyric acid (molar amount 6%) was excreted, 95% having the R-configuration as determined according to van Gennip *et al.* (1981).

DHPDH activity values measured in leukocytes are given in Table 1. All three patients had an almost complete absence of enzyme activity. The parents of R.E. are within, and those of M.S. and B.B. below, the normal range.

DISCUSSION

From the results described above we conclude that all three patients have a generalised DHPDH deficiency. The high basal excretory values for both thymine and uracil are already highly suggestive of a defect localised at the level of DHPDH. The oral loading tests, proximal and distal to the enzyme block, confirmed this hypothesis and indicated a DHPDH deficiency in the liver. At the enzyme level the deficiency has been proven in the leukocytes of all three patients.

The parents' urinary pyrimidine excretion is not elevated. DHPDH activity of their leukocytes is within or just below the normal range. Therefore we conclude

that DHPDH deficiency is inherited in an autosomal recessive mode.

Thymine-uraciluria has been described before in a 2-year-old child with a malignant tumour of the brain (Berglund *et al.*, 1979). The question arises whether the pyrimidines originated from the tumour, as the authors concluded, or whether the patient had an inherited DHPDH deficiency. Very recently another patient with transient epilepsy and generalised seizures was described (Bakkeren *et al.*, 1984) and we know about another one with neurological problems and liver disease (B. Wilcken, personal communication, 1984). The number of patients with DHPDH deficiency is still too small to conclude whether there is a characteristic clinical picture or not.

References

Bakkeren, J. A. J. M., De Abreu, R. A., Sengers, R. C. A., Gabrëls, F. J. M., Maas, J. M. and Renier, W. O. Elevated urine, blood and cerebrospinal fluid levels of uracil and thymine in a child with dihydrothymine dehydrogenase deficiency. *Clin. Chim. Acta* 140 (1984) 247–256

Berglund, G., Greter, J., Lindstedt, S., Steen, G., Waldenström, J. and Wass, U. Urinary excretion of thymine and uracil in a two-year-old child with a malignant tumour of the brain. *Clin. Chem.* 25 (1979) 1325–1328

van Gennip, A. H., Kamerling, J. P., de Bree, P. K. and Wadman, S. K. Linear relationship between R- and S-enantiomers of β-aminoisobutyric acid in human urine. *Clin. Chim. Acta* 116 (1981) 261–267

van Gennip, A. H., Van Noordenburg-Huistra, D. Y., de Bree, P. K. and Wadman, S. K. Two-dimensional thin-layer chromatography for the screening of disorders of purine and pyrimidine metabolism. *Clin. Chim. Acta* 86 (1978) 7–20

Goedde, H. W., Hoffbauer, R. and Blume, K. G. Reduction of thymine by leucocytes. *Biochem. Genet.* 2 (1968) 93–99

Piper, A. A., Tattersall, M. H. N. and Fox, R. M. The activities of thymidine metabolising enzymes during the cell cycle of a human lymphocyte cell line LAZ-007 synchronised by centrifugal elutriation. *Biochim. Biophys. Acta* 633 (1980) 400–409

Wadman, S. K., Beemer, F. A., de Bree, P. K., Duran, M., van Gennip, A. H. and van Sprang, F. J. New defects of pyrimidine metabolism in man. In de Bruyn, C. H. M. M., Simmonds, H. A. and Müller, M. M. (eds.) *Purine Metabolism in Man IV, Part A: Clinical and Therapeutic Aspects; Regulatory Mechanisms*, Plenum Press, New York, 1984, pp. 109–114

Table 1   DHPDH activity in leukocytes

	nmol h^{-1} (mg protein)$^{-1}$
Patient R.E.	0.04
Father	1.43
Mother	1.45
Healthy sibling	1.66
Patient M.S.	0.01
Father	0.69
Mother	0.62
Patient B.B.	<0.01
Father	0.87
Mother	0.31

Four controls: mean 2.27; range 1.01–4.46

J. Inher. Metab. Dis. 8 Suppl. 2 (1985) 115–116

Short Communication

Dihydropyrimidine Dehydrogenase Deficiency — A Further Case

B. Wilcken and J. Hammond
Oliver Latham Laboratory, N.S.W. Department of Health, Sydney, Australia

R. Berger
Department of Pediatrics, University of Groningen, Oostersingel 59, Groningen, The Netherlands

G. Wise
Prince of Wales Children's Hospital, Sydney, Australia

C. James
Royal Alexandra Hospital for Children, Sydney, Australia

Dihydropyrimidine dehydrogenase (EC 1.3.1.2.) deficiency has recently been described in two separate reports of four patients, all of whom excreted large quantities of thymine and uracil in the urine. Bakkeren *et al.* (1984) described a girl who developed grand-mal epilepsy at 3 years of age, and had microcephaly, but normal intelligence. Berger *et al.* (1984) reported on three patients, a boy with transient petit-mal and behavioural abnormalities developing at 18 months, a mentally retarded girl aged 14 years with solitary behaviour and petit-mal, and a boy with microcephaly, mental retardation and probable growth retardation, whose symptoms first appeared at 9 months. A further report of excretion of thymine and uracil was made by Berglund *et al.* (1979) in a 2-year-old with a medulloblastoma. However, severe deficiency of dihydropyrimidine dehydrogenase could not be demonstrated in this patient, in studies of cultured fibroblasts.

CASE REPORT

M.M., a male baby, was the first child of Lebanese parents who are first cousins once removed. Pregnancy and labour were normal and the baby's Apgar scores at 1 and 5 min were 7 and 10. He had a retrousse chin and single palmar transverse line, but no other dysmorphic features. Increased tone was present from day one. Over the next weeks he remained stiff, required tube feeding and had several episodes of aspiration. He developed a slightly enlarged but firm liver. Liver transaminases were elevated and coagulation was impaired, but other pathology investigations, including serum electrolytes, urea, glucose, uric acid, amylase, calcium, magnesium, amino acids, and a full blood count, were normal. A urinary metabolic screen performed on day three and repeated on several occasions revealed excretion of thymine and uracil, compounds not normally detected in urine by the method used.

A barium swallow showed neuromuscular in-coordination and tracheal aspiration, and abdominal ultrasound showed increased echogenicity of the liver, without focal lesions, and an enlarged spleen.

His parents discharged him from hospital, but he was readmitted to another hospital at 7 weeks. His weight was then below the 3rd centile, and his head circumference at the 25th. He had generalised hypertonia and hyperreflexia, was not fixing or following, and had an uncertain response to sound. High resolution CT scans of head, thorax, and abdomen revealed only an unusually dense but uniform liver. Thymine and uracil were present in the urine, together with increased levels of 4-hydroxyphenylacetic, 4-hydroxyphenyllactic and 4-hydroxyphenylpyruvic acids and cystathionine. He suffered several episodes of aspiration and ultimately died during one of these. Before death a sample of liver was obtained by needle biopsy and stored at $-80°C$.

Postmortem examination, including detailed examination of the brain, revealed no abnormality except a large, pale liver, in which most of the parenchymal cells were grossly enlarged and contained large and small fat droplets. No other storage material could be identified. There was no evidence of any neural crest tumour.

METHODS AND RESULTS

Acidified urine was extracted using ethyl acetate. Trimethylsilyl derivatives were prepared and separated using a 3% SE-30 gas–liquid chromatography column heated from 80 to 250°C at 6°C min^{-1}. This system was interfaced with a Dupont 491B mass spectrometer for positive identification.

Urinary thymine and uracil were detected during routine organic acid profile analysis. The methylene units were 13.30–13.35 for uracil and 13.95–14.00 for thymine. The urinary organic acids on day 3 are shown in Figure 1.

Dihydropyrimidine dehydrogenase in liver biopsy material was measured as described by Piper *et al.* (1980). Homogenates were incubated with [*methyl*-^{3}H]thymine and the reaction products, dihydrothymine and β-aminoisobutyric acid, separated by paper

Journal of Inherited Metabolic Disease. ISSN 0141-8955. Copyright © SSIEM and MTP Press Limited, Queen Square, Lancaster, UK.

chromatography and the radioactivity of the fractions counted.

Dihydropyrimidine dehydrogenase activity was almost completely absent, being $<0.05\,\text{nmol}\,\text{h}^{-1}$ (mg protein)$^{-1}$ compared with control values of 4.7 and 1.8 ($<2\,\text{nmol}\,\text{h}^{-1}$ (g wet wt)$^{-1}$, control values 234 and 102).

DISCUSSION

The clinical presentation of our patient was quite different from that of the other patients described by Bakkeren *et al.* (1984) and by Berger *et al.* (1984) and much more severe. None of the other patients had suffered the striking alterations in tone and neuromuscular co-ordination that we saw, and there are no reports of hepatomegaly. Nor do the patients described closely resemble each other clinically, and it is possible that the clinical findings are unrelated to the deficient activity of dihydropyrimidine dehydrogenase. The enzyme activity in our patient was measured in liver, whereas in the other patients measurements were made in fibroblasts (Bakkeren *et al.*, 1984), and leukocytes (Berger *et al.*, 1984). It is possible that the other patients described did not have such completely deficient activity in liver as did our patient.

Thymine and uracil are not efficiently extracted from urine by ethyl acetate or ether and, because of this, greatly increased excretion of these compounds could easily be missed by the usual GLC screening for organic aciduria.

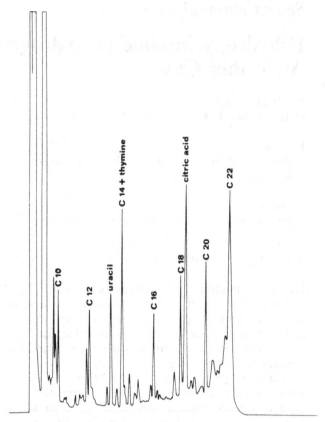

Figure 1 Gas–liquid chromatography of urinary organic acids on day 3, with added hydrocarbons (see text)

References

Bakkeren, J. A. J. M., DeAbreu, R. A., Sengers, R. C. A., Gabreëls, F. J. M., Maas, J. M. and Renier, W. O. Elevated urine, blood and cerebrospinal fluid levels of uracil and thymine in a child with dihydrothymine dehydrogenase deficiency. *Clin. Chim. Acta* 140 (1984) 247–256

Berger, R., Stoker-de Vries, S. A., Wadman, S. K., Duran, M., Beemer, F. A., de Bree, P. K., Weits-Binnerts, J. J., Penders, T. J. and van der Woude, J. K. Dihydropyrimidine dehydrogenase deficiency leading to thymine-uraciluria. An inborn error of pyrimidine metabolism. *Clin. Chim. Acta* 141 (1984) 227–234

Berglund, G., Greter, J., Lindstedt, S., Steen, G., Waldestrom, J. and Weiss, Ü. Urinary excretion of thymine and uracil in a two year old child with a malignant tumour of the brain. *Clin. Chem.* 25 (1979) 1325–1328

Piper, A. A., Tattersall, M. H. N. and Fox, R. M. The activities of thymidine metabolising enzymes during the cell cycle of a human lymphocyte cell line LAZ-007 synchronised by centrifugal elutriation. *Biochim. Biophys. Acta* 633 (1980) 400–409

J. Inher. Metab. Dis. 8 Suppl. 2 (1985) 117–118

Short Communication

Combined Deficiency of Xanthine Oxidase and Sulphite Oxidase: Diagnosis of a New Case Followed by an Antenatal Diagnosis

P. Desjacques, B. Mousson, C. Vianey-Liaud, R. Boulieu, C. Bory, P. Baltassat, P. Divry, M. T. Zabot and J. Cotte
Laboratoire de biochimie, Hôpital Debrousse, 69322 Lyon Cedex 05, France

P. Lagier
Service de réanimation néonatale, Hôpital Nord, 13326 Marseille Cedex 15, France

N. Philip
Service de génétique médicale, CHU La Timone, 13385 Marseille Cedex 5, France

Combined deficiency of xanthine oxidase (XO, EC 1.2.3.2) and sulphite oxidase (SO, EC 1.8.2.1), ("molybdenum cofactor" deficiency) is a very rare disorder. Up to now, only seven cases have been published (Duran *et al.*, 1978; Munnich *et al.*, 1983; Wadman *et al.*, 1983). In these patients, a metabolic defect at the level of the "molybdenum cofactor" common to the two enzymes (Johnson *et al.*, 1980) appeared to be responsible for the loss of both enzyme activities. The clinical symptoms include axial hypotonia with peripheral hypertonicity, tonic–clonic seizures refractory to all therapy, feeding difficulties, eye lens dislocation and deep mental retardation. Most of the clinical abnormalities are already present in the neonatal period. The prognosis is very poor and the patients who survived the neonatal period present very severe neurological disturbances. So far, all therapeutic attempts have been unsuccessful. We report here biochemical and enzymatic study of a new case, which led to an antenatal diagnosis.

CASE REPORT

G.D. was the first child of non-consanguineous parents, born after an uncomplicated pregnancy and delivery. Hypotonia and seizures refractory to all therapy appeared on the 24th hour of life and the baby was referred to the intensive care unit at day 3.

On examination he was found to have severe axial hypotonia, peripheral hypertonicity, tonic–clonic seizures, myoclonic jerks. Routine laboratory investigation showed normal results except low plasma and urine uric acid concentrations. EEG was strikingly abnormal and CT scan showed cerebral and cerebellar atrophy. The child died on the ninth day of life.

BIOCHEMICAL INVESTIGATION IN BODY FLUIDS

Cystine, sulphocysteine and taurine were quantitated by conventional automated ion exchange chromatography, routinely used for amino acids determination. Uric acid was measured by a routine enzymatic method. Hypoxanthine and xanthine were measured by a previously described HPLC procedure (Boulieu *et al.*, 1982).

Biochemical diagnosis of combined XO and SO deficiency was suspected on the third day of life on the view of a positive sulphite test in urine (test strip Merckoquant 10013 Sulfit test, Merck), associated with high concentrations of sulphocysteine, hypoxanthine and xanthine, both in plasma and urine and low concentration of cystine in plasma and of uric acid in plasma and urine (Table 1).

ENZYMATIC STUDIES

XO activity was measured on liver and jejunal tissues, using a very sensitive radioisotopic assay (Mousson *et al.*, 1983). SO (sulphite-dependent cytochrome *c* reductase) activity was assayed in liver using the procedure described by Johnson and Rajagopalan (1976) slightly modified. The medium contained cytochrome *c* type III (Sigma; $40 \mu mol \, l^{-1}$), EDTA ($100 \mu mol \, l^{-1}$), sodium sulphite ($400 \mu mol \, l^{-1}$) and liver homogenate (1:10 w:v; $15 \mu l$ for a final volume of $1250 \mu l$). The reaction was started by addition of sulphite and specific cytochrome *c* reduction was followed at 550 nm at 30°C, in a Beckman DU-8B spectrophotometer.

For assay of SO in fibroblasts and amniotic fluid cells, owing to a very high non-specific cytochrome *c* reductase activity, the lysate had to be centrifuged at 20 000 g for 10 min (Johnson *et al.*, 1980), and then the supernatant fluid was desalted by exclusion diffusion chromatography on polyacrylamide agarose gel (IBF Ultrogel ACA 202). The excluded protein fraction was concentrated by ultrafiltration and assayed for sulphite-dependent cytochrome *c* reductase activity using the same medium as reported above with the addition of sodium deoxycholate ($0.4 \, g \, l^{-1}$) and sodium cyanide ($0.5 \, mmol \, l^{-1}$), in a final volume of $200 \mu l$ containing $150 \mu l$ of concentrated supernatant.

XO activity measured on a jejunal biopsy and SO activity on both liver and fibroblasts were undetectable in our patient (Table 1). It should be noticed that for measurement of SO activity in liver, sodium deoxy-

Journal of Inherited Metabolic Disease. ISSN 0141-8955. Copyright © SSIEM and MTP Press Limited, Queen Square, Lancaster, UK.

Table 1 Biochemical results in molybdenum cofactor deficiency; enzyme activity is in μkat (kg protein)$^{-1}$

	Uric acid	Hypoxanthine	Xanthine	S-sulphocysteine	Half cystine	Sulphite
Plasma (μmol l^{-1})						
Patient G.D.	40	13	40	60	1	
Normal values	230 ± 50	2.5 ± 1	1.4 ± 0.7	ND[1]	42 ± 12	
Urine (μmol 24 h^{-1})						
Patient G.D.	42	73	195	24	1.3	+ + +
Normal values	2500 ± 500	48 ± 28	68 ± 42	ND	15 ± 5	ND
Amniotic fluid (μmol l^{-1})						
Patient's mother[2]	220	<0.25	<0.5	ND	70	
Normal range	192–228	0.25–0.7	0.5–0.9 (n = 12)	ND	68–87	

	Xanthine oxidase		Sulphite oxidase	
	Patient	Normal range	Patient	Normal range
Jejunum	<2	18–40 (n = 10)		
Liver			<1	60–170 (n = 8)
Fibroblasts			<1	2–10 (n = 10)
Amniotic cells			6.8[2]	2–5 (n = 4)

[1]ND, not detectable
[2]Second pregnancy giving normal baby

cholate and sodium cyanide addition could be omitted. Fibroblast and amniotic cells were cultivated in HAM F 10 medium, supplemented with fetal calf serum (10–15 %); this culture medium is sufficiently rich in trace elements that the addition of molybdenum, as proposed by Shih *et al.* (1977), is unnecessary.

DISCUSSION

This new case of molybdo-enzyme deficiency is very similar to those previously described. Biochemical results emphasize the possibility of diagnosis of this severe disease by simple and/or routine laboratory investigation such as a sulphite test strip and uric acid determination in body fluids. However, the occurrence of a false positive sulphite test has to be considered (mucolytic treatment, with drugs containing mercapto-ethane sulfonate). So diagnosis must be confirmed by plasma amino acid analysis; the typical pattern is characterized by a sulphocysteine peak and a very low cystine value. Absolute confirmation can be obtained by enzymatic studies of XO and SO.

As SO activity is expressed in fibroblast and amniotic fluid cells it allows antenatal diagnosis. In this family, the second pregnancy was monitored by our laboratory. The cultivated amniotic cells obtained at the 17th week exhibited normal SO activity; this was confirmed in J. Johnson's laboratory. Moreover, amniotic fluid analysis revealed undetectable levels of sulphocysteine, xanthine, hypoxanthine and normal values of cystine and uric acid (Table 1). These results are in agreement with a normal baby. Recently a new case of combined deficiency has been diagnosed in München; so this metabolic disorder may be not so rare and must be systematically considered in acute neonatal neurological trouble. Although the diagnosis of this disease does not lead to an efficient treatment, it is highly important as it permits genetic counselling and antenatal diagnosis.

References

Boulieu, R., Bory, C., Baltassat, P. and Gonnet, P. High performance liquid chromatographic determination of hypoxanthine and xanthine in biological fluids. *J. Chromatogr.* 233 (1982) 131–140

Duran, M., Beemer, F. A., Heiden, C. V. D., Korteland, J., de Bree, P. K., Brink, M. and Wadman, S. K. Combined deficiency of xanthine and sulphite oxidase: a defect of molybdenum metabolism or transport? *J. Inher. Metab. Dis.* 1 (1978) 175–178

Johnson, J. L. and Rajagopalan, K. V. Purification and properties of sulphite oxidase from human liver. *J. Clin. Invest.* 58 (1976) 543–560

Johnson, J. L., Waud, W. R., Rajagopalan, K. V., Duran, M., Beemer, F. A. and Wadman, K. Inborn errors of molybdenum metabolism: combined deficiencies of sulphite oxidase and xanthine dehydrogenase in a patient lacking the molybdenum cofactor. *Proc. Natl. Acad. Sci. USA* 77 (1980) 3715–3719

Mousson, B., Desjacques, P. and Baltassat, P. Measurement of xanthine oxidase activity in some human tissues. An optimized method. *Enzyme* 29 (1983) 32–43

Munnich, A., Saudubray, J. M., Charpentier, C., Ogier, H., Coudé, F. X., Frézal, J., Yacoub, L., Harbi, A. and Snoussi, S. Multiple molybdoenzyme deficiencies due to an inborn error of molybdenum cofactor metabolism: two additional cases in a new family. *J. Inher. Metab. Dis.* 6, Suppl. 2 (1983) 95–96

Shih, V. E., Abroms, J. F., Johnson, J. L., Carney, M., Mandell, R., Robb, R., Cloherty, J. P. and Rajagopalan, K. V. Sulphite oxidase deficiency. *N. Engl. J. Med.* 297 (1977) 1022–1028

Wadman, S. K., Duran, M., Beemer, A. F., Cats, B. P., Johnson, J. L., Rajagopalan, K. V., Saudubray, J. M., Ogier, H., Charpentier, C., Berger, R., Smit, G. P. A., Wilson, J. and Krywawych, S. Absence of hepatic molybdenum cofactor: an inborn error of metabolism leading to a combined deficiency of sulphite oxidase and xanthine dehydrogenase. *J. Inher. Metab. Dis.* 6, Suppl. 1 (1983) 78–83

J. Inher. Metab. Dis. 8 Suppl. 2 (1985) 119

Short Communication

An Abnormal Amino Acid Pattern in Adenosine Deaminase Deficiency

C. Borrone and M. Di Rocco
III Pediatria, Istituto "G. Gaslini", Via 5 Maggio 39, 16148 Genova, Italy

U. Caruso
Clinica Pediatrica II, Università di Genova, Genova, Italy

S. Reali
Cattedra di Genetica Umana, Ospedali "Galliera", Genova, Italy

Heritable adenosine deaminase (ADA; EC 3.5.4.4) deficiency (McKusick 10270) results in purine nucleoside accumulation and subsequent lymphoid toxicity. ADA deficient patients show a severe combined immunodeficiency and several additional nonimmunological abnormalities. The improvement of the neurological abnormalities after enzyme replacement therapy suggests that they may be an integral part of the ADA deficiency syndrome (Hirschhorn *et al.*, 1980). Given the relationship between adenosine metabolism and sulfur amino acid metabolism, we have studied amino acid patterns in biological fluids of a patient with ADA deficiency and neurological symptoms. Preliminary results of this original study are reported.

CASE REPORT

A 3-month-old girl, daughter of related parents, was admitted to our hospital because of failure to thrive, respiratory distress, hypotonia, developmental delay and seizures. Severe combined immunodeficiency was diagnosed after demonstration of respiratory, intestinal and urinary candidosis, absolute lymphopenia, absence of thymic shadow on X-rays, very low levels of immunoglobulins, absent response to *in vitro* stimulation with phytohaemagglutinin, B and T cell deficiency and absence of ADA activity in red blood cells. An increased protein content (289 mg%) was found in cerebrospinal fluid (CSF), while cells and glucose were normal.

Plasma, urine and CSF amino acids were assayed by ion exchange chromatography. Increased levels of methionine were found in plasma and in CSF. In urine there were high levels of homocyst(e)ine. In CSF glutamine and ammonia were also increased (Table 1). Hepatic function was normal.

The girl died at the age of 4 months despite attempts at enzyme replacement therapy with irradiated red blood cells.

DISCUSSION

An increase in adenosine concentration, as would occur from a lack of ADA, is accompanied by high levels of *S*-adenosyl-homocysteine and by some degree of transsulfuration pathway inhibition (Kredich and Hershfield,

Table 1 Amino acid concentrations in adenosine deaminase deficiency (μmol l^{-1})

Plasma	
Methionine	231 (controls: 27 ± 5)
Urine	
Homocyst(e)ine	22 (controls: not detectable)
CSF	
Methionine	30 (controls: 11–23; no 5)
Glutamine	1518 (controls: 535–860; no 5)

1983). Therefore the finding of an abnormal sulfur amino acid pattern in our patient suggests another secondary metabolic derangement in ADA deficiency, beside purine nucleoside accumulation.

It is interesting to speculate whether in ADA deficient patients this abnormal amino acid pattern plays a pathogenetically important role in the central nervous system dysfunction. High levels of intracellular ADA have recently been demonstrated in specific neuronal populations, which probably release adenosine as a neurotransmitter (Nagy *et al.*, 1984). Thus it also seems possible that neurological impairment is more directly due to central nervous system ADA deficiency.

Finally we emphasize that, beside cystathionine-β-synthase deficiency and 6-azauridine administration, the biochemical pattern of hypermethioninaemia and homocystinuria may be caused by ADA deficiency.

References

Hirschhorn, R., Papageorgiou, P. S., Kesarwala, H. and Taft, L. T. Amelioration of neurological abnormalities after "enzyme replacement" in adenosine deaminase deficiency. *N. Engl. J. Med.* 303 (1980) 377

Kredich, N. M. and Hershfield, M. S. Immunodeficiency diseases caused by adenosine deaminase deficiency and purine nucleoside phosphorylase deficiency. In Stanbury, J. B., Wyngaarden, J. B., Fredrickson, D. S., Goldstein, J. L. and Brown, M. S. (eds.) *The Metabolic Basis of Inherited Disease*, 5th edn., McGraw Hill, New York, 1983, pp. 1157–1183

Nagy, J. I., Labella, L. A., Buss, M. and Daddona, P. E. Immunochemistry of adenosine deaminase: implication for adenosine neurotransmission. *Science* 224 (1984) 166

Journal of Inherited Metabolic Disease. ISSN 0141-8955. Copyright © SSIEM and MTP Press Limited, Queen Square, Lancaster, UK.

J. Inher. Metab. Dis. 8 Suppl. 2 (1985) 121–122

Short Communication

Amino Acidaemias and Brain Maturation: Interference with Sulphate Activation and Myelin Metabolism

F. A. HOMMES

Department of Cell and Molecular Biology, Medical College of Georgia, Augusta, GA 30912, USA

Several studies have provided evidence that inborn errors in the metabolism of some of the amino acids may result in a decrease in central nervous system myelin. Examples are phenylketonuria (McKusick 26160), maple syrup urine disease (McKusick 24860; for reviews see Gaull *et al.*, 1975; Hommes, 1984), ornithine transcarbamylase deficiency (McKusick 31125; see Harding *et al.*, 1984) and non-ketotic hyperglycinaemia (McKusick 23830; see Shurman *et al.*, 1978). In addition to this common feature, each of these diseases presents with its own specific clinical symptoms, many of which are acute effects caused by the specific toxicity of the compounds accumulating.

It has recently been shown that hyperphenylalaninaemia results in an increased turnover of part of the central nervous system myelin, which is not compensated by an increased synthesis. The overall result is a decrease in myelin (Berger *et al.*, 1979, 1980; Hommes *et al.*, 1982a,b; Taylor and Hommes, 1983). Chase and O'Brien (1970) have furthermore shown that a hyperphenylalaninaemic condition inhibits the incorporation of sulphate into sulphatides at the level of sulphate activation, while London *et al.* (London and Vossenberg, 1973; London *et al.*, 1973) demonstrated that myelin basic protein not complexed with acidic glycolipids, especially cerebroside sulphate, is rather vulnerable to proteolytic attack. To explore this as a possible explanation for the increased turnover of myelin, the sulphate activating system (SAS) was studied.

METHODS

Rat brain fractions were prepared according to Whittaker and Barker (1972). Rat liver was homogenized in 0.25 M sucrose. ATP-sulphurylase (EC 2.7.7.4) and APS-kinase (EC 2.7.1.25) were measured as described by Conrad and Woo (1980). Results are expressed as total flux through ATP-sulphurylase and APS-kinase. Protein was measured according to Lowry *et al.*

RESULTS AND DISCUSSION

The $100\,000\,g$ supernatant of young adult rat liver showed an SAS-activity of 2591 ± 87 nmol h^{-1} (g wet weight)$^{-1}$ ($n = 6$). Phenylalanine, up to 5 mmol l^{-1}, did not inhibit this activity. The $100\,000\,g$ supernatant of the brain of these rats yielded an activity of 94.6 ± 8.9 nmol h^{-1} (g wet weight)$^{-1}$ ($n = 6$) which decreased to 73.8 ± 3.3 nmol h^{-1} (g wet weight)$^{-1}$ ($n = 6$) in the presence of 2 mmol l^{-1} phenylalanine. The maximum inhibition observed was 22%. This maximum rate of inhibition could be obtained at 0.45 mmol l^{-1} phenylalanine, which is well within the range of phenylalanine levels of the untreated PKU patient. The brain enzyme can therefore be partly inhibited by phenylalanine, while the liver enzyme cannot. This points to a different enzyme system for the brain as compared to the liver, in agreement with the findings of Sugahara and Schwartz (1982a,b) in their study of the brachymorphic mouse. It could explain why PKU patients demonstrate severe neuropathology but virtually no hepatopathology.

The development of the SAS of the cytosol of the brain is shown in Figure 1. The development of the species of SAS which can be inhibited by phenylalanine closely parallels the rate of myelination, but there is still a considerable amount of that species present at the young adult stage (i.e. rats of 175–200 g body weight), decreasing to low values in senescent rats. The phenylalanine-inhibitable species of SAS is a transient species. The soluble, phenylalanine-inhibitable, SAS constitutes about 50% of the total amount of this species, the other 50% being equally distributed over the

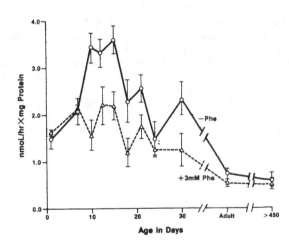

Figure 1 Activity of SAS of the $100\,000\,g$ supernatant of brain homogenates as a function of age. The assays were carried out in the absence or presence of 3 mmol l^{-1} phenylalanine. Mean values $\pm$ SD ($n = 3$) are given

Journal of Inherited Metabolic Disease. ISSN 0141-8955. Copyright © SSIEM and MTP Press Limited, Queen Square, Lancaster, UK.

mitochondrial fraction and the myelin fraction. The particulate bound SAS can be completely inhibited by $2\,\text{mmol}\,l^{-1}$ phenylalanine. The inhibition is not specific for phenylalanine. Leucine, glycine, ammonium ions, and phenyllactate at a concentration of $5\,\text{mmol}\,l^{-1}$, yielded inhibitions of 75, 51, 25, and 48 %, respectively. None of these compounds inhibited the SAS of liver.

These amino acids and ammonium ions can, therefore, like phenylalanine, inhibit sulphate activation in brain. As in PKU, these compounds decrease the availability of sulphatides (c.f. Chase and O'Brien, 1970) and thus leave myelin basic protein more vulnerable to proteolytic attack, resulting in the degradation of the myelin sheath. This mechanism of myelin instability provides a common basis for the loss of myelin observed in a number of amino acidaemias. It might also explain why the growing brain is vulnerable to such imbalances in the level of some amino acids only during a limited period of time. The species of SAS which can be inhibited by these amino acids is a transient species, only expressed during the period of active myelination.

In addition to this long-term effect of an imbalance in a specific amino acid, each of the inhibitory compounds may cause acute effects, giving rise to the specific clinical symptoms. Such acute effects may be life-threatening, especially in maple syrup urine disease, non-ketotic hyperglycinaemia and hyperammonaemia, but less so in hyperphenylalaninaemia. The long-term effect only becomes apparent after a longer period of time of exposure to a high concentration of these amino acids.

References

Berger, R., Dias, Th. and Hommes, F. A. Developmental aspects of brain protein and myelin metabolism in hyperphenylalaninemic rats. In Hommes, F. A. (ed.) *Models for the Study of Inborn Errors of Metabolism*, Elsevier, Amsterdam, 1979, pp. 111–122

Berger, R., Springer, J. and Hommes, F. A. Brain protein and myelin metabolism in young hyperphenylalaninemic rats. *Molec. Cell Biol.* 26 (1980) 31–36

Chase, H. P. and O'Brien, D. Effects of excess phenylalanine and other amino acids on brain development in the infant rat. *Pediatr. Res.* 4 (1970) 96–102

Conrad, G. W. and Woo, M. J. Synthesis of 3'-phospho-adenosine-5'-phosphosulfate (PAPS) increases during corneal development. *J. Biol. Chem.* 225 (1980) 3086–3091

Gaull, G. E., Tallan, H. H., Lajtha, A. and Rassin, D. K. Pathogenesis of brain dysfunction in inborn errors of metabolism. In Gaull, G. E. (ed.) *Biology of Brain Development*, Vol. 3, Plenum Press, New York, 1975, pp. 47–143

Harding, B. N., Leonard, J. V. and Erdohasi, M. Ornithine carbamoyl transferase deficiency: a neuropathological study. *Eur. J. Pediatr.* 141 (1984) 215–220

Hommes, F. A. Amino aciduria and brain dysfunction, in Lajtha, A. (ed.) *Handbook of Neurochemistry*, Plenum Publ. Corp., New York, 1984, Vol. 10, pp. 15–41

Hommes, F. A., Eller, A. G. and Taylor, E. H. The effect of phenylalanine on myelin metabolism in adolescent rats. In Cockburn, F. and Gitzelmann, R. (eds.) *Inborn Errors of Metabolism in Humans*, MTP Press, Lancaster, 1982a, pp. 193–199

Hommes, F. A., Eller, A. G. and Taylor, E. H. Turnover of the fast component of myelin and myelin protein in experimental hyperphenylalaninaemia. Relevance to termination of dietary treatment in human PKU. *J. Inher. Metab. Dis.* 5 (1982b) 21–27

London, Y. and Vossenberg, F. G. A. Specific interactions of central nervous systems myelin basic protein with lipids. Specific regions of the protein sequence protected from the proteolytic action of trypsin. *Biochim. Biophys. Acta* 307 (1973) 478–490

London, Y., Demul, R. A., Geurts van Kessel, W. S. M., Vossenberg, F. G. A. and Van Deenen, L. L. M. The protection of A_1 myelin basic protein against the action of proteolytic enzymes after interaction of the protein with lipids at the air–water interface. *Biochim. Biophys. Acta* 311 (1973) 520–530

Shuman, R. M., Leech, R. W. and Scott, C. R. The neuropathology of the non ketotic and ketotic hyperglycinemias: Three cases. *Neurology* 28 (1978) 139–146

Sugahara, K. and Schwartz, N. B. Defect in 3'-phospho-adenosine 5'-phosphosulfate synthesis in brachymorphic mice. I: Characterization of the defect. *Arch. Biochem. Biophys.* 214 (1982a) 589–601

Sugahara, K. and Schwartz, N. B. Defect in 3'-phospho-adenosine 5'-phosphosulfate synthesis in brachymorphic mice. II: Tissue distribution of the defect. *Arch. Biochem. Biophys.* 214 (1982b) 602–609

Taylor, E. H. and Hommes, F. A. The effect of experimental hyperphenylalaninemia on myelin metabolism at later stages of brain development. *Int. J. Neurosci.* 20 (1983) 217–228

Whittaker, J. P. and Barker, L. A. The subcellular fractionation of brain tissue with special reference to the preparation of synaptosomes and their component organelles. In Fried, R. (ed.) *Methods of Neurochemistry*, Vol. 2, Marcel Dekker, New York, 1972, pp. 1–52

J. Inher. Metab. Dis. 8 Suppl. 2 (1985) 123–124

Short Communication

Juvenile Non-ketotic Hyperglycinaemia in Three Siblings

D. E. C. Cole and D. C. Meek
*Departments of Paediatrics, Dalhousie University, Halifax, Nova Scotia and
Saint John Regional Hospital, Saint John, New Brunswick, Canada*

Non-ketotic hyperglycinaemia (NKH; McKusick 23830) is an inherited disorder of glycine metabolism that classically presents in the newborn as hypotonia, generalized myoclonic seizures, and respiratory distress. In the few survivors of infancy, severe retardation and intractable seizures are the rule (Carson, 1982). We describe three male siblings who first presented in middle childhood with a distinctive clinical syndrome that we call juvenile NKH.

CASE REPORTS

Sibling 1 (12 years old) was developmentally delayed and has always had a "speech impediment". In September 1983, he developed a fever and persistent cough; a chest film indicated viral pneumonia. He became irritable and ataxic, and displayed marked asterixis on examination; EEG showed prominent high voltage 2–3 Hz waves which obscured background activity. Intravenous diazepam induced marked somnolence but led to an improvement in the EEG pattern; hypsarrhythmia was never observed. At present, fine motor co-ordination is poor but the neurological examination is otherwise unremarkable.

Sibling 2 (10 years old) is of nearly normal intelligence, although there is significant difference between his receptive and expressive verbal abilities on psychological testing. He is hyperactive and shows some deficit of fine motor co-ordination.

Sibling 3 (8 years old) showed a marked delay in speech development. At 6 years, he is still not forming complete sentences. Motor development is delayed and hyperactivity is a major behavioural problem.

METHODS AND RESULTS

Amino acid chromatography of plasma, urine and cerebrospinal fluid (CSF) was performed on a Beckman 6300 High Performance Analyzer; the results are shown in Table 1. Gas chromatography–mass spectrometry for organic acids was performed on two separate urine samples from the children by Dr Orval Mamer (MRC Mass Spectroscopy Unit, McGill University, Montreal). Results were uniformly negative. Oral glycine was administered to parents and children at a dosage of 150 mg kg^{-1} to a maximum of 12 g. Subjects were fasting at the beginning of the test but ate a light lunch at about 4 h. The effects on plasma glycine and serine are shown in Figure 1. No changes in the EEG or the clinical state were observed during the test. Long-term benzoate therapy (5 g day^{-1}) left plasma or urine glycine concentrations unchanged in all three siblings. However, attention span and behaviour improved significantly, as evidenced by parents' accounts, clinical observation and psychological testing.

DISCUSSION

The clinical features of our patients bear a striking resemblance to those reported by Ando *et al.* (1978), Frazier *et al.* (1978), and Flannery *et al.* (1983), especially with respect to the expressive speech deficit and the aberrant neurological response to intercurrent infection (cf. Frazier *et al.*, 1978). The defect in overall glycine catabolism and in conversion to serine is clearly manifested in all three siblings. In the mother, glycine excretion was somewhat elevated and conversion to serine after a glycine load was reduced. Whether these abnormalities reflect an unusual heterozygous genotype is not known, but the possibility of X-linkage cannot be ignored. However, further family studies and other case reports do not support this interpretation. The apparent efficacy of benzoate therapy on the clinical status is gratifying, but, as Matalon *et al.* (1983) observed in their patients with the infantile form, it need not be accompanied by a biochemical improvement.

Table 1 Glycine and serine concentrations in the juvenile NKH family

	Normal*	Mother	Father	Sib 1†	Sib 2	Sib 3
Plasma glycine	<400	376	257	606 (530)	604	579
Plasma serine	<200	146	144	127 (92)	117	96
Urine glycine	<0.2	0.69	0.17	4.77 (5.76)	6.45	2.79
CSF glycine	6 ± 3			32 (62)	25	42
Plasma/CSF glycine ratio	55 ± 26			19 (8.5)	24	14

Plasma and CSF amino acids are in µmol l^{-1}, urine glycines in µmol (µmol creatinine)$^{-1}$
* Normals from Carson (1982)
† Values in parentheses were obtained during an intercurrent infection

Journal of Inherited Metabolic Disease. ISSN 0141-8955. Copyright © SSIEM and MTP Press Limited, Queen Square, Lancaster, UK.

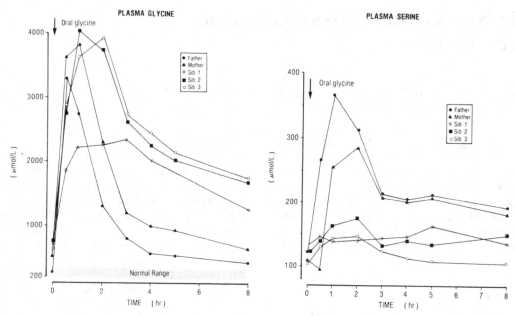

Figure 1   The response of plasma glycine and serine to an oral glycine load in three siblings with juvenile NKH and their parents

References

Ando, T., Nyhan, W. L., Bicknell, J., Harris, R. and Stern, J. Non-ketotic hyperglycinaemia in a family with an unusual phenotype. *J. Inher. Metab. Dis.* 1 (1978) 79–83

Carson, N. A. J. Non-ketotic hyperglycinaemia — A view of 70 patients. *J. Inher. Metab. Dis.* 5, Suppl. 2 (1982) 126–128

Flannery, D. B., Pellock, J., Bousonis, D., Hunt, P., Nance, C. and Wolf, B. Non-ketotic hyperglycinemia in two retarded adults: A mild form of infantile non-ketotic hyper-glycinemia. *Neurology* 33 (1983) 1064–1066

Frazier, D. M., Summer, G. K. and Chamberlin, H. R. Hyperglycinuria and hyperglycinemia in two siblings with mild developmental delays. *Am. J. Dis. Child.* 132 (1978) 777–781

Matalon, R., Naidu, S., Hughes, J. R. and Michals, K. Non-ketotic hyperglycinemia: Treatment with diazepam — a competitor for glycine receptors. *Pediatrics* 71 (1983) 581–584

J. Inher. Metab. Dis. 8, Suppl. 2 (1985) 125–126

Short Communication

Amino Acid Loading Tests in a Patient with Non-ketotic Hyperglycinaemia

T. Palmer
Department of Life Sciences, Trent Polytechnic, Nottingham NG11 8NS, UK

V. G. Oberholzer
Clinical Chemistry Department, Queen Elizabeth Hospital for Children, London E2 8PS, UK

Non-ketotic hyperglycinaemia (NKH) (McKusick 23830) was first described by Gerritsen *et al.* (1965) in a child who failed to thrive from birth and had episodes of seizures. A defect of serine formation from glycine (glycine cleavage) was indicated by isotope and amino acid loading studies in the original patient and another, and the same defect was demonstrated in a third patient by enzyme assay following liver biopsy (de Groot *et al.*, 1970). NKH is distinct from hyperglycinaemia with ketosis, which appears to be secondary to propionic acidaemia, methylmalonic acidaemia and possibly other primary disorders.

We have used amino acid loading tests to investigate the defect in our patient. Findings from this case have been incorporated into a review (Carson, 1982), but are given here in more detail in response to a suggestion by Krieger and Nigro (1983) that the defect in glycine cleavage in NKH could be secondary to a defect in threonine dehydratase, which converts threonine to α-ketobutyrate.

CASE REPORT

The patient, a boy born to healthy, unrelated West Indian negroes weighed 3.3 kg at birth. He was well for 3 months but then developed bronchitis and 2 days later had generalised convulsions. He was admitted to hospital. His convulsions could not be controlled with phenobarbitone, but were reduced with valium. Raised amounts of glycine were found in plasma and urine specimens.

He was well nourished, but persistently irritable with momentary twitching movements of the eyelids, face and limbs. These occurred at about 2 min intervals. He did not follow light, had poor head control and increased tone in limbs. All peripheral reflexes were increased. His liver was palpable 2 cm below the costal margin. His length was on the 25th percentile and his weight on the 90th percentile. He was treated with valium and withdrawal of this for a series of amino acid loading tests led to momentary twitching. His EEG showed a very slow activity in all areas with a very high voltage of up to 200 μV. He died aged 9 months; no autopsy was performed.

During the time he was being investigated he had intermittent respiratory acidosis. No ketosis was ever detected. Plasma and urine levels of methylmalonic acid and propionic acid were within normal limits.

METHODS AND RESULTS

Amino acid levels were determined as previously described (Palmer *et al.*, 1973). Glycine levels were always in excess of normal in plasma, urine and CSF ($64 \mu mol \, l^{-1}$). Threonine and hydroxyproline levels were occasionally high. All other amino acid levels were always normal.

The plasma glycine level was always in excess of $730 \mu mol \, l^{-1}$. A milk load giving 1 g protein kg^{-1} raised the glycine level from a fasting one of $760 \mu mol \, l^{-1}$ to one of $827 \mu mol \, l^{-1}$ 2 h after the load. Plasma glycine levels remain unchanged or fall slightly in normal subjects under these conditions (Palmer *et al.*, 1973).

Several L-amino acid loading tests ($0.25 \, g \, kg^{-1}$) were performed (Table 1). A glycine loading test showed a delayed return of plasma glycine to the fasting level as compared with controls (Childs *et al.*, 1961). Plasma serine steadily decreased with time throughout the test, whereas it normally rises following a glycine load. In contrast, plasma levels of both glycine and serine rose following a serine load. The rise was abnormally great, resembling that found in Gerritsen's patient with NKH. There was a normal response to a leucine load, as found in Gerritsen's patient, and in contrast to an abnormal response found in a patient with ketotic hyperglycinaemia and propionic acidaemia (Nyhan *et al.*, 1961). The

Table 1 Plasma amino acid levels ($\mu mol \, l^{-1}$) in the patient following L-amino acid loads ($0.25 \, g \, kg^{-1}$)

	Fasting	*1 h*	*2 h*	*4 h*
Glycine load				
Glycine	855	2065	2800	2335
Serine	210	180	185	160
Threonine	185	185	170	145
Serine load				
Glycine	975	1120	1095	1145
Serine	220	885	505	375
Threonine	185	160	150	125
Leucine load				
Glycine	960	865	905	880
Serine	155	115	135	125
Threonine	145	93	88	73
Threonine load				
Glycine	805	840	840	815
Serine	235	250	220	165
Threonine	145	965	725	410
α-Aminobutyrate	24	89	110	135

Journal of Inherited Metabolic Disease. ISSN 0141-8955. Copyright © SSIEM and MTP Press Limited, Queen Square, Lancaster, UK.

observed rise in the plasma threonine level after a threonine load was prolonged compared to that in normal subjects (Childs and Nyhan, 1964). Plasma serine fell, in contrast to the rise obtained in a patient with ketotic hyperglycinaemia and propionic acidaemia (Nyhan *et al.*, 1961).

DISCUSSION

The main pathway of glycine catabolism is via serine. However, it may also be converted to glyoxylate, or condense with acetyl-CoA to form aminoacetone, which can reform acetyl-CoA via 2-oxopropanal and pyruvate. Threonine may be catabolised via glycine, α-ketobutyrate or aminoacetone. Serine may be converted to glycine, probably by means of the same enzyme which converts threonine to glycine (Krieger and Nigro, 1983).

The results of the loading tests of the present study are entirely consistent with a defect in serine formation from glycine. The occasionally raised threonine level and the rise in glycine following the threonine load could both be explained by the fact that threonine can be catabolised via glycine. The possibility of a defect in threonine dehydratase, as found in the patients of Krieger and Nigro (1983), seems to be excluded by the considerable

rise in plasma α-aminobutyrate levels following the threonine load. However, the results do not exclude the possibility of a defect in the aminoacetone pathway.

References

Carson, N. A. J. Non-ketotic hyperglycinaemia — a review of 70 patients. *J. Inher. Metab. Dis.* 5, Suppl. 2 (1982) 126–128

Childs, B. and Nyhan, W. L. Further observations of a patient with hyperglycinemia. *Pediatrics* 33 (1964) 403–412

Childs, B., Nyhan, W. L., Borden, M., Bard, L. and Cooke, R. E. Idiopathic hyperglycinemia: a new disorder of amino acid metabolism. *Pediatrics* 27 (1961) 522–538

Gerritsen, T., Kaveggia, E. and Waisman, H. A. A. A new type of idiopathic hyperglycinemia with hypo-oxaluria. *Pediatrics* 36 (1965) 882–891

de Groot, C. J., Troelstra, J. A. and Hommes, F. A. The enzymatic defect of the nonketotic form of hyperglycinemia. *Pediatr. Res.* 4 (1970) 238–243

Krieger, I. and Nigro, M. Evidence for defective threonine metabolism in non-ketotic hyperglycinaemia. *J. Inher. Metab. Dis.* 6 (1983) 40–43

Nyhan, W. L., Borden, M. and Childs, B. Idiopathic hyperglycinemia: a new disorder of amino acid metabolism. *Pediatrics* 27 (1961) 539–550

Palmer, T., Rossiter, M. A., Levin, B. and Oberholzer, V. G. The effect of protein loads on plasma amino acid levels. *Clin. Sci. Mol. Med.* 45 (1973) 827–832

J. Inher. Metab. Dis. 8 Suppl. 2 (1985) 127–128

Short Communication

Plasma Selenium Levels in Treated Phenylketonuric Patients

A. Rottoli, G. Lista, G. Zecchini, C. Butté and R. Longhi
V Pediatric Department, University of Milan, S. Paolo Hospital, 8 di Rudini, 20142 Milan, Italy

While in the last few years many basic congenital defects of trace element metabolism have been discovered, only very recently has emphasis also been placed on the possible pathologies due to trace element deficiency, secondary to the dietary restrictions of patients with inborn errors of metabolism (Lombeck *et al.*, 1978; Acosta *et al.*, 1981; Longhi *et al.*, 1983). For this reason, plasma selenium (Se) levels were measured in 16 treated phenylketonuric (PKU) children, as a part of the program of nutritional control undertaken by the V Pediatric Department of the University of Milan, in order to point out the pathologies caused by marginal or selective malnutrition in patients on a restricted diet.

MATERIALS AND METHODS

Sixteen PKU children, 2 months–12 years old, 15 of which were diagnosed as classic PKU and one as tetrahydrobiopterin deficiency (dihydropteridine reductase (EC 1.6.99.7) deficiency (McKusick 26163)) have been studied. All patients had been on a phenylalanine (Phe) restricted diet for at least 9 months, with a single exception (1 month). The diet is based on a Phe-free protein substitute to cover most of the protein requirements and unlimited amounts of low Phe products to cover the various nutritional needs. The children were divided into two groups on the basis of the mean plasma Phe value of the previous year: the first group with plasma Phe $< 8 \, \text{mg} \, \text{dl}^{-1}$ (good metabolic control); the second group with plasma Phe $> 12 \, \text{mg} \, \text{dl}^{-1}$ (poor metabolic control). None had a mean plasma Phe between 8 and $12 \, \text{mg} \, \text{dl}^{-1}$. No clinical signs of Se deficiency (Raptis *et al.*, 1983) were evident in any of the patients. The control population included 22 subjects (11 males, 11 females) apparently healthy, of comparable age, on a "normal" diet. In all children, blood was drawn after a 12 h fast. Plasma Se determinations were done by atomic absorption spectrophotometry with electrothermal atomization

(Edinger, 1975). For the statistical analysis, Student's *t*-test was utilized. To obviate the exiguity of the groups a non-parametric test (Wilcoxon's test) was also employed.

RESULTS

In Table 1 mean ($\overline{\text{M}}$), standard deviation (SD) and statistical analysis of plasma Se values of patients and controls are reported.

The evaluation of the results shows a statistically significant difference ($p < 0.01$) between the plasma Se values of all the PKU patients and the controls. The significance is even more evident ($p < 0.005$) if the comparison is made only with the patients on good metabolic control. Finally, plasma Se values of the patients in poor metabolic control were compared with the Se levels of the normal population and of the patients in good metabolic control: no significant differences were present.

The negative correlation between severity of diet control and plasma Se values is also made evident by the linear regression between plasma Phe and Se ($r = 0.5$ for all PKU patients and $r = 0.83$ for PKU patients in good metabolic control).

DISCUSSION

Diet represents the only source of Se in man. For this reason, patients on severely restricted diet, because of inborn errors of metabolism, are at risk for Se deficiency. The difference in plasma Se values between the two groups of patients can be explained by the consideration that a "good metabolic control" is obtained only when the diet is strictly followed. As an obvious consequence, the diet our patients were following did not cover the Se daily requirements. Utilizing tables of composition of foodstuffs (Thompson *et al.*, 1975; Raptis *et al.*, 1983), we calculated the approximate Se daily intake allowed by

Table 1 Mean ($\overline{\text{M}}$), standard deviation (SD) and statistical analysis of plasma Se values of PKU patients and controls (values in $\mu\text{g} \, \text{dl}^{-1}$)

Population	n	$\overline{\text{M}}$	SD	Student's t-test			Wilcoxon's test	
(1) Controls	22	9.88	3.33	(1) vs. (2)	$t = 2.85$	$p < 0.01$	$T = 399$	$p < 0.01$
(2) PKU	16	6.91	2.91	(1) vs. (3)	$t = 1.20$	p NS	$T = 149$	p NS
(3) PKU (Phe $> 12 \, \text{mg} \%$)	8	8.24	3.22	(1) vs. (4)	$t = 3.43$	$p < 0.005$	$T = 185$	$p < 0.01$
(4) PKU (Phe $< 8 \, \text{mg} \%$)	8	5.59	1.94	(3) vs. (4)	$t = 2.00$	p NS	$T = 53$	p NS

Journal of Inherited Metabolic Disease. ISSN 0141-8955. Copyright © SSIEM and MTP Press Limited, Queen Square, Lancaster, UK.

standard PKU diets. The intake, calculated in excess, varies, in relation to age, between 7.2 and 9.5 µg day^{-1}, figures clearly lower than the recommended (RDA: 20–200 µg day^{-1}) (Committee on Dietary Allowances, 1980). In fact, the Se present in the foods offered *ad libitum* to PKU patients represents only 3–7% of the Se intake with a regular diet. While plasma Se level is a "static" parameter of Se metabolism, red cell Se-dependent glutathione peroxidase activity is an excellent index of the biological availability of this trace element. Studies are now in progress in our laboratory to correlate plasma Se values of our PKU patients with their erythrocyte glutathione peroxidase activity.

We conclude that: (1) A low Phe diet does not guarantee a sufficient supply of Se. For this reason, PKU patients are at risk for Se deficiency. (2) Se supplementation, as selenomethionine or sodium selenite, is suggested, either by fortification of the protein substitute or separately. (3) In the case of Se supplementation, frequent monitoring of the urinary excretion of Se metabolites, to avoid overdosage, is indicated.

References

Acosta, P. B., Fernhoff, P. M., Warshaw, H. S., Hambridge, K. M., Ernest, A., McCobe, E. R. B. and Elsos II, L. J. Zinc and copper status of treated children with phenylketonuria. *J. Parent. Ent. Nutr.*, 5 (1981) 406–409

Committee on Dietary Allowances. Food and Nutritional Board. *Recommended Dietary Allowances*, 9th Revised Edn., National Academy of Sciences, Washington D.C., 1980

Edinger, R. D. Atomic absorption analysis with the graphite furnace using matrix modification. *At. Absorpt. Newsl.* 14 (1975) 127

Lombeck, I., Kaspareck, K., Harbish, H. D., Becker, K., Schumann, E., Scrhoter, W., Feinendegen, L. E. and Bremer, H. I. The selenium state of children. II: Selenium content of serum, whole blood, hair and the activity of erythrocyte glutathione peroxidase in dietetically treated patients with phenylketonuria and maple syrup urine disease. *Eur. J. Pediatr.* 128 (1978) 213–223

Longhi, R., Riva, E., Turrini, G., Fiocchi, A., Rottoli, A. and Giovannini, M. Controllo nutrizionale nei fenilchetonurici in dietoterapia: gli oligoelementi. *Riv. Ital. Ped.* 9 (1983) 363–370

Raptis, S. E., Kaiser, G. and Tolg, G. A survey of selenium in the environment and a critical review of its determination of trace levels. *Fresenius Z. Anal. Chem.* 316 (1983) 105–123

Thompson, J. N., Erdy, P. and Smith, D. C. Selenium content of food consumed by Canadians. *J. Nutr.* 105 (1975) 274–277

J. Inher. Metab. Dis. 8 Suppl. 2 (1985) 129

Short Communication

Plasma Lipid Concentrations in 42 Treated Phenylketonuric Children

C. R. Galluzzo, M. T. Ortisi, L. Castelli, C. Agostoni and R. Longhi
V Pediatric Department, University of Milan, S. Paolo Hospital, 8 di Rudimi 20142 Milan, Italy

A low phenylalanine diet is the only therapy for classic phenylketonuria (PKU) (Berry *et al.*, 1967). This diet is based on a reduced intake of natural proteins replaced, to a great extent, by synthetic protein substitutes, such as very low phenylanine protein hydrolysates or phenyl-alanine-free amino acid mixtures. The remaining protein requirements are generally met by vegetable proteins with a reduced content of phenylalanine (Schurrle and Bickel, 1971; Giovannini *et al.*, 1979). Such a diet can be defined as "non-atherogenic" as the reduction of animal proteins (meat, milk, eggs) involves a decreased intake of animal lipids, cholesterol, saturated fatty acids (with consequent increased plasma polyunsaturated/saturated fatty acids ratio), decreased plasma lysine/arginine ratio and increased intake of dietary fibres (Vahouny, 1982). All these factors have well-known effects on the control of plasma cholesterol, while the reduced plasma levels of sulphur amino acids seem to lower the presence of circulating mono- and disulphurated compounds. These chemicals have been implicated in the atheromasic process, because of their damaging effects on the endothelium (Carrol, 1982).

SUBJECTS AND METHODS

The 42 PKU patients were males and females, 1–13 years of age, on a low phenylanine diet, in good health, without clinical or laboratory signs of malnutrition and with normal liver function tests. Dietetic compliance was monitored by frequent Guthrie tests. Controls were 150 healthy children, of comparable age and sex distribution, seen in our day hospital for a physical and biochemical check-up, without clinical or laboratory signs of malnutrition.

Plasma total cholesterol, HDL cholesterol and triglycerides were all measured by enzymatic-colorimetric assay. For the statistical analysis Student's *t*-test was utilized.

RESULTS AND CONCLUSIONS

PKU patients showed significantly lower plasma total cholesterol values than the controls, while there were no statistically significant differences for plasma HDL cholesterol and triglyceride levels (Table 1). Thus treated PKU subjects have a better lipidaemic profile than children of comparable age and sex, in good health.

Acosta *et al.* (1973) and Barashnev *et al.* (1982) have previously found alterations of serum lipids in PKU patients. Barashnev, studying an untreated PKU population, suggested that they were indicative of a

Table 1 Plasma lipid concentrations (mg $100\,ml^{-1}$)

Lipids	PKU patients			Control			Student's t-test
	n	$\bar{x}$	SD	n	$\bar{x}$	SD	p
Total cholesterol	42	145.00	25.46	150	177.70	33.16	<0.001
HDL cholesterol	41	45.10	11.75	150	42.87	10.11	<0.30
Triglycerides	30	92.73	34.29	150	82.47	39.69	<0.20

defect in hepatic lipid synthesis, due to liver damage secondary to the high plasma phenylalanine and/or phenylalanine metabolites. This is not the case of our patients in which there were no clinical or biochemical signs of liver malfunction and in which the low phenylalanine diet was started early, before any significant liver damage could possibly occur. For this reason, we believe that the dietary modifications to which PKU patients are submitted have a relevant role in modifying their plasma lipid pattern. The role of diet in modifying the lipidaemic profile is therefore emphasized.

We point out that an abnormal lipidic pattern is strongly implicated in the pathogenesis of the athero-sclerotic disease, which is the main cause of death and morbidity in the western countries (Lewis, 1980).

References

Acosta, P. B., Alfin-Stater, R. B. and Koch, R. Serum lipids in children with phenylketonuria (PKU). *J. Am. Diet. Assoc.* 63 (1973) 631–635

Barashnev, Y. I., Korneichuk, V. V., Klehborsky, A. I. and Klyushina, L. A. Role of the liver in the pathogenesis of cerebral disorders in phenylketonuria. *J. Inher. Metab. Dis.* 5 (1982) 204–210

Berry, H. K., Sutherland, B. S. and Umberger, B. Treatment of phenylketonuria. *Am. J. Dis. Child.* 113 (1967) 2

Carrol, K. K. Hypercholesterolemia and atherosclerosis: effects of dietary proteins. *Fed. Proc.* 41 (1982) 2792–2796

Giovannini, M., Riva, E., Segre, A. and Episcopi, E. A practical approach to the dietary management of phenylketonuria. *Perspect. Med. Dis.* 1 (1979) 117

Lewis, B. Dietary prevention of ischaemic heart disease—a policy for the 80's. *Br. Med. J.* 281 (1980) 177–180

Schurrle, L. and Bickel, J. Practical dietetics. In Bickel, H., Hudson, F. P. and Woolf, L. I. (eds.) *Phenylketonuria*, George Thieme Verlag, Stuttgart, 1971, p. 240

Vahouny, G. V. Dietary fiber, lipid metabolism and atherosclerosis. *Fed. Proc.* 41 (1982) 2801–2806

Journal of Inherited Metabolic Disease. ISSN 0141-8955. Copyright © SSIEM and MTP Press Limited, Queen Square, Lancaster, UK.

J. Inher. Metab. Dis. 8 Suppl. 2 (1985) 130

Short Communication

Speech and Language Disorders in Histidinaemia and other Amino Acid Disturbances

J. HYÁNEK and V. RAISOVÁ

Department of Clinical Chemistry and Foniatric Department, Medical School, Charles University, Prague, Czechoslovakia

The first described "cases" of histidinaemia were accompanied with typical clinical symptoms—speech disturbances. The purpose of this paper is to establish the blood and urine levels of histidine and its metabolites found in patients presenting with speech neuroses.

MATERIALS AND METHODS

We have examined 200 patients (5–48 years) presenting with speech difficulty (stammering and faltering); one histidinaemia patient with high blood histidine ($1037 \mu mol\,l^{-1}$ on the 5th day after birth), positive histidine and imidazoles excretion in urine, negative urocanic acid in sweat, lower skin histidase activity and full-scale IQ score 107, and 60000 healthy newborns screened on the 5th day after birth. Twenty-two healthy school children and 15 adults served as a control group. Thirty-five patients presenting with phenylketonuria, homocystinuria, cystinuria and tyrosinosis on dietary treatment since the newborn period were also examined.

One-dimensional chromatography was used for screening of amino acids with Pauly reagent detection (Efron *et al.*, 1964; Levy *et al.*, 1974). Two-dimensional thin layer chromatography of histidine and imidazoles with the same detection (Wadman *et al.*, 1967) and quantitative estimation with liquid column chromatography on amino acid analyzers using short programmes were used for confirmatory studies. Skin histidase activity was measured according to Kihara and Boggs (1968). In loading test with L-histidine (100 mg kg weight^{-1}) blood and urine were taken at intervals of 0, 60, 120, 180, 240 and 360 mins and changes in speech capacity were evaluated using the Lee effect method 60 min after the load.

RESULTS

Blood and urine concentrations of histidine and its metabolites in patients presenting with speech disorders showed no direct dependence and were within normal limits. Speech in the single detected histidinaemia patient was absolutely without any disturbance. Histidine load did not provoke such deterioration of speech capacity as a clinical response that could be regarded as the result of higher histidine levels in patients with stammering and faultering. The frequency of histidinaemia in the normal population in the region of central Bohemia is about 1:60000. No higher incidence of this disorder was found in the risk population of children and adults with speech disturbances.

In the patients with stammering and faultering the incidence of non-specific hyperaminoaciduria was significantly raised but these findings cannot be considered as being typical of these speech disorders. In a group of patients presenting with phenylketonuria, homocystinuria, cystinuria and tyrosinosis a statistically insignificant difference in the frequency of stammering, in comparison to the normal population, was observed.

Our paper proves that histidinaemia is a rare metabolic disorder in the Slavonic population, without relation to speech defects.

References

Efron, M. L., Young, G. and Moser, W. H. A simple chromatographic test for the detection of disorders of amino acid metabolism. *N. Engl. J. Med.* 270 (1964) 1378–1383

Kihara, H. and Boggs, D. E. Histidinemia: Studies on histidase activity in stratum corneum. *Biochem. Med.* 2 (1968) 243–250

Levy, H. L., Shih, V. E. and Madigan, P. M. Routine newborn screening for histidinemia: clinical and biochemical results. *N. Engl. J. Med.* 291 (1974) 1214–1219

Novák, A. The influence of delayed auditory feedback in stutterers. *Folia Phon.* 30 (1978) 278–285

Wadman, S. K., Van Sprang, F. J. and Van Stekelenberg, G. J. Three new cases of histidinemia: Clinical and biochemical data. *Acta Paediatr. Scand.* 56 (1967) 485–493

Journal of Inherited Metabolic Disease. ISSN 0141-8955. Copyright © SSIEM and MTP Press Limited, Queen Square, Lancaster, UK.

J. Inher. Metab. Dis. 8 Suppl. 2 (1985) 131–132

Short Communication

Early Diagnosis and Dietetic Management in Newborn with Maple Syrup Urine Disease. Birth to Six Weeks

E. R. NAUGHTEN, I. P. SAUL, G. ROCHE and C. MULLINS
The Children's Hospital, Temple Street, Dublin 1, Eire

Maple syrup urine disease (MSUD; McKusick 24860) results from a defect in oxidative decarboxylation of the ketoacids derived from the branched chain amino acids (BCAA) leucine, isoleucine and valine. The outcome is related to early diagnosis and management (Clow *et al.*, 1981; Naughten *et al.*, 1982; Leonard *et al.*, 1984). The diagnosis can be made in the first 48 h (Di George *et al.*, 1982). We describe the early diagnosis and dietetic management of a neonate.

MATERIALS AND METHODS

Amino acids were measured using the Locarte amino acid analyser. Blood levels were monitored daily. We aim to keep the plasma leucine $100-700 \mu mol\,l^{-1}$, isoleucine and valine $50-400 \mu mol\,l^{-1}$, and to achieve normal growth and development.

DIAGNOSIS AND TREATMENT

A newborn female at risk for MSUD was diagnosed following a high risk screen. Branched chain amino acids were measured in cord blood and in samples taken at 2 h, 7 h and 14 h. She was fed with a modified milk formula (Osterfeed $60\,ml\,kg^{-1} = 0.15$ g protein (kg body wt)$^{-1}$, 4-hourly). Alloisoleucine was detected in plasma at 7 h and increased at 14 h. No alloisoleucine was detected in the control sample and the control plasma leucine remained below $130\,\mu mol\,l^{-1}$ (Figure 1).

Dietary treatment commenced at 26 h. Blood amino acids were monitored daily and the diet adjusted accordingly. The diet consisted of:

(a) Low natural protein intake as modified milk formula to provide low BCAA intake (100 ml = 1.45 g protein: leucine 144 mg: isoleucine 84 mg: valine 94 mg).

(b) Synthetic protein intake as BCAA-free amino acid mixture MSUD Aid (3 g kg^{-1}).

(c) Carbohydrate as glucose and glucose polymer (Caloreen).

(d) Fat as arachis oil emulsion (Prosparol).

(e) Mineral and trace element supplement (Aminogran mineral mixture 1.5 g kg^{-1}).

(f) Vitamin (Ketovite tablets and liquid).

(g) Supplements of L-isoleucine and L-valine as indicated by plasma levels.

The daily natural protein intake varied from 0.14 to 1.07 g (kg body wt)$^{-1}$ during growth (leucine intake = 58–432 mg day^{-1} or 13–105 mg kg^{-1} day^{-1}). The total protein (synthetic and natural) varied from 2.40 to 3.24 g kg^{-1} day^{-1}. Supplements of L-valine varied from 0 to 35 mg kg^{-1} day^{-1} and L-isoleucine from 0 to 53 mg kg^{-1} day^{-1}. The calorie intake varied from 106 to 123 kg^{-1} day^{-1}, mean 116 kg^{-1} day^{-1}. The weight is above and parallel to the 50th centile. The patient is developmentally normal at 8 months.

DISCUSSION

The alloisoleucine which was detected at 7 h, after the first feed, confirmed the diagnosis of MSUD in this newborn infant whose 6 year old male sibling is on a diet for this condition.

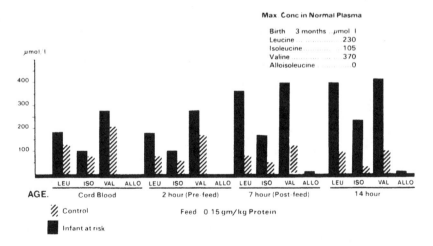

Figure 1 BCAA levels in newborn at risk for MSUD and in control

131

Journal of Inherited Metabolic Disease. ISSN 0141-8955. Copyright © SSIEM and MTP Press Limited, Queen Square, Lancaster, UK.

We found that meticulous attention to the amino acid balance gave good weight gain and growth in the newborn. Supplements of the L-isoleucine and L-valine prevented gross imbalance of the BCAA and contributed to keeping the leucine level down.

References

Clow, C. L., Reade, T. M. and Scriver, C. R. Outcome of early and long-term management of classical maple syrup urine disease. *Pediatrics* 68 (1981) 856–861

Di George, A. M., Rezvani, I., Garibaldi, L. R. and Schwartz, M. Prospective study of maple-syrup urine disease for the first four days of life. *N. Engl. J. Med.* 307 (1982) 1492–1495

Leonard, J. V., Daish, P., Naughten, E. R. and Bartlett, K. The management and long term outcome of organic acidaemias. *J. Inher. Metab. Dis.* 7, Suppl. 1 (1984) 13–17

Naughten, E. R., Jenkins, J., Francis, D. E. M. and Leonard, J. V. Outcome of maple syrup urine disease. *Arch. Dis. Child.* 57 (1982) 918–921

J. Inher. Metab. Dis. 8 Suppl. 2 (1985) 133–134

Short Communication

α-Aminoadipic and α-Ketoadipic Aciduria: Detection of a New Case by a Screening Program using Two-dimensional Thin Layer Chromatography of Amino Acids

C. Vianey-Liaud, P. Divry and J. Cotte
Laboratoire de Biochimie, Hôpital Debrousse, 69322 Lyon Cedex 05, France

G. Teyssier
Clinique de Pédiatrie, Hôpital Bellevue, 42023 Saint Etienne Cedex, France

α-Aminoadipic acid and α-ketoadipic acid are intermediates of lysine catabolism; they are synthetized mainly via the saccharopine pathway, although the pipecolic acid pathway may be significant in some tissues, such as the central nervous system. α-Ketoadipic acid may be produced also via tryptophan catabolism. Since 1974, 10 patients with α-aminoadipic aciduria (McKusick 20475) have been described but seven of them (Przyrembel *et al.*, 1975; Wilson *et al.*, 1975; Gray *et al.*, 1979; Fischer and Brown, 1980; Duran *et al.*, 1984) were reported to also present α-ketoadipic aciduria (McKusick 24513), suggesting that the enzymatic defect might be located either at the level of α-aminoadipate aminotransferase (α-aminoadipic aciduria only) or at the level of α-ketoadipate dehydrogenase (α-amino- and α-ketoadipic aciduria). In one case (Przyrembel *et al.*, 1975), Wendel *et al.* (1975) showed that conversion of ^{14}C-labelled α-ketoadipate to $^{14}CO_2$ was decreased, although glutaryl-CoA dehydrogenase activity was normal. Clinically, most of the patients described are slightly to deeply mentally retarded with hypotonia or seizures. One was reported to have an immune deficiency (Gray *et al.*, 1979). However, normal siblings of these patients have been reported to also excrete excessive amounts of α-amino- and α-ketoadipic acids (Wilson *et al.*, 1975; Fischer and Brown, 1980). We report here a new patient with α-aminoadipic aciduria and α-ketoadipic aciduria in association with respiratory infections and mild hypotonia.

CASE REPORT

The patient (N.H.), a 7 year-old girl, is the fourth child of consanguineous Moroccan parents. The three other children are in good health. She was born after an uneventful pregnancy and delivery. Psychomotor development was normal until 6 months when she developed repeated infections of the respiratory tract. At 13 months, she was noticed to be hypotrophic and slightly hypotonic with delayed motor development. She began to walk at 21 months and her walk always remained peculiar: clumsy and with apparent cerebellar ataxia. Deep tendon reflexes were absent. Muscle enzymes and electromyography were normal. She was

reinvestigated in February 1984: analysis of amino acids and organic acids revealed excessive amounts of α-aminoadipic and α-ketoadipic acid.

MATERIALS AND METHODS

Two-dimensional thin layer chromatography of urinary amino acids, after desalting, was performed according to Wadman *et al.* (1975). Amino acids were quantitatively determined by classical automated ion exchange chromatography. GLC of urinary organic acids was performed as previously described (Divry *et al.*, 1981), except that a 25 m capillary column filled with SE-54 was used. For GLC analysis of urinary ketoacids, *O*-TMS quinoxalinol derivatives were prepared according to Langenbeck *et al.* (1977), and analysed on the same SE-54 25 m capillary column with a programmed temperature from 150 to 300°C. α-Ketoadipic acid was quantitatively determined by electron impact selected ion monitoring gas chromatography–mass spectrometry (EI SIM GC/MS) using a Hewlett-Packard 5970A mass detector.

Oral loading tests with L-lysine (100 mg kg^{-1}) and L-tryptophan (100 mg kg^{-1}) were performed according to the protocol of Przyrembel *et al.* (1975) and Casey *et al.* (1978).

RESULTS

Two-dimensional TLC urinary amino acids revealed a spot overlapping glutamic acid, which might be either α-aminoadipic acid or formimino glutamic acid, as glutamine was normal. Quantitative chromatography confirmed the occurrence of excessive amounts of α-aminoadipic acid both in plasma (118 μmol l^{-1}—normal range <5 μmol l^{-1}) and urine (249 mmol (mol creatinine)$^{-1}$—normal range <17 mmol (mol creatinine)$^{-1}$. Lysine concentrations were normal and neither saccharopine nor pipecolic acid could be detected. GC–MS analysis revealed excessive amounts of α-ketoadipic acid (112 mmol (mol creatinine)$^{-1}$) with a moderate increase of glutaric (174 μmol l^{-1}) and α-ketoglutaric acids.

Compared to a normal subject, oral loading tests with

133

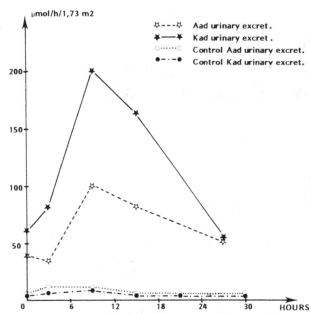

Figure 1 Oral L-lysine load: α-aminoadipic (Aad) and α-ketoadipic (Kad) excretion in urine of patient N.H. and in urine of a normal control

either L-lysine (Figure 1) or L-tryptophan (data not shown) resulted in a large increase in both α-aminoadipic and α-ketoadipic acids.

DISCUSSION

The biochemical abnormalities observed in our patient are in agreement with an α-ketoadipic aciduria with α-aminoadipic aciduria. The failure to detect significant increases of lysine, saccharopine, pipecolic and glutaric acids excludes other defects of lysine catabolism (urinary glutaric acid levels are much lower than those found in glutaric aciduria type I). The slight increase of urinary glutaric and α-ketoglutaric acids observed is difficult to explain: it may be due to non-enzymatic degradation of α-ketoadipic acid urine.

Compared to a normal subject, oral L-lysine load resulted in a marked increase of α-aminoadipic acid both in plasma (reaching $185 \mu mol\,l^{-1}$) and urine (Figure 1) but did not modify lysine excretion. These results are in good agreement with those previously published (Przyrembel *et al.*, 1975; Casey *et al.*, 1978), except for lysine excretion which was found to be abnormally high in the patient of Przyrembel *et al.* (1975). Moreover, in

our case, a three-fold increase of urinary ketoadipate was observed (Figure 1). Oral tryptophan load was attempted as tryptophan is a precursor of α-ketoadipic acid but not of α-aminoadipic acid. It also resulted in an increased excretion of the substituted adipates. These two loading tests seem to prove that the enzymatic defect involves a lack of α-ketoadipate dehydrogenase.

To our knowledge, it is the 11th reported case of α-aminoadipic aciduria–α-ketoadipic aciduria. As in the previously described cases, the clinical symptoms of our patient were not indicative of the metabolic defect. α-Aminoadipic acid was detected by an amino acid screening test motivated by the parents' consanguinity. This new case emphasizes the clinical heterogeneity of this metabolic disorder.

References

Casey, R. E., Zaleski, W. A., Philip, M., Mendelson, I. S. and MacKenzie, S. L. Biochemical and clinical studies of a new case of α-aminoadipic aciduria. *J. Inher. Metab. Dis.* 1 (1978) 129–135

Divry, P., Rolland, M. O., Teyssier, J., Cotte, J., Formosinho Fernandez, M. C., Tavares de Almeida, I. and Da Silveira, C. 3-Hydroxy-3-methylglutaric aciduria combined with 3-methylglutaconic aciduria: a new case. *J. Inher. Metab. Dis.* 4 (1981) 173–174

Duran, M., Beemer, A., Wadman, S. K., Wendel, U. and Janssen, B. A patient with α-ketoadipic and α-aminoadipic aciduria. *J. Inher. Metab. Dis.* 7 (1984) 61

Fischer, M. H. and Brown, R. R. Tryptophan and lysine metabolism in α-aminoadipic aciduria. *Am. J. Med. Genet.* 5 (1980) 35–41

Gray, R. G. F., O'Neil, E. M. and Pollitt, R. J. α-Aminoadipic aciduria: Chemical and enzymatic studies. *J. Inher. Metab. Dis.* 2 (1979) 89–92

Langenbeck, V., Mohring, H. V., Hinney, B. and Spiteller, M. Quinoxalinol derivatives. *Biomed. Mass Spectrom.* 4 (1977) 197–203

Przyrembel, H., Bachmann, D., Lombeck, I., Becker, K., Wendel, U., Wadman, S. K. and Bremer, H. J. α-Ketoadipic aciduria, a new inborn error of lysine metabolism; biochemical studies. *Clin. Chim. Acta* 58 (1975) 257–269

Wadman, S. K., de Bree, P. K., Van Sprang, F. J., Kamerling, J. P., Haverkamp, J. and Vliegenthart, J. F. G. Nξ-(carboxymethyl) lysine, a constituent of human urine. *Clin. Chim. Acta* 59 (1975) 313–320

Wendel, U., Rudiger, H. W., Pzryrembel, H. and Bremer, H. J. Alpha-ketoadipic aciduria: degradation studies with fibroblasts. *Clin. Chim. Acta* 58 (1975) 271–276

Wilson, R. W., Wilson, S. M., Gates, S. C. and Higgins, J. V. α-Ketoadipic aciduria: a description of a new metabolic error in lysine–tryptophan degradation. *Pediatr. Res.* 9 (1975) 522–526

J. Inher. Metab. Dis. 8 Suppl. 2 (1985) 135–136

Short Communication

The Diagnosis and Biochemical Investigation of a Patient with a Short Chain Fatty Acid Oxidation Defect

M. J. Bennett
Department of Chemical Pathology, Sheffield Children's Hospital, Sheffield S10 2TH, UK

R. G. F. Gray
Sub-Department of Medical Genetics, University of Sheffield, Sheffield S10 5DN, UK

D. M. Isherwood and N. Murphy
Departments of Biochemistry and Paediatrics, Alder Hey Children's Hospital, Liverpool L12 2AP, UK

R. J. Pollitt
Neonatal Screening Laboratory and University Department of Psychiatry, Middlewood Hospital, Sheffield S6 1TP, UK

Though the clinical and biochemical features of medium chain acyl-CoA dehydrogenase deficiency are now becoming well established we have much less experience of defects in short chain acyl-CoA dehydrogenation. The patient described here demonstrated defective oxidation of butyrate and hexanoate by cultured fibroblasts but normal oxidation of both medium and long chain fatty acid substrates, indicating a specific short chain abnormality. In keeping with this the urine contained excessive ethylmalonic acid.

CASE REPORT

A female infant N.A., the first child of unrelated Yemeni parents was observed over a 15 month period, in which there were four hospital admissions. She had no neonatal problems and her first hospital admission was at 5 months old with rotavirus gastroenteritis. At that time there was a degree of developmental delay and failure to thrive. She was not acidotic and there was no hypoglycaemia. At 11 months of age she was admitted with otitis media, her weight was below the tenth centile and she had developmental delay with signs of mild spastic diplegia. Despite a normal platelet count, there were petechiae on the face and upper trunk. She was ill with tachypnoea, and was found to have a lactic acidosis but no hypoglycaemia. For 2 weeks there were lapses into semi-coma and periods of convulsive movements, followed by a slow recovery over 3 weeks. At 13 months she was again admitted with diarrhoea and vomiting, she had a lactic acidosis and ketonuria with a maximum base deficit of $-18\,\mathrm{mmol\,l^{-1}}$ but no hypoglycaemia. Petechiae were again noted with a positive Hess test but platelets were normal. An infectious cause was not found for the diarrhoea and she slowly recovered following IV fluids and regrading on milk. She became less acidotic on bicarbonate supplements but remained hypocapnoeic. She was relatively well for 3 months before her final admission at 19 months with campylobacter gastroenteritis. On admission the patient had Kussmaul breathing and neurological examination showed truncal hypotonia with signs of spastic diplegia. She was unable to sit unaided and motor and cognitive developmental assessment placed on her at a 9–10 month level. Petechiae were again noted on the face and upper trunk. Following an initial improvement on IV fluids there was marked deterioration. In the final 2 weeks she developed a massive non-selective proteinuria and died in renal failure at the age of 20 months.

BIOCHEMICAL INVESTIGATIONS

A sweat test and xylose absorption test performed at $4\frac{1}{2}$ months were normal, as were blood and urine amino acids. Blood glucose measured on a total of 32 occasions was consistently normal. Acid base studies revealed a persistent base deficit (mean deficit $4.5\,\mathrm{mmol\,l^{-1}}$) and there was a compensated respiratory alkalosis with a mean $p\mathrm{CO_2}$ of $3.7\,\mathrm{kPa}$. A persistent lactic acidaemia (1.5–$6.7\,\mathrm{mmol\,l^{-1}}$) led to the investigation of enzymes of pyruvate metabolism and gluconeogenesis in cultured fibroblasts which gave normal results. The leukocyte lysosomal hydrolases were normal. GC–MS analysis of organic acids in two urine samples collected in the terminal stages showed ethylmalonate as the major peak and the presence of methylsuccinate and butyrylglycine. The adipate peak was quite small and there was no appreciable excess of other dicarboxylic acids. An octenoic acid and smaller amounts of octanoic acid were present in both samples but, as the patient was on a high-fat diet (Prosparol) at the time, the significance of this is unclear.

The oxidation of labelled fatty acids of various chain lengths was measured using fibroblast monolayers (Bennett *et al.*, 1984). This revealed a specific defect in short chain fatty acid oxidation (Table 1). The oxidation

Journal of Inherited Metabolic Disease. ISSN 0141-8955. Copyright © SSIEM and MTP Press Limited, Queen Square, Lancaster, UK.

Table 1 Fatty acid oxidation rates of various chain length substrates in cultured fibroblasts [pmol CO_2 min^{-1} (mg protein)$^{-1}$]

Substrate	Patient			Controls		
	Mean	SD	N[1]	Mean	SD	N[2]
[1-^{14}C]Oleic acid	0.30	0.02	3	0.39	0.015	7
[1-^{14}C]Palmitic acid	0.32	0.07	3	0.43	0.14	5
[1-^{14}C]Octanoic acid	4.20	1.76	3	3.55	0.71	5
[1-^{14}C]Hexanoic acid	9.42	1.54	3	20.2	4.5	6
[1-^{14}C]Butyric acid	0.88	0.21	5	2.25	0.56	9

[1] Number of assays
[2] Number of lines

of oleic, palmitic and octanoic acids was within the normal range whilst that of hexanoate and butyrate was significantly reduced.

DISCUSSION

The major clinical features in this patient with a defect in short chain fatty acid oxidation were developmental delay and repeated severe infections. There was a persistent lactic acidaemia and base deficit but hypoglycaemia was never observed. This contrasts with the findings in other acyl-CoA dehydrogenase defects [medium chain acyl-CoA dehydrogenase deficiency (McKusick 22274), glutaric aciduria type II (McKusick 23168) and ethylmalonic adipic aciduria (EMA; McKusick 22717)] where acidosis tends to be intermittent and accompanied by severe hypoglycaemia. EMA appears to be a generalised defect in acyl-CoA dehydrogenation, probably due to defective electron transport, affecting predominantly the oxidation of butanoyl and hexanoyl CoA (Mantagos *et al.*, 1979; Green *et al.*, 1985) and might give rather similar biochemical results to those found in N.A. However, while EMA may show ethylmalonic and methylsuccinic acids as the only urinary abnormality during clinical remission, very large amounts of adipic acid are excreted during illness. Though only two urine samples from N.A. were examined in detail both were collected whilst she was extremely ill and excessive adipic acid was not detected in either. Other metabolites, such as isovaleryl-glycine and hexanoylglycine, which are sometimes found in EMA, were not detected in either of the samples from N.A. Taking all the findings together, particularly the absence of hypoglycaemia, it seems most likely that N.A. had a specific deficiency of short chain acyl-CoA dehydrogenase activity. Though the fibroblasts show a high residual activity with both C_4 and C_6 substrate this may in part be due to overlapping activity of the medium chain dehydrogenases.

The only case of short chain acyl-CoA dehydrogenase deficiency so far fully reported was a 46-year-old woman who presented with muscle weakness. There was a severe lipid myopathy and a deficiency of short chain acyl-CoA dehydrogenase (using butyryl CoA) was demonstrated in muscle mitochondria (Turnbull *et al.*, 1984). This patient showed excessive lactic acidosis on exercise and increased ketone body concentrations and turnover. Cultured fibroblasts oxidised [U-^{14}C]palmitate at a normal rate and it was suggested that the disorder was confined to skeletal muscle. However, the fibroblast results from our patient suggest that such an assay would not be particularly sensitive in detecting short chain acyl-CoA dehydrogenase deficiency. The severe disease in N.A. suggests a generalised enzyme deficiency. A rather similar patient with severe neurological problems and an ethylmalonic aciduria but no hypoglycaemia has been described in abstract by Boujet *et al.* (1983).

References

Bennett, M. J., Curnock, D. A., Engel, P., Shaw, L., Gray, R. G. F., Hull, D., Patrick, A. D. and Pollitt, R. J. Glutaric aciduria type II: Biochemical investigations and treatment of child diagnosed prenatally. *J. Inher. Metab. Dis.* 7 (1984) 57–61

Boujet, C., Joannard, A. and Favier, A. A case of ethylmalonic aciduria. *Proc. 21st Symposium S.S.I.E.M. Lyon* (1983) 55A

Green, A., Marshall, T. G., Bennett, M. J., Gray, R. G. F. and Pollitt, R. J. Riboflavin-responsive ethylmalonic–adipic aciduria. *J. Inher. Metab. Dis.* 8 (1985) 67–70

Mantagos, S., Genel, M. and Tanaka, K. Ethylmalonic–adipic aciduria. *In vivo* and *in vitro* studies indicating deficiency of activities of multiple acyl-CoA dehydrogenases. *J. Clin. Invest.* 64 (1979) 1580–1589

Turnbull, D. M., Bartlett, K., Stevens, D. L., Alberti, K. G. M. M., Gibson, G. J., Johnson, M. A., McCulloch, A. J. and Sherratt, H. S. A. Short-chain acyl-CoA dehydrogenase deficiency associated with a lipid-storage myopathy and secondary carnitine deficiency. *N. Engl. J. Med.* 311 (1984) 1232–1236

J. Inher. Metab. Dis. 8 Suppl. 2 (1985) 137–138

Short Communication

Multiple Acyl-CoA Dehydrogenase Deficiency: A Neonatal Onset Case Responsive to Treatment

Z. H. Verjee and W. G. Sherwood
Department of Clinical Biochemistry and the Research Institute, Hospital for Sick Children, Toronto, Ontario M5G 1X8, Canada

The complex organic acidopathy known as multiple acyl-CoA dehydrogenase deficiency (MACD) appears to involve a spectrum of clinical severity with the more severe phenotypes being represented by glutaric aciduria type II (GAII; McKusick 23168) (Goodman *et al.*, 1982) and the less severe phenotypes being represented by ethylmalonic–adipic aciduria (EMAuria McKusick 22717) (Mantagos *et al.*, 1979). Survival beyond the newborn period in GAII cases is rare. The molecular defect appears to involve deficient electron transferring flavoprotein (ETF) or its dehydrogenase (Goodman *et al.*, 1983). In contrast, cases of EMAuria do survive with treatment. The exact molecular defect remains unclear, but some cases appear to respond to riboflavin (Gregerson *et al.*, 1982).

The purpose of this preliminary communication is to report biochemical findings and our clinical experiences with the treatment aspects of a clinically severe case of EMAuria.

CASE REPORT AND METHODS

A 6 month old female presented with a 3–4 month history of failure to thrive, poor feeding and a 3 day history of increasing lethargy, vomiting and irritability. She was pale, wasted (weight 5.6 kg), hypertonic and semiconscious. Her liver was 3.4 cm enlarged below the right costal margin. At admission, she had hypoglycaemia (blood glucose, $0.5 \, \mathrm{mmol \, l^{-1}}$) with metabolic acidosis (blood pH 7.33, pCO_2 23 mmHg and HCO_3^- $12 \, \mathrm{mmol \, l^{-1}}$) and moderate ketonuria. Electrolytes were normal. She responded to IV glucose and the blood parameters returned to normal. Urinary organic acids were analyzed by gas chromatography–mass spectroscopy, as described by Goodman and Markey (1981). Quantitation was achieved by SIM technique, on Hewlett–Packard GC/MS 5992 B. Urine and serum amino acids were quantitated on Durrum 500 (Dionex Corporation, Sunnyvale, CA). Free and total carnitine were quantitated in plasma as described by McGarry and Foster (1976). Short chain fatty acids were analyzed by the methods of Mamer and Gibbs (1973).

RESULTS AND CLINICAL MANAGEMENT

Urine organic acid profile at admission (Figure 1(a)) showed an abnormal excretion of the following, expressed as mg (mg creatinine)$^{-1}$: ethylmalonate, 3.76; glutarate, 7.53; adipate, 1.08. As treatment commenced, these values decreased with ethylmalonic acid as the predominant urinary organic acid (Figure 1(b)). During subsequent treatment, there were episodes of hypoglycaemia with metabolic acidosis, during which the excretion of glutaric acid and ethylmalonic acid was high accompanied with abnormal excretion of *n*-butyrylglycine, adipic, 2-hydroxyglutaric, suberic, sebacic and dodecanedioic acids. Short chain fatty acid analysis revealed the presence of butyric acid. Plasma amino acids were normal except for the raised levels of sarcosine (13 and $54 \, \mu\mathrm{mol \, l^{-1}}$). Thus a diagnosis of ethylmalonic–adipic aciduria was made at 6 months of age.

Between 6 and 13 months of age, various dietary modifications were attempted. Weight gain was eventually achieved with a milk formula that provided $110–120 \, \mathrm{kcal \, kg^{-1} \, day^{-1}}$ with $1.25 \, \mathrm{g}$ protein $\mathrm{kg^{-1}} \, day^{-1}$. The caloric distribution was carbohydrate 75 %, fat 15 % and protein 10 %. Riboflavin, $200 \, \mathrm{mg \, day^{-1}}$, had no apparent effect upon urinary organic acid excretion. Complete feed refusal and persistent regurgitation necessitated the use of continuous nasogastric tube feeds. Weight increased from 5.6 to 7.5 kg. Episodes of metabolic decompensation occurred, which were promptly treated with IV glucose.

However, persistent gagging and vomiting presented an extremely difficult management problem. At 13 months of age, a gastrostomy tube was inserted and all forms of therapy were administered by that route. This improved weight gain and at 24 months of age weight was 12 kg, all caloric intake was by mouth and the gastrostomy tube was removed.

At 10 months of age the patient's plasma free and total carnitine levels were 4 and $15 \, \mu\mathrm{mol \, l^{-1}}$ (normal 40 and $60 \, \mu\mathrm{mol \, l^{-1}}$), respectively. Urinary carnitine levels were almost undetectable. With carnitine therapy at approximately $30 \, \mathrm{mg \, kg^{-1} \, day^{-1}}$, her plasma free and total carnitine levels were normal.

At her present age of 3 years, she is on the 50th percentile for both somatic and neurological development, having been less than 3rd percentile at 6 months of age.

DISCUSSION

The diagnosis in this case points to the EMAuria variant of MACD. The urinary organic acid profiles revealed persistent ethylmalonic aciduria, whereas adipic aciduria and glutaric aciduria were intermittent. The adipic aciduria appears to synchronize with the glutaric aciduria rather than the ethylmalonic aciduria. Periods of increased glutaric aciduria were not necessarily

Journal of Inherited Metabolic Disease. ISSN 0141-8955. Copyright © SSIEM and MTP Press Limited, Queen Square, Lancaster, UK.

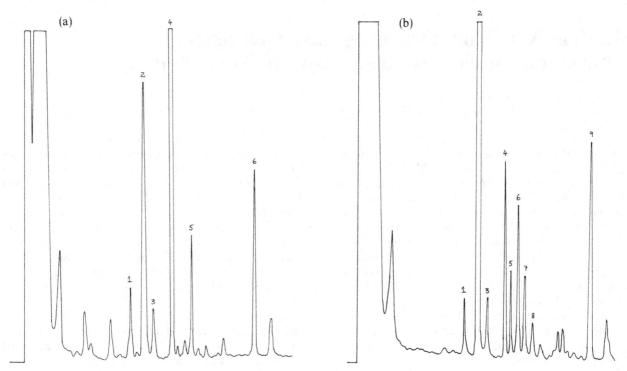

Figure 1   Gas chromatography separation of urinary organic acids: (a) at admission, 6 months of age (1) malonic acid (internal standard), (2) ethylmalonic acid, (3) 5-OH-hexanoic acid, (4) glutaric acid, (5) adipic acid, (6) eicosan (external standard); (b) at 10 months of age (1) malonic acid (internal standard), (2) ethylmalonic acid, (3) 5-OH-hexanoic acid, (4) glutaric acid, (5) unidentified, (6) n-butyrylglycine, (7) adipic acid, (8) 2-OH-glutaric acid, (9) eicosan (external standard)

associated with periods of increased ethylmalonic aciduria. This is a strange observation in that one might expect increased ethylmalonate and adipate excretion to synchronize during metabolic crisis in that both metabolites are derived from fatty acid. One might speculate that the ethylmalonic aciduria represents the expression of defective short chain fatty-acyl-(butyryl-)-CoA dehydrogenase activity, whereas adipic aciduria represents the expression of defective medium chain fatty-acyl-CoA dehydrogenase activity, a function that might be interfered with by glutaryl-CoA that accumulates with increased lysine degradation. That some sort of association between lysine metabolism and fatty acid metabolism exists has recently been found in: (a) virus-associated Reye's syndrome, in which hyperlysinaemia is characteristic (Verjee and Sherwood, 1984); and (b) mitochondrial malonyl-CoA decarboxylase deficiency in which lysine administration results in increased malonate excretion (Danks *et al.*, 1984). The exact nature of this association remains unclear. Interestingly acyl-CoA derivatives of branched chain amino acids were never found although mild hypersarcosinaemia and hypersarcosinuria were noted. Preliminary laboratory results (data not provided) indicate: (1) half normal oxidation of [1-^{14}C]butyrate and [1-^{14}C]octanoate by cultured skin fibroblasts; and (2) presence of both ETF and ETF-dehydrogenase by immunoprecipitation of [^{35}S]methione-labelled fibroblast proteins. In conjunction with the clinical features, the diagnosis of EMAuria is indicated and thus riboflavin responsiveness was sought. There was no evidence that this case is riboflavin-responsive.

References

Danks, D. M., Brown, G. K., Haan, E. A., Hunt, S. and Schloem, R. Malonyl-CoA decarboxylase deficiency—a further case with an unusual pattern of organic acids in the urine. *22nd Annual Symposium of Society for the Study of Inborn Errors of Metabolism*, Newcastle-upon-Tyne, 5–7 September 1984, Abstract. P-83.

Goodman, S. I. and Markey, S. P. *Diagnosis of Organic Acidemias by Gas Chromatography—Mass Spectrometry*, Alan R. Liss, New York, 1981, pp. 105–114

Goodman, S. I., Stene, D. O., McCabe, E. R. B., Norenberg, M. D., Shikes, R. H., Stumpf, D. A. and Blackburn, G. K. Glutaric acidemia type II: Clinical, biochemical, and morphologic considerations. *J. Pediatr.* 100 (1982) 946–950

Goodman, S. I., Reale, M. and Berlow, S. Glutaric acidemia type II: A form with deleterious intrauterine effects. *J. Pediatr.* 102 (1983) 411–413

Gregerson, N., Wintzensen, H., Kolvraa, S., Christensen, E., Christensen, M. F., Brandt, N. J. and Rasmussen, K. C_6–C_{10}-Dicarboxylic aciduria: Investigations of a patient with riboflavin responsive multiple acyl-CoA dehydrogenation defects. *Pediatr. Res.* 16 (1982) 861–868

Mamer, O. A. and Gibbs, B. F. Simplified gas chromatography of trimethylsilyl esters of C_1 through C_5 fatty acids in serum and urine. *Clin. Chem.* 19 (1973) 1006–1009

Mantagos, S., Genel, M. and Tanaka, K. Ethylmalonic–adipic aciduria: *In vivo* and *in vitro* studies indicating deficiency of activities of multiple acyl-CoA dehydrogenases. *J. Clin. Invest.* 64 (1979) 1580–1589

McGarry, J. D. and Foster, D. W. An improved and simplified radioisotopic assay for the determination of free and esterified carnitine. *J. Lipid Res.* 17 (1976) 277–280

Verjee, Z. H. and Sherwood, W. G. Plasma amino acids in Reye's syndrome. *Clin. Chem.* 30 (1984) 944, Abstract 24

J. Inher. Metab. Dis. 8 Suppl 2 (1985) 139–140

Short Communication

Metabolic Effects of Carnitine Medication in a Patient with Multiple Acyl-CoA Dehydrogenation Deficiency

N. GREGERSEN
Research Laboratory for Metabolic Disorders, University Department of Clinical Chemistry, Aarhus kommunehospital, D K-8000 Aarhus C, Denmark

M. FJORD CHRISTENSEN
Department of Pediatrics, Herning Hospital, Herning, Denmark

S. KØLVRAA
Institute of Human Genetics, University of Aarhus, Denmark

In 1982 we described a patient with riboflavin responsive multiple acyl-CoA dehydrogenation deficiency (Gregersen *et al.*, 1982). Free carnitine concentration in plasma was $6\,\mu mol\,l^{-1}$ (control $26–74\,\mu mol\,l^{-1}$) and esterified carnitine was $32\,\mu mol\,l^{-1}$ (control $17–32\,\mu mol\,l^{-1}$). It was suggested that the low carnitine was caused by a sequestration of free carnitine as short and medium chain acylcarnitines.

As carnitine is necessary for the transport of fatty acids into the mitochondria, carnitine medication could be expected to alter the metabolic picture, an alteration that could be reflected in the urine. The present communication is the result of such a trial in the patient.

TREATMENT

During the carnitine medication trial, for which informed consent from the parents was obtained, the boy P.J. received 100 mg riboflavin three times daily, as reported elsewhere (Gregersen *et al.*, 1982). Before the trial one 24 h urine sample was collected. During one week the dosage of DL-carnitine was increased from 200 to 1200 mg (three times 400 mg) daily given perorally. After 3 days on $1200\,mg\,day^{-1}$ another 24 h urine sample was collected. The urines were kept frozen at $-20°C$ until analysed.

METHODS

Organic acids were analysed by gas chromatography and gas chromatography–mass spectrometry as described previously (Gregersen *et al.*, 1980, 1982). Free and esterified (perchloric acid soluble) carnitine were quantitated by the radiochemical method of Pace *et al.* (1978), and the individual acylcarnitines were separated chromatographically as described by Choi and Bieber (1977), and measured after alkaline hydrolysis by selected ion monitoring gas chromatography–mass spectrometry on a 10% NPGS, 1% H_3PO_4 column.

RESULTS AND DISCUSSION

The urinary output of key metabolites reflecting the acyl-CoA dehydrogenation deficiency in fatty acid β-oxidation, branched chain amino acid oxidation and lysine, 5-hydroxylysine and tryptophan oxidation are depicted in Figure 1. The excretion of these metabolites reflects the accumulation of acyl-CoA esters, which in turn is the result of a dynamic balance between production and disappearance rates. The metabolites reflecting the β-oxidation, i.e. the dicarboxylic and 5-hydroxyhexanoic acids, ethylmalonic and methylsuccinic acids, hexanoylglycine, butyryl-, hexanoyl- and octanoylcarnitines, change their excretion rate very little after the ingestion of 1200 mg carnitine. Therefore, at the present stage of our knowledge, the conclusion must be that the accumulated amounts of acyl-CoA esters in the β-oxidation pathway have not changed significantly.

This does not necessarily imply that the flow through β-oxidation has not changed. An increase in the production rate of acyl-CoA esters could be outweighed by a corresponding increase in β-oxidation of these compounds. 3-Hydroxybutyric acid and acetylcarnitine excretion reflect accumulation of the β-oxidation end-product acetyl-CoA. The excretion of 3-hydroxybutyric acid changed very little during the treatment, but acetylcarnitine increased greatly. From Figure 1 it can be seen that acetylcarnitine output was approximately $15\,\mu mol\ (mmol\ creatinine)^{-1}$ before and $260\,\mu mol\ (mmol\ creatinine)^{-1}$ (80% of all the esterified carnitine) after the carnitine ingestion. Although acetyl-CoA also originates from carbohydrate and amino acid metabolism and is the substrate for fatty acid synthesis, part of the increased production of acetylcarnitine during the carnitine medication may reflect an increased β-oxidation activity.

Unlike the β-oxidation-derived metabolites, some of the compounds derived from the oxidation of the branched chain amino acids did change their excretion rate during the carnitine ingestion. As the biochemical mechanism for the production of 3-hydroxyisovaleric acid is not known with certainty no rational explanation for the increase in the excretion of this compound can be offered. The five-fold increase in excretion of isovaleryl-carnitine and 2-methylbutyrylcarnitine and the tendency to an increase in isobutyrylcarnitine can, on the other hand, be looked upon as a corroboration that carnitine is involved in the metabolism of the branched chain amino acids, as suggested by Choi *et al.* (1977) and by van Hinsberg *et al.* (1980). Despite these small

Journal of Inherited Metabolic Disease. ISSN 0141-8955. Copyright © SSIEM and MTP Press Limited, Queen Square, Lancaster, UK.

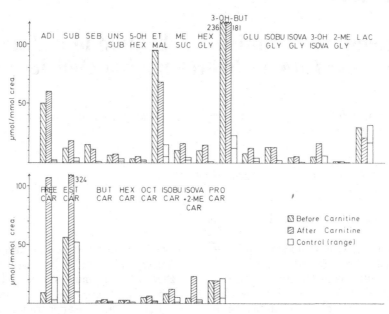

Figure 1 Urinary excretion of organic acids, free and esterified carnitine in 24 h urine samples before (29 April 1981) and after (8 May 1981) carnitine medication. The symbols are: ADI, adipic acid; SUB, suberic acid; SEB, sebacic acid; UNS SUB, unsaturated suberic acid; 5-OH HEX, 5-hydroxyhexanoic acid; ET MAL, ethylmalonic acid; ME SUC, methylsuccinic acid; HEX GLY, hexanoylglycine; 3-OH BUT, 3-hydroxybutyric acid; GLU, glutaric acid; ISOBU GLY, isobutyrylglycine; ISOVA GLY, isovalerylglycine; 3-OH ISOVA, 3-hydroxyisovaleric acid; 2-ME GLY, 2-methylbutyrylglycine; LAC, lactic acid; FREE CAR, free carnitine; EST CAR, esterified carnitine; BUT CAR, butyrylcarnitine; HEX CAR, hexanoylcarnitine; OCT CAR, octanoylcarnitine; ISOBU CAR, isobutyrylcarnitine; ISOVA + 2-ME CAR, isovaleryl- plus 2-methylbutyrylcarnitine; PRO CAR, propionylcarnitine

changes the conclusion of the present investigation must be that the effects of carnitine on acyl-CoA ester metabolism are remarkably small and that the excessive carnitine given is excreted either unchanged as free carnitine or as acetylcarnitine.

We thank the technicians Mrs Vibeke S. Winter, Inge Knudsen and Anne Marie Holm for their contribution to the study, which was supported by The Danish Medical Research Council.

References

Choi, Y. R. and Bieber, L. L. A method for the isolation and quantitation of water-soluble aliphatic acylcarnitines. *Analyt. Biochem.* 79 (1977) 413–418

Choi, Y. R., Fogle, P. J., Clarke, P. R. H. and Bieber, L. L. Quantitation of water-soluble acylcarnitines and carnitine acyltransferases in rat tissues. *J. Biol. Chem.* 252 (1977) 7930–7931

Gregersen, N., Rosleff, F., Kølvraa, S., Hobolth, N., Rasmussen, K. and Lauritzen, R. Non-ketotic C_6–C_{10}-dicarboxylic aciduria: Biochemical investigations of two cases. *Clin. Chim. Acta* 102 (1980) 179–189

Gregersen, N., Wintzensen, H., Kølvraa, S., Christensen, E., Christensen, M. F., Brandt, N. J. and Rasmussen, K. C_6–C_{10}-dicarboxylic aciduria: Investigation of a patient with riboflavin responsive multiple acyl-CoA dehydrogenation defect. *Pediatr. Res.* 16 (1982) 861–868

van Hinsbergh, V. W. M., Veerkamp, J. H. and Cordewener, J. H. G. Effect of carnitine and branched chain acylcarnitines on the 2-oxo acid dehydrogenase activity in intact mitochondria of rat muscle. *Int. J. Biochem.* 12 (1980) 559–565

Pace, J. A., Wannemacher, R. W. and Neufeld, H. A. Improved radiochemical assay for carnitine and its derivatives in plasma and tissue extracts. *Clin. Chem.* 24 (1978) 32–35

J. Inher. Metab. Dis. 8 Suppl. 2 (1985) 141–142

Short Communication

L-Carnitine and Glycine Therapy in Isovaleric Acidaemia

R. A. CHALMERS, C. DE SOUSA, B. M. TRACEY and T. E. STACEY
Paediatric Research Group, MRC Clinical Research Centre, Harrow HA1 3UJ, UK

C. WEAVER and D. BRADLEY
Department of Child Health and Medicine, University Hospital of Wales, Cardiff, UK

Isovaleric acidaemia (McKusick 24350) is a disorder of leucine catabolism characterized clinically by episodes of acidosis and coma with consequent mild psychomotor retardation. Biochemically, the disorder is caused by deficient activity of isovaleryl-CoA dehydrogenase associated with accumulation of isovaleryl-CoA and its metabolites, isovalerylglycine and 3-hydroxyisovalerate.

Some patients may present with life-threatening episodes in the first weeks of life, associated with overwhelming sepsis and pancytopenia. This latter presentation is said to have been characterized by the urinary excretion of other abnormal metabolites (methylsuccinate, methylfumarate, 4-hydroxy-isovalerate, 3-hydroxyisoheptanoate, isovalerylglutamate and isovalerylglucuronide) (Truscott *et al.*, 1981; Wysocki *et al.*, 1983) and the concept of "chronic" and "acute neonatal" forms of the disease has developed. Glycine therapy has been advocated for the regular treatment of such patients and for the management of acute ketoacidotic episodes (Krieger and Tanaka, 1976; Yudkoff *et al.*, 1978). We have shown previously that such patients have an insufficiency of L-carnitine and have proposed supplemental L-carnitine in their treatment (Chalmers *et al.*, 1983). We report here a girl with isovaleric acidaemia, presenting at $2\frac{1}{2}$ years with the full metabolite pattern previously associated with the acute neonatal form of the disease. The results of L-carnitine challenges and of glycine, L-carnitine and reduced dietary protein therapy have provided the basis for optimal treatment of this patient.

METHODS

Urine and plasma organic acids were measured and identified after quantitative DEAE-Sephadex extraction as their trimethylsilyl (TMS) and TMS-ethoxime derivatives, using capillary gas chromatography and GC–MS on fused silica columns. Urine and plasma L-carnitine and acylcarnitines were measured using a radioenzymatic assay based on the use of [1-^{14}C]acetyl-CoA and L-carnitine acetyltransferase. Acylcarnitines were identified in urine after chromatography on Dowex 2, using fast atom bombardment (FAB) mass spectrometry with high resolution mass measurements (Roe *et al.*, 1983).

PATIENT AND RESULTS

K.P. is a girl who presented at $2\frac{1}{2}$ years with a short history of vomiting following a mild upper respiratory tract infection, becoming rapidly unwell with lethargy and irritability. She became dehydrated with a "cheesy" odour to her breath; blood pH was 7.22, base excess was 18.7 meq l^{-1}. Her previous history included hospitalization at 12 days of age for poor feeding and constipation; referral at 17 months for delayed development (mild spastic diplegia) and at 2 years for diarrhoea and vomiting requiring intravenous rehydration. She had previously had chicken-pox and measles at 1 year, both with mild courses. Her parents were unrelated and she had one older healthy female sibling. GC–MS studies of plasma and urine at $2\frac{1}{2}$ years revealed the diagnosis of isovaleric acidaemia. Identifications and concentrations of organic acids are detailed in Table 1. Her plasma and urine free carnitine concentrations were low and acylcarnitine concentrations increased with an increased acylcarnitine/free carnitine ratio (Table 1), indicative of carnitine insufficiency.

Metabolic studies were made 1 month after diagnosis when she was clinically well. On admission she was alert and well but developmentally delayed in language acquisition and fine motor skills. An oral challenge with L-carnitine (200 mg (kg body wt)$^{-1}$) resulted in a rise in acylcarnitine excretion with a much smaller increase in free carnitine in both urine and plasma. The major acylcarnitine involved was identified as isovalerylcarnitine consistent with an accumulation of isovaleryl-CoA and indicative of the ability of L-carnitine to conjugate and remove isovaleryl groups. Hippurate excretion also rose during this challenge. During a second challenge carried out while she was receiving glycine therapy, isovalerylglycine excretion also rose dramatically (by about 70%)

Glycine therapy (300 mg (kg body wt)$^{-1}$ day^{-1} in four divided doses) was attempted during a trial period of 5 days. Plasma glycine rose to a maximum of 1.68 µmol ml^{-1} and isovalerylglycine excretion rose by about 20% over 4 days. However, she developed increasing lethargy and ataxia during this period and glycine administration was stopped after 5 days.

The patient was maintained on a reduced protein diet (2 g kg^{-1} day^{-1}, corresponding to a leucine intake of 185 mg kg^{-1} day^{-1}) with low dose L-carnitine

141

Journal of Inherited Metabolic Disease. ISSN 0141-8955. Copyright © SSIEM and MTP Press Limited, Queen Square, Lancaster, UK.

Table 1 Organic acids and carnitines in isovaleric acidaemia at diagnosis (2½ years of age) and on admission for metabolic studies 1 month later

| | Urine (mmol (mol creatinine)$^{-1}$) | | Plasma (μmol l^{-1}) | |
	Diagnosis	Admission	Diagnosis	Admission
Acid				
Lactic	118	68	1892	1610
3-Hydroxybutyric	2553	11	1579	138
Acetoacetic	1117	ND*	77	28
3-Hydroxyisovaleric	1611	6	189	8
4-Hydroxyisovaleric	160	ND	54	3
Methylsuccinic	183	ND	2	ND
Methylfumaric (mesaconic)	149	ND	2	ND
Isovalerylglycine	2716	3865	73	ND
Isovalerylglutamate	109	39	<1	ND
Isovalerylglucuronide	49	ND	ND	ND
Carnitines				
Free carnitine	2.2	1.7	2.8	7.9
Acylcarnitines	24.1	8.5	7.7	7.1
Acyl/free ratio	11.0	5.0	2.8	0.9

* ND = not detected
† Normal (mean $\pm$ SD) in urine 12.2 $\pm$ 7.6, in plasma 29.5 $\pm$ 4.3
‡ Normal (mean $\pm$ SD) in urine 15.1 $\pm$ 3.2, in plasma 4.6 $\pm$ 3.4

(40 mg kg^{-1} day^{-1} in three divided doses). She has remained clinically well on this regimen and has tolerated a further episode of acidosis associated with a respiratory infection without clinical intervention. Equally important, her speech development was normal on reassessment after 9 months of this treatment.

DISCUSSION AND CONCLUSIONS

The presentation of this girl with concomitant clinical features of the "chronic form" of isovaleric acidaemia and biochemical features of the "acute neonatal form" demonstrates that isovaleric acidaemia is a single disease entity with *onset* at birth and with differing presentations modulated by environmental factors, the amount of residual enzyme activity and by the effects of differing enzymatic phenotypes in different individuals. This is supported by the results of complementation studies on cultured skin fibroblasts from such patients when only a single complementation group is observed (Truscott *et al.*, 1981; Dubiel *et al.*, 1983). The clinical response to glycine therapy cautions against its indiscriminate use without careful monitoring of possible encephalopathic side-effects. The response to L-carnitine challenges provides further evidence for the proposed mechanisms of action, removal of accumulating acyl moieties from the mitochondrion with release of free CoA, restoration of intramitochondrial metabolic homoeostasis with normalization of ATP synthesis, thereby promoting arylglycine (hippurate) and acylglycine (isovaleryl-glycine) synthesis (Chalmers *et al.*, 1983; Roe *et al.*, 1983). The combination of a moderate reduction in dietary protein intake, together with low dose L-carnitine, has provided the optimal treatment for this patient and may, in addition, be preferred for other patients with isovaleric acidaemia.

These studies were approved by the Harrow Health District Ethical Committee. We are grateful to Miss M. Jones and Mrs S. Bartlett for excellent technical assistance and collaboration and to Dr A. M. Lawson for access to mass spectrometry facilities. We are indebted to Sigma-Tau s.p.a., Rome for provision of L-carnitine for these studies.

References

Chalmers, R. A., Roe, C. R., Tracey, B. M., Stacey, T., Hoppel, C. L. and Millington, D. S. Secondary carnitine insufficiency in disorders of organic acid metabolism: modulation of acyl CoA/CoA ratios by L-carnitine *in vivo*. *Biochem. Soc. Trans.* 11 (1983) 724–725

Dubiel, B., Dabrowski, C., Wetts, R. and Tanaka, K. Complementation studies of isovaleric acidemia and glutaric aciduria type II using cultured skin fibroblasts. *J. Clin. Invest.* 72 (1983) 1543–1552

Kreiger, I. and Tanaka, K. Therapeutic effects of glycine in isovaleric acidemia. *Pediatr. Res.* 10 (1976) 25–29

Roe, C. R., Hoppel, C. L., Stacey, T. E., Chalmers, R. A., Tracey, B. M. and Millington, D. S. Metabolic response to carnitine in methylmalonic aciduria. An effective strategy for elimination of propionyl groups. *Arch. Dis. Child.* 58 (1983) 916–920

Truscott, R. J. W., Malegan, D., McCairns, E., Burke, D., Hicks, L., Sims, P., Halpern, B., Tanaka, K., Sweetman, L., Nyhan, W. L., Hammond, J., Bumack, C., Haan, E. A. and Danks, D. M. New metabolites in isovaleric acidemia. *Clin. Chim. Acta* 110 (1981) 187–203

Wysocki, S. J., French, N. P. and Grauaug, A. Organic aciduria associated with isovaleric aciduria. *Clin. Chem.* 29 (1983) 1002–1003

Yudkoff, M., Cohn, R. M., Puschak, R., Rothman, R. and Segal, S. Glycine therapy in isovaleric acidemia. *J. Pediatr.* 92 (1978) 813–817

J. Inher. Metab. Dis. 8 Suppl. 2 (1985) 143–144

Short Communication

The Identification of Acylcarnitines by Desorption Chemical Ionization Mass Spectrometry

M. Duran, D. Ketting, L. Dorland and S. K. Wadman
University Children's Hospital, "Het Wilhelmina Kinderziekenhuis", Nieuwe Gracht 137, 3512 LK Utrecht, The Netherlands

Several organic acidaemias are accompanied by a decreased availability of free carnitine, probably as a result of excessive urinary losses of acylcarnitine (Allen *et al.*, 1982). The identification of urinary carnitine (3-hydroxy-4-(trimethylamino)butyric acid), and its esters is a cumbersome task. Direct chromatographic procedures have not been published because: (a) there does not exist a specific staining reagent which allows the unequivocal detection after thin layer or column liquid chromatography, and (b) derivatization in order to make gas chromatography possible has proven to be unsuccessful.

Indirect methods for the analysis of short chain acylcarnitines involve separation from other acyl-containing compounds by gel filtration, followed by anion- and cation-exchange chromatography. The esters are then saponified and the liberated acids quantitated by using gas chromatography (Bieber and Lewin, 1981). The first method for the identification of propionylcarnitine in the urine of a patient with methylmalonic aciduria by using fast atom bombardment and B/E linked mass spectrometry was described recently (Roe *et al.*, 1983). Here we describe a technique for the identification of acylcarnitines by desorption chemical ionization–mass spectrometry (DCI–MS) with ammonia as the reactant gas.

MATERIALS AND METHODS

The carnitine esters were obtained from the following sources: L-acetylcarnitine, DL-propionylcarnitine and L-palmitoylcarnitine from P-L Biochemicals Inc. (Milwaukee, WI, USA), and L-carnitine, DL-hexanoyl-carnitine, DL-octanoylcarnitine, DL-decanoylcarnitine, DL-lauroylcarnitine and DL-myristoylcarnitine from Sigma (St. Louis, MO, USA).

Experiments were performed using a Ribermag R 10-10 C quadrupole mass spectrometer (NERMAG, Reuil-Malmaison, France) in the positive ionization mode. The recording and calculation of spectra were done using a PDP 11/23 computer coupled to the spectrometer. Typical analytical conditions were: source temperature 180°C, the probe filament (Tungsten wire 60 μm, nine turns) current was switched to 350 mA, upon which desorption started. Mass spectra were recorded every second (mass range 50–700) for a period up to 1 min. Aqueous samples were applied to the probe filament with a microliter syringe and dried at ambient temperature. Ammonia was used as the reactant gas at a pressure of 10^{-1} torr.

The urinary acylcarnitines were prefractionated by the method of Bieber and Lewin (1981) with exception of the gel filtration step, or by the paper chromatographic technique as described earlier (Duran *et al.*, 1983). Either procedure was followed by thin layer chromatography on 10 × 10 cm alumina sheets coated with silica (Merck, Darmstadt, FRG, art no. 5553). The eluting agent was chloroform–methanol–conc. ammonia; 50:30:8 v:v:v (Bohmer and Bremer, 1968). The relevant bands were scraped off and the acylcarnitines were eluted with water.

RESULTS AND DISCUSSION

The technique of desorption chemical ionization mass spectrometry can also be regarded as "slow filament pyrolysis in a chemical ionization source". As such the method is well suited for the study of thermolabile compounds and of macromolecules, which decompose into smaller subunits in the process of pyrolysis (Virelizier *et al.*, 1983).

When using ammonia as reactant gas, the NH_4^+ ion will act as ionizing species. This will theoretically lead to the formation of $(M + 1)^+$-ion and $(M + 18)^+$-ion as parent ions in the mass spectrum. The mass spectra that we obtained are summarized in Table 1. Only the most abundant ions are given. All substances except palmitoylcarnitine showed the $(M + 1)^+$-ion as the parent ion, the $(M + 18)^+$-ion was not observed. The mass spectra showed remarkable similarities: ions at $M + 1$, $M - 13$ and $M - 41$ were virtually always present. This was also true for free carnitine itself. In addition all mass spectra showed identical peaks in the lower mass range at m/z values of 60, 85, 102, 130 and 144. The base peak in all mass spectra was at $m/z = 60$, representing the protonated trimethylamine ion. The latter ion is cleaved very easily from the carnitine molecule.

This type of mass spectrometry was applied to the urine of patients with a defective oxidation of medium chain fatty acids. It was shown previously that five patients with this defect excreted abnormal amounts of bound octanoic acid in their urine (Duran *et al.*, 1984). A substance which was thought to be identical with octanoylcarnitine was isolated from the urine by means of paper chromatography and thin layer chromatography. Its mass spectrum matched completely that of authentic octanoylcarnitine, which was also taken through the thin layer chromatography step. This is the

143

Table 1 Fragmentation pattern of carnitine and its esters subjected to desorption chemical ionization mass spectrometry (NH_3); characteristic fragments are in italic type

Compound	Mol. wt.	Fragments (m/z)
Carnitine	161.2	*162, 148, 144, 130, 120,* 103, *102, 85, 60*
Acetylcarnitine	203.2	*204, 190, 186, 162, 144, 130,* 122, *102, 85, 60,* 58
Propionylcarnitine	217.2	*218, 204, 186, 176, 159, 144, 130, 102, 85, 60*
Hexanoylcarnitine	259.3	*260, 246, 228, 218, 214,* 201, 200, 186, *144, 130, 102,* 77, *60*
Octanoylcarnitine	287.4	*288, 274, 246,* 229, 214, 196, 186, 157, *144, 130, 102, 85, 60*
Decanoylcarnitine	315.5	*316, 302, 274,* 257, 190, 186, 157, *144, 130,* 119, *102, 85,* 77, *60*
Lauroylcarnitine	343.5	*344, 330, 302,* 285, 241, 213, 200, 183, 157, *144, 130, 120, 85, 60*
Myristoylcarnitine	371.6	*372, 358, 330, 313,* 269, 228, 213, 199, 185, 157, *144, 130,* 111, *102,* 98, *85, 60*
Palmitoylcarnitine	399.6	*386, 358, 341,* 274, 256, 238, 213, 199, 186, 182, 168, 157, *144, 130, 102, 85, 60*

first direct evidence for the excessive urinary loss of octanoylcarnitine in medium chain acyl-CoA dehydrogenase deficiency which could well contribute to the carnitine insufficiency, a frequent observation in patients with this disorder. Although this technique requires extensive purification of the biological sample, the identification is very easy with a mass spectrometer equipped with a desorption chemical ionization probe.

Attempts to identify other acylcarnitines in the urines of patients accumulating various acyl-CoA esters are currently in progress.

References

Allen, R. J., Hansch, D. B. and Wu, H. L. C. Hypocarnitinaemia in disorders of organic acid metabolism. *Lancet* 2 (1982) 500–501

Bieber, L. L. and Lewin, L. Measurements of carnitine and *O*-acylcarnitines. *Methods Enzymol.* 72 (1981) 276–287

Bohmer, T. and Bremer, J. Propionylcarnitine. Physiological variations *in vivo. Biochim. Biophys. Acta* 152 (1968) 559–567

Duran, M., de Klerk, J. B. C., van Pelt, J., Wadman, S. K., Scholte, H. R., Beekman, R. P. and Jennekens, F. G. I. The analysis of plasma and urinary organic acids during prolonged fasting differentiates between systemic carnitine deficiency and a defect of fatty acid oxidation. *J. Inher. Metab. Dis.* 6, Suppl. 2 (1983) 121–122

Duran, M., de Klerk, J. B. C., Wadman, S. K., Bruinvis, L. and Ketting, D. Differential diagnosis of dicarboxylic aciduria. *J. Inher. Metab. Dis.* 7, Suppl. 1 (1984) 48–51

Roe, C. R., Hoppel, C. L., Stacey, T. E., Chalmers, R. A., Tracey, B. M. and Millington, D. S. Metabolic response to carnitine in methylmalonic aciduria. *Arch. Dis. Child.* 58 (1983) 916–920

Virelizier, H., Hagemann, R. and Jankowski, K. Systematic analysis of desorption chemical ionization (DCI) mass spectra of nucleic acids—7. *Biomed. Mass Spectrom.* 10 (1983) 559–566

J. Inher. Metab. Dis. 8 Suppl. 2 (1985) 145–146

Short Communication

The Prenatal Diagnosis of Glutaric Aciduria Type II, using Quantitative GC–MS

R. A. Chalmers and B. M. Tracey
Paediatric Research Group, MRC Clinical Research Centre, Harrow, Middlesex, UK

G. S. King and B. Pettit
Queen Charlotte's Maternity Hospital, London, UK

F. Rocchiccioli and J.-M. Saudubray
Departement de Pediatrie, Hôpital Necker-Enfants Malades, Paris, France

R. G. F. Gray
University Sub-Department of Medical Genetics, Sheffield, UK

J. Boué
Centre de Etudes Biologiques Prenatales, Paris, France

J. W. Keeling
John Radcliffe Hospital, Oxford, UK

R. H. Lindenbaum
Churchill Hospital, Oxford, UK

Glutaric aciduria type II (multiple acyl-CoA dehydrogenase deficiency) (McKusick 23168) is an inherited metabolic disease associated clinically with severe hypoglycaemia, metabolic acidosis, hepatomegaly, hypotonia, neurological symptoms and death in the neonatal period. Biochemically it is characterised by increased urinary excretion of several organic acids, particularly glutarate, 2-hydroxyglutarate, 3-hydroxyisovalerate, adipate and other dicarboxylic acids, and isovalerylglycine and other acylglycines. Pathologically, there is fatty infiltration of the liver and heart and a number of cases have been described in which grossly enlarged polycystic kidneys occur together with severe dysmorphic features. We report here prenatal diagnosis for severe neonatal dysmorphic glutaric aciduria type II using both chemical analysis of amniotic fluid supernatant with quantitative selected ion monitoring (SIM) on GC–MS and also enzymology on cultured amniocytes. Affected and unaffected fetuses have been correctly predicted with results being duplicated in three independent laboratories.

PROPOSITUS AND CASE HISTORY

The parents are unrelated and in their twenties. During the mother's first pregnancy (1982), a raised α-fetoprotein (AFP) at 17 weeks' gestation led to referral: amniocentesis yielded fluid with a normal AFP and amniocytes showed a normal 46,XY karyotype. Repeat renal scans showed the very slow development of moderate cystic changes and the pregnancy continued to term. At term a 2.58 kg boy was delivered normally. He developed pallor and respiratory distress at 30 min with rapidly developing severe metabolic acidosis. He showed dysmorphic features including a large head (circumference 36 cm), deepset eyes, sunken nasal bridge, wide mouth, abnormal tragus, coronal hypospadias and prominent heels. Kidneys were easily palpable and there was an odour of 'sweaty feet'. The baby died at 50 h and histology of kidneys showed a medulla replaced by dilated tubular cysts, primitive ducts and blurring of the cortico–medullary junction. GC–MS of urine showed a raised glutaric acid ($5230 \, \text{mmol mol creatinine}^{-1}$), adipic acid ($407 \, \text{mmol mol}^{-1}$) and 3-hydroxyisovaleric acid ($340 \, \text{mmol mol}^{-1}$), consistent with a diagnosis of glutaric aciduria type II (Dr J. Leonard, Institute of Child Health, London). GC–MS of stored amniotic fluid supernatant at the CRC and QCMH showed greatly increased concentrations of glutaric acid and 2-hydroxyglutaric acid (Table 1), confirming the diagnosis and providing the basis for future prenatal diagnosis by direct chemical analysis.

METHODS

Organic acids were extracted from amniotic fluid using DEAE Sephadex and glutarate quantified by selected ion monitoring (SIM) on GC–MS of the trimethylsilyl (TMS) ester against a 3-methylglutarate internal standard added to the fluid before extraction or by addition of the internal standard, lyophilisation and direct preparation of *n*-butyl esters. 2-Hydroxyglutarate was quantified as the TMS derivative against a C_{24}-hydrocarbon internal standard using a response factor determined with an authentic standard. Adipic, suberic and sebacic acids were quantified by SIM GC–MS

145

Journal of Inherited Metabolic Disease. ISSN 0141-8955. Copyright © SSIEM and MTP Press Limited, Queen Square, Lancaster, UK.

Table 1 Organic acid concentrations in amniotic fluid (μmol l^{-1})

Acid		Pregnancy 1 (stored fluid)	Pregnancy 2	Pregnancy 3	Normal ranges
Glutaric	H	9.3, 10.1, 9.3	23.1, 21.5	0.76, 0.61, 0.57	0.6–1.1
	L	9.8	21	0.6	1.4 ± 0.2
	P		25.9	0.63	0.87 ± 0.01
2-Hydroxyglutaric	H	6.1	9.0	3.3, 3.2	1.6–4.9
Adipic	H		0.53		0.13–0.18
Suberic	H		0.12		0.16–0.17
Sebacic	H		0.20		<0.05–0.12

H = Clinical Research Centre, Harrow; L = Queen Charlotte's Hospital, London; P = Hôpital Necker-Enfants Malades, Paris

against 3-methylglutarate internal standard. Enzymology was carried out on cultured amniocytes and fetal skin fibroblasts by measurement of the oxidation of [1-^{14}C]-labelled oleate, octanoate and butyrate by intact cells in monolayers with collection and measurement of the $^{14}CO_2$ evolved.

RESULTS

The second pregnancy (1983) was monitored at 16 weeks' gestation. Serum AFP was normal and ultrasound showed no clear renal defect. Amniocentesis at 17 weeks 5 days revealed a normal amniotic fluid AFP and acetylcholinesterase gel electrophoresis. GC–MS analysis of amniotic fluid supernatant gave results within 3 days of amniocentesis and showed greatly increased concentrations of glutarate and 2-hydroxyglutarate (Table 1). Adipate and sebacate concentrations were slightly increased but suberate concentrations were within the normal range (Table 1). Termination was carried out at 19 weeks and 5 days by prostaglandin administration and a female fetus was delivered which showed grossly enlarged kidneys and some dysmorphic features. Renal histology showed cystically dilated tubules in the cortex and medulla. Fetal blood plasma, collected by fetoscopy just prior to termination showed elevated concentrations of glutarate (12.9 μmol l^{-1}) and 2-hydroxyglutarate (4.7 μmol l^{-1}) compared to control fetal plasma (glutarate <4 μmol l^{-1}; 2-hydroxyglutarate <4 μmol l^{-1}). Cultured amniocytes showed, 3–4 weeks after amniocentesis, reduced oxidation of [1-^{14}C]butyrate at 4.43 $\pm$ 0.26 pmol CO_2 produced min^{-1} (mg protein)$^{-1}$ compared to controls of 48.1 $\pm$ 15.8. Cultured fetal skin fibroblasts showed reduced oxidation of butyrate, octanoate and oleate at 17.1, 4.9 and 9.7% of normal control lines, respectively, confirming the diagnosis.

A third pregnancy (1984) was again monitored at 16–17 weeks' gestation, showing normal plasma AFP and ultrasound. Amniotic fluid supernatant showed a normal pattern and concentrations of organic acids (Table 1), indicating an unaffected fetus. The pregnancy was allowed to continue to term. Subsequent analysis of cultured amniocytes showed normal oxidation of [1-^{14}C]butyrate at 9.29 and 9.87 pmol CO_2 min^{-1} (mg protein)$^{-1}$ compared to simultaneous controls of 12.7 $\pm$ 1.9. Karyotype was 46,XX.

DISCUSSION AND CONCLUSIONS

The prenatal diagnosis of glutaric aciduria type II at 16–18 weeks' gestation has only recently been reported (Mitchell *et al.*, 1983; Boué *et al.*, 1984; Jakobs *et al.*, 1984; Bennett *et al.*, 1984) based on enzymology of cultured amniocytes or GC–MS of amniotic fluid supernatant. Enzymology is dependent upon culture of sufficient cells for assay and both this and the assays themselves are time-consuming, some 4 weeks being required from amniocentesis for adequate results. The present work has confirmed the reliability of prenatal diagnosis of glutaric aciduria type II by direct chemical analysis both on the basis of glutaric acid and of 2-hydroxyglutaric acid concentrations. Results were available within 3 days of amniocentesis, were unambiguous and reproducible between three independent laboratories and both affected and unaffected fetuses have been correctly predicted. The occurrence of both an affected male and an affected female in this family provides evidence for autosomal recessive inheritance of acute dysmorphic glutaric aciduria type II. Glutarate concentrations provide the most reliable index and 2-hydroxyglutarate provides the differential diagnosis, but other dicarboxylic acids such as adipate (Jakobs *et al.*, 1984) may be insufficiently elevated to provide reliable diagnoses. This study has again demonstrated the reliability of prenatal diagnosis of selected organic acidurias by direct chemical analysis of amniotic fluid supernatant.

R.A.C. and B.M.T. are grateful to Mr D. Watson and Mr M. Madigan for excellent technical collaboration during parts of this work and to Dr A. M. Lawson for access to mass spectrometry facilities.

References

Bennett, M. J., Curnock, D. A., Engel, P. C., Shaw, L., Gray, R. G. F., Hull, D., Patrick, A. D. and Pollitt, R. J. Glutaric aciduria type II: Biochemical investigation and treatment of a child diagnosed prenatally. *J. Inher. Metab. Dis.* 7 (1984) 57–61

Boué, J., Chalmers, R. A., Tracey, B. M., Watson, D., Gray, R. G. F., Keeling, J. W., King, G. S., Pettit, B. R., Lindenbaum, R. H., Rocchiccioli, F. and Saudubray, J.-M. Prenatal diagnosis of dysmorphic neonatal-lethal type II glutaric aciduria. *Lancet* 1 (1984) 846–847

Jakobs, C., Sweetman, L., Wadman, S. K., Duran, M., Saudubray, J.-M. and Nyhan, W. L. Prenatal diagnosis of glutaric aciduria type II by direct chemical analysis of dicarboxylic acids in amniotic fluid. *Eur. J. Pediatr.* 141 (1984) 153–157

Mitchell, G., Saudubray, J.-M., Benoit, Y., Rocchiccioli, F., Charpentier, C., Ogier, H. and Boué, J. Antenatal diagnosis of glutaric aciduria type II. *Lancet* 1 (1983) 1099

J. Inher. Metab. Dis. 8 Suppl. 2 (1985) 147–148

Short Communication

3-Methyladipate Excretion in Animals Fed a Phytol Supplement with Reference to Refsum's Disease

S. KRYWAWYCH, D. P. BRENTON, M. J. JACKSON, C. FORTE and D. K. WALKER
Department of Medicine, University College London School of Medicine, The Rayne Institute, London WC1E 6JJ, UK

A. M. LAWSON
M.R.C. Clinical Research Centre Mass Spectrometry Unit, Harrow HA1 3UJ, UK

In Refsum's disease (McKusick 26650) impaired hepatic α-hydroxylase activity results in the accumulation of a branched chain fatty acid, phytanate, which is the substrate for this enzyme. In man phytanate is formed to a small extent from ingested phytol (Baxter *et al.*, 1967), a component of chlorophyll. The remainder is ingested as phytanate bound in the triglycerides of animals which themselves have formed it from phytol.

Treatment of this disease by restricting dietary phytol and phytanate intake not only arrests further increase in plasma and tissue phytanate accumulation, but also results in the slow reduction of the phytanate concentration (Steinberg *et al.*, 1970; Sahgal and Olsen, 1975; personal observation).

The oxidation of phytanate proceeds either by residual enzyme activity of the α-hydroxylation system, or by an alternative oxidation pathway. Brenton and Krywawych (1982) have reported the excretion of elevated quantities of 3-methyladipate in the urine from a patient with Refsum's disease. They suggested that it was formed from phytanate by ω-oxidation followed by β-oxidation. ω-Oxidation of fatty acids is a regulated process occurring in the microsomal and cytosolic compartments of hepatic cells (Pettersen, 1972; Bjorkhem, 1976). The quantities of 3-methyladipate excreted in this patient varied between 9 and 82 μmol (g creatinine)$^{-1}$, which was equivalent to the degradation of 2–30 mg phytanate. These lower quantities occurred during treatment when the patient's plasma phytanate concentration decreased.

This report describes the effects of feeding phytol upon the urine and plasma 3-methyladipate concentration in rats.

METHODS

Two-month-old female Wistar rats were fed either (a) a diet of 25% yeast (Distillers Co. Ltd, London), 10% corn oil, 36% starch, 24% sucrose and 4% salt, mineral and vitamin mix, or (b) the same diet with added 1% phytol. After the animals were maintained on these diets for 1 month specimens were collected for measurement of plasma and urine organic acids and fatty acids.

A third group of 2-month-old female Wistar rats were first maintained on the phytol-free diet and then changed to the phytol-containing diet. Plasma and urine organic acids and fatty acids were analysed whilst the animals were fed the phytol-free diet and then for a duration of 28 days whilst on the phytol-supplemented diet.

Blood samples were collected from the tail vein.

Organic acids were isolated from urine using the method of Chalmers and Watts (1972), with minor modifications. Plasma organic acids were isolated by filtration through Amicon CF50 cones. The filtrate was then treated as for urine. Plasma was also saponified in a boiling water bath for 30 min to hydrolyse the esterified fatty acids. The liberated fatty acids were extracted into ether from a sodium chloride saturated acidified aqueous phase.

The organic and fatty acids were measured as their trimethylsilyl esters by gas liquid chromatography, using a 25 m long BP10 capillary column with an internal diameter of 0.22 mm, and temperature programming from 80–250°C at 5°C min^{-1}. The identity of 3-methyladipate was confirmed by mass spectrometry using a Finnigan MAT-731 gas chromatograph–mass spectrometer operated at 70 eV ionisation voltage, 8 kV accelerating voltage and the resolution of 1000.

RESULTS

The mass spectrum produced by the trimethylsilylated derivative of the compound isolated from rat urine suspected of being 3-methyladipate was identical to that of authentic bis(trimethylsilyl)3-methyladipate.

Animals fed phytol excreted greater quantities of 3-methyladipate in urine, 185–274 μmol (g creatinine)$^{-1}$ (mean 225, $n = 6$), than those not fed phytol, 9–27 μmol (g creatinine)$^{-1}$ (mean 17, $n = 6$). 3-Methyladipate excretion increased at the time when phytol was introduced into the diets of these animals (Figure 1). Phytanate was present in the plasma only from the animals receiving phytol (Figure 1). The excretion of other even chain dicarboxylic acids was not influenced by dietary phytol intake.

Phytol supplementation did not increase the plasma 3-methyladipate concentration in the plasma from the animals.

DISCUSSION

Phytol supplementation resulted in the accumulation of phytanate in the plasma triglycerides of the animals. This is consistent with the findings of Baxter *et al.* (1967), who demonstrated that 10–20% of ingested phytol is

147

Journal of Inherited Metabolic Disease. ISSN 0141-8955. Copyright © SSIEM and MTP Press Limited, Queen Square, Lancaster, UK.

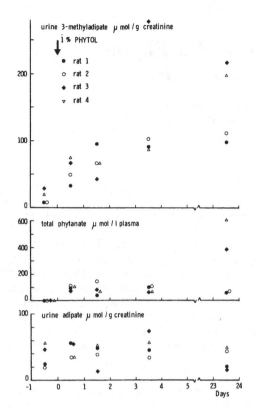

Figure 1 The excretion of adipate and 3-methyladipate and plasma phytanate concentrations in rats fed phytol

elevated in patients with enzyme defects in fatty acid metabolism, on the occasions when they were excreting raised quantities of even chain dicarboxylic acids (personal observation). In the present study it is most unlikely that increased 3-methyladipate excretion in the phytol-fed rats resulted from a non-specific stimulation of ω-oxidation, since the concentration of other ω-oxidation products, e.g. adipate, was not raised. It is more probable that 3-methyladipate production was accelerated because of the increased availability of its precursor, phytol. Phytol would first be converted to phytanate and then by ω-oxidation proceeded by β-oxidation phytanate would be oxidised to 3-methyladipate.

This finding further implicates phytanate as a precursor of 3-methyladipate.

converted to phytanate. This reaction occurs endogenously in the animals and is independent of bacterial metabolism in the gut.

The animals fed phytol excreted significantly larger quantities of 3-methyladipate in urine compared to those not fed phytol. Furthermore, the excretion of increased quantities of 3-methyladipate coincided with the administration of phytol.

Apart from the reported patient with Refsum's disease, urine 3-methyladipate excretion was also

References

Baxter, J. H., Steinberg, D., Mize, C. E. and Avigan, J. Absorption and metabolism of uniformly ^{14}C labeled phytol and phytanic acid by the intestine of the rat studied with thoracic duct canulation. *Biochim. Biophys. Acta* 137 (1967) 227–290

Bjorkhem, I. On the mechanism of ω-oxidation of fatty acids. *J. Biol. Chem.* 251 (1976) 5219–5266

Brenton, D. P. and Krywawych, S. 3-Methyladipate excretion in Refsum's disease. *Lancet* 1 (1982) 624

Chalmers, R. A. and Watts, R. W. E. The quantitative extraction and gas liquid chromatographic determination of organic acids in urine. *Analyst* 97 (1972) 958–967

Pettersen, J. E. Formation of *n*-hexandioic acid from hexadecanoic acid by initial ω-oxidation in ketotic rats. *Clin. Chim. Acta* 41 (1972) 231–237

Sahgal, V. and Olsen, W. O. Heredopathia atactica polyneuritiformis (phytanic acid storage disease). A new case with special reference to treatment. *Arch. Int. Med.* 135 (1975) 585–587

Steinberg, D., Mize, C. E., Herndon Jr, J. H., Fales, H. M., Engel, W. K. and Vroom, F. Q. Phytanic acid in patients with Refsum's syndrome and response to dietary treatment. *Arch. Int. Med.* 125 (1970) 75–87

J. Inher. Metab. Dis. 8 Suppl. 2 (1985) 149–150

Short Communication

Difficulties in Assessing Biochemical Properties of Abnormal Muscle Mitochondria

H. R. SCHOLTE, I. E. M. LUYT-HOUWEN and H. F. M. BUSCH
Departments of Biochemistry I, Neurology and Pathology, Medical Faculty, Erasmus University, Rotterdam, PO Box 1738, 3000 DR Rotterdam, The Netherlands

The study of oxidative phosphorylation in mitochondria is hampered by many obvious and less evident matters. We encountered several problems during the study of 162 preparations of isolated human muscle mitochondria from 1979 until May 1984.

METHODS

The methods are described by Barth *et al.* (1983). Muscle biopsies of 0.2–2 g were taken from M.biceps, quadriceps or gastrocnemius under local analgesia, from patients with persisting muscular problems, like hypotonia, weakness, stiffness, cramps and/or exercise intolerance. The isolation of mitochondria started within 15 min after biopsy. The isolation took $1\frac{1}{2}$ h.

RESULTS

We study oxidative phosphorylation with substrates entering the respiratory chain before NAD^+ (pyruvate + malate, glutamate + malate), at NAD^+ and CoQ (palmitoylcarnitine + malate), at CoQ (succinate + rotenone) and at cytochrome *c* (ascorbate + N,N,N',N'-tetramethyl-*p*-phenylenediamine). In the presence of glucose and hexokinase we determine oxygen uptake, stimulation of respiration by ADP, P/O ratios and uncoupler stimulation of Mg^{2+}-ATPase. We found many patients with apparent defects in the dehydrogenases (of pyruvate and long and medium chain acyl-CoA), in the respiratory chain (mainly NADH-CoQ reductase and, to a smaller extent, CoQ-cytochrome *c* reductase or cytochrome *c* oxidase), and in energy conservation. We will now list some problems encountered during this study.

The problems of latency

Often we found latency in the oxidation of one of the NAD^+-linked substrates or succinate. The latency of the former substrates was abolished by storage of the mitochondria for several hours at 0°C. The latency of palmitoylcarnitine oxidation could also be overcome by a substrate-free preincubation of the mitochondria for 10 min at 25°C. The succinate latency persisted. We deduced the latency from the fact that the antimycin-sensitive succinate-cytochrome *c* reductase activity in freeze-thawed mitochondria was normal. The most likely explanation of this "succinate paradox" is a defect in succinate transport, due to absence of counter-ions in the mitochondrial matrix, which could also explain the low oxidation rates with the NAD^+-linked substrates

that are often seen in these patients. However, only some of them showed an increase in succinate oxidation after freezing and thawing of the mitochondria. In these patients therapy aiming at replenishment of Krebs cycle intermediates could be considered.

The problem of a decreasing oxygen uptake with time

Slow diffusion of inhibitors (rotenone, antimycin) from the oxygen electrode or connecting rubber or plastic must be excluded. A deflection with the NAD^+-linked substrates may be due to lack of NAD^+ or CoA in the matrix. A deflection of succinate + rotenone was found in patients with low oxidation rates with pyruvate or palmitoylcarnitine, and was prevented by acetyl-carnitine or more rotenone. This suggests that endogenous acetyl-CoA, normally trapping the small amount of oxaloacetate which is formed in spite of the presence of rotenone, is lacking. Deflection in ascorbate oxidation is probably due to a lowered affinity of cytochrome aa_3 for O_2 (e.g. Barth *et al.*, 1983).

The problem of apparently loose coupling

Low stimulation of respiration by ADP was found with all substrates when the O_2 uptake fell below 30 natoms O_2 min^{-1} (mg protein)$^{-1}$. No stimulation was found with substrates which are poorly oxidized by muscle mitochondria like glycerol-3-P, citrate, isocitrate and 3-hydroxybutyrate.

The stimulation of respiration by ADP decreased when the amount of mitochondria was too small (<120 µg of protein/0.55 ml).

The problem of high P/O ratios at low oxygen uptake velocities

Very high P/O ratios were found under these conditions. It was found that the ATP-trapping system (glucose, hexokinase and Mg^{2+}) formed a considerable amount of glucose-6-P before ADP was added. Reliable P/O ratios were obtained when a sample was taken just before the addition of ADP, to correct for this. In this way we were able to identify patients lacking energy conservation at sites 1, 2 and/or 3.

Problems of mitochondrial lability

In some patients we observed a gradual decrease in O_2 uptake upon storage of the mitochondria at 0°C. In others we found a sudden collapse of the respiratory capacity after several hours, but sometimes within 2 h after beginning the assays.

Journal of Inherited Metabolic Disease. ISSN 0141-8955. Copyright © SSIEM and MTP Press Limited, Queen Square, Lancaster, UK.

The problem of secondary mitochondrial defects

In CoA-sequestration (e.g. Mooy et al., 1984), and in anoxia, secondary changes may cover the primary defect. Fortunately, in CoA-sequestration when the liver is also involved, the urinary organic acid pattern suggests the defect. By courtesy of Prof. Dr B. van Linge, we were able to study biopsies from surgical patients after $1\frac{1}{2}$ h of general anaesthesia, and we found decreased oxidation rates (to 31–45%).

The problem of transient mitochondrial defects

In young children it is conceivable that the mitochondrial defect interferes with protein synthesis, post-translational modifications and differentiation. DiMauro et al. (1983) described a child with a transient cytochrome aa_3 deficiency. In an adult patient we encountered a transient defect in the oxidation of ascorbate (with K. V. Toyka and U. Trockel, unpublished). In a baby we found a complete cytochrome c_1 deficiency (Scholte et al., 1983). Later the defect was partly abolished (with H. Przyrembel, unpublished). In the majority of patients the defects were permanent.

The problem of H_2O_2 production

Accidentally we discovered a patient who produced significant amounts of H_2O_2 with glutamate. The addition of catalase led to a considerable decrease in O_2 uptake. In other patients we found the same with ascorbate. This phenomenon gives rise to an underestimation of the P/O ratio.

The problem of control patients

All investigated mitochondria were from patients with muscular problems. As controls we used patients without morphological (including histochemical) abnormalities. In this group, however, mitochondrial defects were found. These patients were deleted from the control group. On the other hand, in patients with morphological abnormalities, we often found normal mitochondrial functioning.

The problem of small biopsy size

A small amount of mitochondria implies fewer tests, and a smaller chance to detect the lesion. In that case we prefer combined assays (e.g. buffer, mitochondria, pyruvate + malate, ADP, rotenone, succinate, 2-thenoyltrifluoroacetone, durohydroquinone, antimycin, see Barth et al., 1983).

DISCUSSION

We are aware of the fact that our method may not be adequate to identify the defect precisely. The control strength on mitochondrial oxidation is exerted by more than one component, as follows from elegant titration studies with inhibitors (Tager et al., 1983), but these studies require a relatively high amount of mitochondria. In some patients this type of investigation may be necessary to identify the ultimate lesion.

With our relatively simple set-up we found more than 50 patients with more or less defined mitochondrial lesions. This high number stresses the involvement of the mitochondria in the pathogenesis of muscle disease (Busch et al., 1981).

We are very grateful to our clinical colleagues for referring patients, to Professor Willem C. Hülsmann for stimulating interest, and to "De Willem H. Kröger Stichting, Rotterdam" for financial support.

References

Barth, P. G., Scholte, H. R., Berden, J. A., van der Klei-van Moorsel, J. M., Luyt-Houwen, I. E. M., van't Veer-Korthof, E. Th., van der Harten, J. J. and Sobotka-Plojar, M. A. An X-linked mitochondrial disease affecting cardiac muscle, skeletal muscle and neutrophil leucocytes. *J. Neurol. Sci.* 62 (1983) 327–355

Busch, H. F. M., Jennekens, F. G. I. and Scholte, H. R. (eds.) *Mitochondria and Muscular Diseases*, Mefar B. V., Beesterzwaag, The Netherlands, 1981

DiMauro, S., Nicholson, J. F., Hays, A. P., Eastwood, A. B., Papadimitriou, A., Koenigsberger, R. and DeVivo, D. C. Benign infantile mitochondrial myopathy due to reversible cytochrome c oxidase deficiency. *Ann. Neurol.* 14 (1983) 226–234

Mooy, P. D., Giesberts, M. A. H., van Gelderen, H. H., Scholte, H. R., Luyt-Houwen, I. E. M., Przyrembel, H. and Blom, W. Glutaric aciduria type II: multiple defects in isolated muscle mitochondria and deficient beta-oxidation in fibroblasts. *J. Inher. Metab. Dis.* 7, Suppl. 2 (1984) 101–102

Scholte, H. R., Busch, H. F. M., Barth, P. G., Beekman, R. P., Berden, J. A., Duran, M., Luyt-Houwen, I. E. M., Przyrembel, H., Roth, B. and de Vries, S. Carnitine deficiency and mitochondrial respiratory chain blockade. In Scarlato, G. and Cerri, C. (eds.) *Mitochondrial Pathology in Muscle Diseases*, Piccin Medical Books, Padua, 1983, pp. 215–228

Tager, J. M., Wanders, R. J. A., Groen, A. K., Kunz, W., Bohnensack, R., Küster, U., Letko, G., Böhme, G., Duszynski, J. and Wojtczak, L. Control of mitochondrial respiration. *FEBS Lett.* 151 (1983) 1–9

J. Inher. Metab. Dis. 8 Suppl. 2 (1985) 151–152

Short Communication

Peroxisomal Matrix Enzymes in Zellweger Syndrome: Activity and Subcellular Localization in Liver

R. J. A. WANDERS and R. B. H. SCHUTGENS
*Department of Pediatrics, Academic Medical Centre, University of Amsterdam, Meibergdreef 9,
1105 AZ Amsterdam, The Netherlands*

J. M. TAGER
*Laboratory of Biochemistry, University of Amsterdam, Plantage Muidergracht 12,
1012 TV Amsterdam, The Netherlands*

The cerebro–hepato–renal (Zellweger) syndrome (McKusick 21410) can be considered as the prototype of a newly recognized group of inherited diseases, the peroxisomopathies, in which one or more peroxisomal functions are impaired. In contrast to earlier suggestions, it is now clear that peroxisomes fulfil an essential role in a number of metabolic processes, including ether phospholipid biosynthesis, oxidation of very long chain fatty acids, bile acid synthesis and oxidation of dicarboxylic acids (reviewed in Borst, 1983; Kelley, 1983). The absence of peroxisomes in Zellweger syndrome is accompanied by a generalized impairment of these peroxisomal functions.

Dihydroxyacetonephosphate acyltransferase (DHAP-AT; EC 2.3.1.42), a membrane bound peroxisomal enzyme that catalyzes the first step in plasmalogen biosynthesis, is deficient in tissues and fibroblasts from Zellweger patients (Schutgens *et al.*, 1984). In contrast, the soluble peroxisomal matrix enzymes catalase (EC 1.11.1.6), D-aminoacid oxidase (EC 1.4.3.3) and L-α-hydroxyacid oxidase (EC 1.1.3.15) are not deficient in livers from the patients (Wanders *et al.*, 1984). Here we show that these peroxisomal matrix enzymes, which are particle-bound in fresh liver from control subjects, are present in the soluble cytoplasm in fresh liver from Zellweger patients.

MATERIALS AND METHODS

Samples of fresh liver were obtained from two patients with the Zellweger syndrome and, as controls, two patients with unrelated disorders. After gentle homogenization of the tissue in 0.25 M sucrose, 0.1 mmol l^{-1} EGTA and 5 mmol l^{-1} Tris–HCl (pH = 7.5), a postnuclear supernatant was prepared by centrifugation at 800 g for 5 min. An aliquot of the postnuclear supernate was subjected to centrifugation at 140 000 g for 10 min. After removal of the supernatant, the pellet was resuspended.

Enzyme activities were measured as described before (Wanders *et al.*, 1984).

RESULTS AND DISCUSSION

In an earlier study (Wanders *et al.*, 1984) we found that the soluble peroxisomal matrix enzymes catalase, D-aminoacid oxidase and L-α-hydroxyacid oxidase are not deficient in liver from patients with the Zellweger syndrome (see also Table 1). Similarly, catalase is not deficient in fibroblasts from the patients. However, whereas at least 70 % of the catalase activity in control fibroblasts is particle-bound, all of the catalase activity in fibroblasts from Zellweger patients is found in the soluble cytoplasm (Wanders *et al.*, 1984). These results raised the question of the intracellular localization of the peroxisomal matrix enzymes in the liver of Zellweger patients. It is clear that this problem cannot be studied in frozen postmortem liver material, in which the ultrastructural integrity is lost upon thawing. We therefore decided to study the subcellular localization of these peroxisomal enzymes in fresh liver material from Zellweger patients and controls. Fresh liver biopsy material was used to obtain a particulate fraction containing mitochondria, lysosomes, peroxisomes, etc. and a supernatant fraction containing cytosolic enzymes. In these fractions lactate dehydrogenase and glutamate dehydrogenase were measured as markers for the cytosolic and mitochondrial compartments, respectively. Furthermore, the activities of D-aminoacid oxidase, L-α-hydroxyacid oxidase and catalase were measured in these fractions. The results (Table 1) indicate that both in control and Zellweger liver glutamate dehydrogenase was almost completely recovered in the particulate fraction, whereas lactate dehydrogenase was found predominantly in the supernatant fraction. However, a clearly different picture emerged with regard to the three peroxisomal enzymes. In control liver the bulk of the activity of D-aminoacid oxidase, L-α-hydroxyacid oxidase and catalase was recovered in the particulate fraction. In contrast, in liver from Zellweger patients D-aminoacid oxidase, L-α-hydroxyacid oxidase and catalase were almost completely recovered in the same fraction as lactate dehydrogenase.

An important distinction between dihydroxyacetonephosphate acyltransferase, which is deficient in Zellweger syndrome, and the three peroxisomal enzymes found to be present in near normal amounts in the patients is that dihydroxyacetonephosphate acyltransferase is a membrane-bound enzyme whereas the other enzymes are soluble peroxisomal matrix enzymes. However, the subcellular fractionation studies show that the soluble enzymes, which are normally present in the peroxisomal matrix in livers from control subjects, are

151

Table 1   Activity and subcellular distribution of D-aminoacid oxidase, L-α-hydroxyacid oxidase and catalase in fresh liver from control subjects and patients with Zellweger syndrome

Liver from: Enzymes	Postnuclear supernatant fraction		140 000 g particulate fraction		140 000 g supernatant fraction	
	1	2	1	2	1	2
Controls						
Lactate dehydrogenase	1550	1905	55	85	1310	1710
Glutamate dehydrogenase	210	180	200	195	25	30
D-aminoacid oxidase	0.51	0.81	0.45	0.71	0.10	0.15
L-α-Hydroxyacid oxidase	2.52	1.41	2.10	1.31	0.40	0.20
Catalase	49	58	28	40	20	17
Zellweger patients						
Lactate dehydrogenase	1310	970	85	45	1410	1010
Glutamate dehydrogenase	185	240	180	225	15	25
D-Aminoacid oxidase	0.41	0.74	0.04	0.10	0.40	0.71
L-α-Hydroxyacid oxidase	1.31	1.71	0.11	0.16	1.30	1.51
Catalase	73	70	6	7	71	65

For experimental details see text. Enzyme activities are expressed as $\mu mol\ min^{-1}$ (catalase) or $nmol\ min^{-1}$ (other enzymes) per mg postnuclear supernatant protein. 1 and 2 refer to separate liver samples from two controls and two Zellweger patients.

present in the soluble cytoplasm in livers from the patients.

Our data support the hypothesis (Borst, 1983) that the primary lesion in the Zellweger syndrome is at the level of the biogenesis of peroxisomes and is due, for example, to the absence of an essential peroxisomal membrane protein or of a component required for the binding or import of peroxisomal proteins.

References

Borst, P. Animal peroxisomes (microbodies), lipid biosynthesis and the Zellweger syndrome. *Trends Biochem. Sci.* 8 (1983) 269–272

Kelley, R. I. The cerebrohepatorenal syndrome of Zellweger, morphological and metabolic aspects. *Am. J. Med. Genet.* 16 (1983) 503–517

Schutgens, R. B. H., Romeyn, G. J., Wanders, R. J. A., van den Bosch, H., Schrakamp, G. and Heymans, H. S. A. Deficiency of acyl-CoA: dihydroxyacetonephosphate acyltransferase in patients with Zellweger (cerebro–hepato–renal) syndrome. *Biochem. Biophys. Res. Commun.* 120 (1984) 179–184

Wanders, R. J. A., Kos, M., Roest, B., Meyer, A. J., Schrakamp, G., Heymans, H. S. A., Tegelaers, W. H. H., van den Bosch, H., Schutgens, R. B. H. and Tager, J. M. Activity of peroxisomal enzymes and intracellular distribution of catalase in Zellweger syndrome. *Biochem. Biophys. Res. Commun.* 123 (1984) 1054–1061

J. Inher. Metab. Dis. 8 Suppl. 2 (1985) 153–154

Short Communication

Prenatal Diagnosis of the Cerebro–hepato–renal (Zellweger) Syndrome by Detection of an Impaired Plasmalogen Biosynthesis

R. B. H. Schutgens, H. S. A. Heymans and R. J. A. Wanders
University Hospital Amsterdam, Department of Pediatrics, Meibergdreef 9, 1105 AZ Amsterdam, The Netherlands

H. van den Bosch and G. Schrakamp
Laboratory of Biochemistry, State University of Utrecht, The Netherlands

The cerebro–hepato–renal (Zellweger) syndrome (ZS, McKusick 21410) is an autosomal recessive disease characterised clinically by severe hypotonia, typical craniofacial dysmorphism, hepatomegaly, disturbances in liver function, renal cysts, failure to thrive and severe psychomotor and sensorial retardation. The disease is usually lethal within the first year of life; no effective treatment is available. Biochemical characteristics are the absence of morphologically distinct peroxisomes (microbodies) in liver and kidney (Goldfischer et al., 1973), an accumulation of very long chain fatty acids (Brown et al., 1982), trihydroxycoprostanoic acid (Hanson et al., 1979) and pipecolic acid (Danks et al., 1975) in blood and urine and the virtual absence of plasmalogens in tissues (Heymans, 1984). Furthermore, we found that the peroxisomal enzyme dihydroxy-acetone phosphate acyltransferase (DHAP-AT; EC 2.3.1.42), which catalyzes the first step in the biosynthetic route of ether phospholipids, is deficient in tissues and cultured skin fibroblasts of ZS patients (Schutgens et al., 1984). Moreover, we recently demonstrated that de novo biosynthesis of plasmalogens is impaired in cultured skin fibroblasts of Zellweger patients (Schrakamp et al., 1985). All these biochemical phenomena probably result from the absence of peroxisomes in cells of Zellweger patients.

The finding that DHAP-AT is clearly expressed in amniotic fluid cells of controls (Schutgens et al., 1984) suggested a prenatal test for Zellweger syndrome. Here we report the outcome of the studies aimed to find specific and sensitive tests to detect Zellweger syndrome prenatally.

METHODS

Dihydroxyacetone phosphate acyltransferase activity was measured as described by Schutgens et al. (1984). The incorporation of [^{14}C]hexadecanol into phospholipids in fibroblasts and amniotic fluid cells was determined as described by Schrakamp et al. (1985). Amniotic fluid cells were obtained after amniocentesis at the 16th week of gestation and cultured in F10 medium supplemented with 25% (v/v) fetal calf serum. Chorionic villi from controls were obtained by ultrasound guided aspiration biopsy at 8–10 weeks of gestation, prior to aspiration curettage for psychosocial indications, by Dr

M. G. J. Johada and Dr R. P. L. Vostus (Department of Obstetrics and Gynaecology, University Hospital Dijkzigt, Rotterdam), visually selected for their fetal origin and stored at −70°C (Dr W. J. Kleijer, Department of Clinical Genetics, Rotterdam).

RESULTS AND DISCUSSION

The activity of DHAP-AT was found to be deficient in amniotic fluid cells from two fetuses affected by Zellweger syndrome (amniocytes obtained by courtesy of Dr H. W. Moser and Dr A. E. Moser). In congruence with this finding, de novo biosynthesis of ether lipids was strongly impaired as manifested by a severely reduced incorporation of a radioactive precursor ([^{14}C]hexa-decanol) of ether phospholipids into plasmalogens (Table 1). In six pregnancies at risk for Zellweger syndrome, both types of analysis in cultured amniotic fluid cells suggested that the fetuses were not affected; five of these pregnancies so far resulted in the birth of a healthy child, one pregnancy is still in progress.

Moser et al. (1984) recently described the successful prenatal detection of Zellweger syndrome by a method based on the measurement of an accumulation of very long chain fatty acids ($>C_{22}$) in patient's cells. An important advantage of the present methods is the much lower amount of fetal amniotic fluid cells required for prenatal detection, usually resulting in culture times of only 1–2 weeks. Moreover, we found that DHAP-AT is also expressed in chorionic villi of controls (Table 1). In these experiments glutamate dehydrogenase activity was also measured to verify retention of enzymatic activities in the biopsy specimens during the visual selection procedure to check for fetal origin. As DHAP-AT is clearly detectable in chorionic villi of controls, we speculate that prenatal detection of Zellweger syndrome in future will even be possible in the first trimester of pregnancy.

This work was financially supported by The Princess Beatrix Fund, The Hague, The Netherlands. We thank Dr H. W. Moser and Dr A. E. Moser, Baltimore for supplying the amniotic fluid cells of the Zellweger fetuses; Dr M. F. Niermeyer and Dr W. J. Kleijer, Rotterdam for supplying the chorionic villi specimens; Dr P. Borst, Dr W. H. H. Tegelaers for their continuous support in this project; Miss P. R. v. d.

Journal of Inherited Metabolic Disease. ISSN 0141-8955. Copyright © SSIEM and MTP Press Limited, Queen Square, Lancaster, UK.

Table 1 Dihydroxyacetone phosphate acyltransferase (DHAP-AT) activity in cultured fibroblasts of Zellweger patients and controls, in cultured amniotic fluid cells of controls and Zellweger fetuses and in chorionic villi specimens of controls and *de novo* biosynthesis of plasmalogens in cultured fibroblasts and amniotic fluid cells of controls and Zellweger fetuses

Tissue	*DHAP-AT activity* (nmol 2 h^{-1} mg protein^{-1}) *Mean ± SD*	[^{14}C]*hexadecanol incorporation*			
		(% *dpm in PE*)†	(% *pPE in PE*)*	(% *dpm in PC*)† *Mean ± SD*	(% *pPC in PC*)*
Fibroblasts					
Controls	9.80 ± 2.10 (n = 27)	57.8 ± 7.7	91.8 ± 5.5	34.5 ± 5.8	22.0 ± 4.2 (n = 6)
Zellweger	0.66 ± 0.50 (n = 9)	17.0 ± 1.6	62.4 ± 9.2	63.0 ± 1.7	2.1 ± 0.7 (n = 6)
Amniotic fluid cells					
Controls	8.52 ± 2.52 (n = 6)	51.5 ± 8.9	92.6 ± 1.7	40.7 ± 7.0	36.2 ± 13.7 (n = 9)
Zellweger fetus AF-K	0.14	16.3	69.7	62.9	2.6
Zellweger fetus AF-B	0.04	11.9	45.3	65.2	1.2

	DHAP-AT activity (nmol 2 h^{-1} mg protein^{-1}) *Mean ± SD*	*Glu-DH*‡ (μmol h^{-1} mg^{-1})	*DHAP-AT/Glu-DH ratio*
Chorion villi (n = 17)	6.6 ± 2.7	9.0 ± 2.5	0.75 ± 0.27

* Radioactivity in dpm incorporated in plasmalogen PE or plasmalogen PC as a percentage of total radioactivity in PE and PC, respectively
† Radioactivity in dpm incorporated in total phosphatidylethanolamine (PE) and total phosphatidylcholine (PC) as a percentage of total radioactivity incorporated in total phospholipids
‡ Glu-DH = glutamate dehydrogenase activity measured as described by Bergmeyer, H. U., In *Methoden der Enzymatische Analyse*, Verlag Chemie, Weinheim, FRG, 1974, p. 2103

Bergh, Miss M. E. Meyboom, G. J. Romeyn and Miss D. E. M. Saelman for expert technical assistance.

References

Brown, F. R., McAdams, A. J., Cumming, J. W., Konkol, R., Singh, I., Moser, A. E. and Moser, H. W. Cerebro–hepato–renal (Zellweger) syndrome and neonatal adrenoleukodystrophy: similarities in phenotype and accumulation of very long chain fatty acids. *Johns Hopkins Med. J.* 151 (1982) 344–361

Danks, D. M., Tippett, P., Adams, C. and Campbell, P. J. Cerebro–hepato–renal syndrome of Zellweger. A report of eight cases with comments upon the incidence, the liver lesion, and a fault in pipecolic acid metabolism. *J. Pediatr.* 86 (1975) 382–387

Goldfischer, S., Moore, C. L., Johnson, A. B., Spiro, A. J., Valsamis, M. P., Wisniewski, H. K., Ritch, R. H., Norton, W. T. and Rapin, I. Peroxisomal and mitochondrial defects in the cerebro–hepato–renal syndrome. *Science* 182 (1973) 62–64

Hanson, R. F., Szczepanik-van Leeuwen, P., Williams, G. C., Grabowski, G. and Sharp, H. L. Defects of bile acid synthesis in Zellweger's syndrome. *Science* 203 (1979) 1107–1108

Heymans, H. S. A. Cerebro–hepato–renal (Zellweger) syndrome. Clinical and biochemical consequences of peroxisomal dysfunction. *Thesis*, University of Amsterdam (1984)

Moser, A. E., Singh, I., Brown III, F. R., Solish, G. I., Kelley, R. I., Benke, P. J. and Moser, H. W. The cerebro–hepato–renal (Zellweger) syndrome. Increased levels and impaired degradation of very long chain fatty acids and their use in prenatal diagnosis. *N. Engl. J. Med.* 310 (1984) 1141–1146

Schrakamp, G., Schutgens, R. B. H., Wanders, R. J. A., Heymans, H. S. A., Tager, J. M. and van den Bosch, H. The cerebro–hepato–renal (Zellweger) syndrome: impaired *de novo* biosynthesis of plasmalogens in cultured skin fibroblasts. *Biochem. Biophys. Acta* 833 (1985) 170–174

Schutgens, R. B. H., Romeyn, G. J., Wanders, R. J. A., van den Bosch, H., Schrakamp, G. and Heymans, H. S. A. Deficiency of acylCoA: dihydroxyacetone phosphate acyltransferase in fibroblasts from patients with Zellweger (cerebro–hepato–renal) syndrome. *Biochem. Biophys. Res. Commun.* 120 (1984) 179–184